Dedication

This book is dedicated to Frederick C. Rimmele, III, MD
(October 3, 1968–September 11, 2001).

Emergency Medicine

Series Editor: Daniel K. Onion

SECOND EDITION

Steven E. Diaz, MD
MaineGeneral Medical Center
Dartmouth Medical School

JONES AND BARTLETT PUBLISHERS
Sudbury, Massachusetts
BOSTON   TORONTO   LONDON   SINGAPORE

World Headquarters

Jones and Bartlett
Publishers
40 Tall Pine Drive
Sudbury, MA 01776
978-443-5000
info@jbpub.com
www.jbpub.com

Jones and Bartlett
Publishers Canada
6339 Ormindale Way
Mississauga, ON L5V 1J2
CANADA

Jones and Bartlett
Publishers
International
Barb House, Barb Mews
London W6 7PA
UK

Jones and Bartlett's books and products are available through most bookstores
and online booksellers. To contact Jones and Bartlett Publishers directly, call
800-832-0034, fax 978-443-8000, or visit our website www.jbpub.com.

Substantial discounts on bulk quantities of Jones and Bartlett's publications are available
to corporations, professional associations, and other qualified organizations. For details
and specific discount information, contact the special sales department at Jones and
Bartlett via the above contact information or send an email to specialsales@jbpub.com.

Library of Congress Cataloging-in-Publication Data
Diaz, Steven E.
    The little black book of emergency medicine / Steven E. Diaz. — 2nd ed.
        p. ; cm.
    Rev. ed. of: Blackwell's primary care essentials. Emergency medicine.
c2002.
    Includes bibliographical references and index.
    ISBN 0-7637-3456-X
    1. Emergency Medicine—Handbooks, manuals, etc.   2. Primary care
    (Medicine)—Handbooks, manuals, etc.   I. Diaz, Steven E.
Blackwell's primary care essentials. Emergency medicine.   II. Title.
    [DNLM: 1. Emergencies—Handbooks.   2. Evidence-Based Medicine
—Handbooks.   WB 39 D542b 2006]
RC86.8.D52 2006
616.02'5—dc22

                                                        2005019334

Production Credits
Executive Publisher: Christopher Davis
Production Director: Amy Rose
Associate Editor: Kathy Richardson
Production Assistant: Alison Meier
Associate Marketing Manager: Laura Kavigian
Manufacturing Buyer: Therese Connell

Composition: ATLIS Graphics
Cover Design: Anne Spencer
Cover Images: © Photos.com
Printing and Binding: Malloy, Inc.
Cover Printing: Malloy, Inc.

Printed in the United States of America
09 08 07 06 05   10 9 8 7 6 5 4 3 2 1

Contents

Preface

The most difficult aspect of medicine is blending the art and science, and knowing the difference. Clinical medicine is undergoing large transformations in the 21st century, and the buzzword is "evidence-based."

The crux of this book is to provide information in a concise, yet complete manner, taking advantage of the available data in the journals that should direct the way that we practice. Unfortunately, evidence-based medicine has many different connotations. Although my application of evidence-based emergency medicine is not unique, I should explain what it means to me.

The availability of data is overwhelming, and as of yet, we cannot rely on journal publications to be entirely correct. Critically evaluating data is a skill that must be practiced continuously in order to maintain expertise, and oftentimes, historical data have not been subject to an appropriate challenge.

In medicine, the scientific grounds that determine diagnostic or therapeutic standards may be weak in methods or statistics. Yet, many times this is all that we have to offer patients. We cannot yet afford to disregard information based on anecdotal, case report, or even flawed studies. It is possible that the conclusions are correct even though the scientific support is weak.

Additionally, some studies are well done, but the authors may be challenged as to having deduced the correct conclusion. Furthermore, it is not uncommon to have a well-designed study with a strongly supported conclusion.

When we evaluate patients, we are relying on pattern recognition to suggest potential disease processes, and this listing gives us our differential diagnoses. Based on what we have been taught and what we have researched, we then give weight to the different possibilities based on history, physical exam, and laboratory data.

As we offer therapies, we again offer interventions that we have been taught and that we have researched. Our interventions after a time also begin resembling standard patterns.

Dan Onion asked me to join his collection of authors and develop this emergency medicine text. Dan has been a mentor and has helped me immensely with different parts of my text. My approach was to blend historical teaching in diagnostics and therapeutics with data available in the medical journals. This is what I consider to be evidence-based, in that it is inherent that some supporting evidence is weaker than others. The key is to know where you stand when you are hypothesizing as to some disease process or offering some intervention.

As mentioned above, some authors may be challenged as to having reached the correct conclusion. If citation abstracts appear to have contrary conclusions to the text, then I believe that the study supports my conclusion. Controversies in medicine will have both "pro" and "con" articles cited.

This book is geared toward those in medical training. It is intended to help teach and sharpen the information that comes at a rapid pace during those formative years. For those in practice, it may provide information and a framework in which to practice emergency medicine. In addition, I would like to see my colleagues become more comfortable with dissecting and interpreting journal articles. I hope that you find this useful.

I had tremendous help from Lawrence Kassman, MD, my mentor, colleague, and boss, who reviewed and improved this writing. Navigating the reams of medical information and obtaining the articles were greatly enhanced with help from Cora Damon, BS in Education and MLS, who is our Health Sciences Librarian at MaineGeneral Medical Center. Despite their assistance, all the errors within this text are solely my own.

Steven E. Diaz, MD

Medical Abbreviations

$\rightarrow$	Leads to
μ	Micron(s)
η	Nanogram(s)
μgm	Microgram(s)
ηL	Nanoliter(s)
ηm	Nanometer(s)
$<$	Less than
$<<$	Much less than
$>$	More than
$>>$	Much more than
5-HIAA	5-Hydroxyindoleacetic acid
5HT	5-Hydroxytryptophan
6MP	6-mercaptopurine
A_2	Aortic (first) component of S_2
AA	Alcoholics Anonymous
AAA	Abdominal Aortic Aneurysm
AADLs	Advanced activities of daily living
ab	Antibodies
Abd	Abdominal
ABGs	Arterial blood gases
ac	Before meals
ACE	Angiotensin-converting enzyme
ACEI	ACE Inhibitor
ACLS	Advanced cardiac life support
ACTH	Adrenocorticotropic hormone
AD	Right ear
ADH	Antidiuretic hormone
ADHD	Attention deficit hyperactivity disorder
AD-HERE	Acute Decompensated Heart Failure National Registry
ADLs	Activities of daily living
AFB	Acid-fast bacillus
Afib	Atrial fibrillation
Aflut	Atrial flutter
AFP	Alpha fetoprotein
ag	Antigen
AGN	Acute glomerular nephritis
AHA	American Heart Association
AI	Aortic insufficiency
AIMs	Abnormal involuntary movements
aka	Also known as
Al	Aluminum
ALA	δ-aminolevulinic acid
ALL	Acute lymphocytic leukemia
ALS	Amyotrophic lateral sclerosis
ALT	SGPT; alanine aminotransferase

am	Ante meridiem	asap	As soon as possible
AMI	Anterior myocardial infarction	ASCVD	Arteriosclerotic cardiovascular disease
AML	Acute myelogeous leukemia	ASD	Atrial septal defect
		ASHD	Asteriosclerotic heart disease
AMS	Acute Mountain Sickness		
ANA	Antinuclear antibody	ASLO/	Antistreptolysin O titer
ANCA	Antineutrophil cytoplasmic autoantibodies	ASO	
		ASO	Anti-streptolysisn-O antibody
ANP	Atrial natriuretic peptide	AST	SGOT; aspartate transferase
anti-HBc	Antibody to Hepatitis B core	asx	Asymptomatic
		AT	Antithrombin
anti-HBe	Antibody to Hepatitis B e antigen	atm	Atmospheres
		ATN	Acute tubular necrosis
anti-HBs	Antibody to Hepatitis B surface antigen	ATP	Adenosine triphosphate
		AU	Both ears
anti-SSA	Extractable nuclear antigen, initially seen in Sjogren's syndrome	AV	Arteriovenous; or atrial-ventricular
		avg	Average
AODM	Adult-onset diabetes mellitus	AVM	Arteriovenous malformation
AOM	Acute Otitis Media	AVNRT	Atrioventricular nodal re-entry tachycardia
AP	Anterior-posterior		
ApoE	apolipoprotein E	AVRT	Atrioventricular re-entry tachycardia
AR	Aldose reductase		
ARA	Angiotensin receptor antagonist	AXR	Abdominal x-ray
ARB	Angiotensin receptor blocker	Ba	Barium
		bact	Bacteriology
ARDS	Adult respiratory distress syndrome	BAFL	Big air, fractured lumbar
		BAL	British anti-Lewisite
ARF	Acute renal failure	BB	Isoform 1 of CPK, mainly found in brain
As	Arsenic		
AS	Aortic stenosis; or left ear	bc	Birth control
ASA	Aspirin	BCG	Bacille Calmette-Guérin

BCLS	Basic cardiac life support
bcp's	Birth control pills
BE	Barium enema
bid	Twice a day
BiPAP	Bi(2)-positive airway pressures
BJ	Bence Jones
BM	Basement membrane
bm	Bowel movement
BMP	Basic metabolic profile
BNP	Brain natriuretic peptide
BP	Blood pressure
BPH	Benign Prostatic Hypertrophy
BS	Blood sugar
BUN	Blood Urea Nitrogen
BVM	Bag valve mask
bx	Biopsy
c + s	Culture and sensitivity
C	Celsius
c/o	Complaining of
C/S	Cesarean section
C'	Complement
CA	Cocaine Anonymous
Ca	Calcium
CABG	Coronary artery bypass graft
CAD	Coronary artery disease
cal	Calories
cAMP	Cyclic AMP
CAPD	Continuous Ambulatory Peritoneal Dialysis
cath	Catheterization
CBC	Complete blood count
CC	Chief complaint
cc	Cubic centimeter

CCK	Cholecystokinin
CEA	Carcinoembryonic antigen
cf	compare
CF	Complement fixation antibodies
CHD	Congenital heart disease
chem	Chemistries
chemo-Rx	Chemotherapy
CHF	Congestive heart failure
CI	Cardiac index
CIN	Cervical intraepithelial neoplasia
CIS	Carcinoma in situ
CK	Creatinine kinase
Cl	Chloride
CLL	Chronic lymphocytic leukemia
CMF	Cytoxan, methotrexate, 5-FU
CML	Chronic myelocytic leukemia
cmplc	Complications
CMV	Cytomegalovirus
CN	Cranial nerve; or cyanide
CNS	Central Nervous System
CO	Cardiac output
col	Colonies
COPD	Chronic obstructive lung disease
COX	Cyclooxygenase
cp	Cerebellar-pontine
CP	Cerebral palsy
CPAP	Continuous positive airway pressure
CPC	Clinical/pathologic conference

CPG	Coproporphyrinogen	DES	Diethylstillbesterol
CPK	Creatine phosphokinase	DHS	Delayed hypersensitivity
CPR	Cardiopulmonary resuscitation	dl	Deciliter
		DI	Diabetes insipidus
cps	Cycles per second	dias	Diastolic
Cr	Creatinine	DIC	Disseminated intravascular coagulation
CREST	Calcinosis, Raynaud's, esophageal reflux, sclerodactyly, telangiectasias		
		Diff Dx	Differential diagnosis
		diff	Differential
		dig	Digoxin
CRF	Chronic renal failure	dip	Distal interphalangeal joint
CRH	Corticotropin-releasing hormone		
		DJD	Degenerative joint disease
crit	Hematocrit	DKA	Diabetic Ketoacidosis
CRP	C reactive protein	DM	Diabetes Mellitus
crs	Course	DMA	Dimethoxyamphetamine
CSF	Cerebrospinal fluid	DMSA	Dimercaptosuccinic acid
CT	Computed tomography	DMT	Dimethyltryptamine
Cu	Copper	DNA	Deoxyribonucleic acid
CVA	Cerebrovasular accident	DOE	Dyspnea on exertion
CVP	Central venous pressure	DPG	Diphosphoglycerate
CXR	Chest x-ray	DPI	Dry powder inhaler
		DPL	Diagnostic peritoneal lavage
d	Day/s		
D + C	Dilatation and curettage	DPN	Diphosphopyridine nucleotide
D + E	Dilatation and evacuation (suction)		
		DPNH	DPN reduced
D_5S	Dextrose 5% in saline	DR	Types of alleles
DAI	Diffuse axonal injury	DRE	Digital rectal exam
DASH	Dietary approach to stop hypertension	DS	Double strength
		DST	Dexamethasone suppression test
DAT	Dementia, Alzheimer's type		
dB	Decibel	dT	Diphtheria, tetanus, adult vaccine
DBCT	Double-blind controlled trial		
		DTaP	Diphtheria, tetanus, acellular pertussis vaccine
DDAVP	Desmopressin		
Decr	Decrease		

DTRs	Deep tendon reflexes	ERCP	Endoscopic retrograde cholangiopancreatography
DTs	Delirium tremens		
DU	Duodenal ulcer		
DUI	Driving under the influence	ERP	Endoscopic retrograde pancreatography
DVT	Deep venous thrombosis	ERT	Estrogen-replacement therapy
E/M	Erythroid/myeloid	ESR	Erythrocyte sedimentation rate
EACA	ϵ-Aminocaproic acid		
EBV	Epstein-Barr virus	et al	And others
ECHO	Echocardiogram	ET	Endotracheal
ECM	Erythema chronicum marginatum	etc	And so forth
		ETOH	Ethanol
ECT	Electroconvulsive therapy	ETT	Exercise tolerance test
ED	Emergency Department		
EDTA	Ethylenediaminetetra-acetate	F	Female; or Fahrenheit
		f/u	Follow up
EEG	Electroencephalogram	FA	Fluorescent antibody; or folic acid
EF	Ejection fraction		
eg	for example	FB	Foreign body
EGD	Esophagogas-troduodenoscopy	FBS	Fasting blood sugar
		FDP	Fibrin degradation products
EIA	Enzyme Immunoassay	Fe	Iron
EKG	Electrocardiogram	FEV_1	Forced expiratory vital capacity in 1 sec
ELISA	Enzyme-linked immunosorbent assay		
		FFA	Free fatty acids
EMG	Electromyogram	FFP	Fresh frozen plasma
EMS	Emergency Medical Services	Fhx	Family history
		FIGLU	Formiminoglutamic acid
EMT	Emergency Medical Technician	fl	Femtoliter
		FMF	Familial Mediterranean fever
Endo	Endoscopy		
EOA	Esophageal obturator airway	freq	Frequency
		FSH	Follicle-stimulating hormone
Epidem	Epidemiology		
ER	Estrogen receptors; or emergency room	FTA	Fluorescent treponemal antibody

FTT	Failure to thrive
FUO	Fever of unknown origin
FVC	Forced vital capacity
fx	Fracture
g	Gauge
GABA	γ-aminobutyric acid
gc	Gonorrhea
GCS	Glasgow Coma Scale
GE	Gastroesophageal
GERD	Gastroesophageal reflux disease
GFR	Glomerular filtration rate
GG	Strain of lactobacillus named for Gorbach and Goldin
GHB	Gamma hydroxy butyrate
GHRH	Growth hormone-releasing hormone
gi	Gastrointestinal
GIK	Glucose-insulin-potassium
gm	Gram
GN	Glomerulonephritis
GnRH	Gonadotropin-releasing hormone
GTT	Glucose tolerance test
gtts	Drops
Gu	Genitourinary
GVHD	Graft versus Host disease
Gyn	Gynecologic
H & E	Hematoxylin and eosin
h	Hour(s)
H. flu	Haemophilus influenzae
h/o	History of
HACE	High Altitude Cerebral Edema
HAPE	High Altitude Pulmonary Edema
HAV	Hepatitis A Virus
HBeAg	Hepatitis B e antigen
HBIG	Hepatitis B immune globulin
HBsAg	Hepatitis B surface antigen
HBV	Hepatitis B Virus
HCG	Human chorionic gonadotropin
HCGrH	HCG-releasing hormone
HCl	Hydrochloric acid
HCO_3	Bicarbonate
hct	Hematocrit
HCV	Hepatitis C Virus
HD	Hemodialysis
HDCV	Human diploid cell vaccine
HDL	High-density lipoprotein
HDV	Hepatitis D Virus
hem	Hematology
Hep A	Hepatitis A Virus
Hep B	Hepatitis B Virus
Hep C	Hepatitis C Virus
Hep D	Hepatitis D Virus
Hep G	Hepatitis G Virus
Hep	Hepatitis
Hg	Mercury
hgb	Hemoglobin
HgbA1C	Hemoglobin A1C level
HGH	Human growth hormone
HGV	Hepatitis G Virus
Hib	Haemophilus influenzae B vaccine
his	Histidine
HIV	Human immunodeficiency virus

HLA	Human leukocyte antigens	IFA	Immunofluorescent antibody
HMG-COA	Hydroxymethylglutaryl-coenzyme A	IgA	Immunoglobulin A
hpf	High power field	IgE	Immunoglobulin E
HPI	History of the present illness	IgG	Immunoglobulin G
		IgM	Immunoglobulin M
HPV	Human papillomavirus	IHSS	Idiopathic hypertrophic subaortic stenosis
hr	hour(s)		
HRIG	Human rabies immune globulin	IL	Interleukin
		im	Intramuscular
hs	At bedtime	incr	Increased
HSP	Henoch-Schönlein purpura	INH	Isoniazid
		INR	International normalized ration (protimes)
HSV	Herpes simplex virus		
HT	Hypertension	IO	Intraosseus
HTLV	Human T-cell lymphocytotropic virus	IP	Interphalangeal
		IPG	Impedance plethysmography
HUS	Hemolytic uremic syndrome	IPPB	Intermittent positive pressure breathing
HVA	Homovanillic acid		
hx	History	IPPD	Intermediate purified-protein derivative
Hz	Hertz		
		IQ	Intelligence quotient
I + D	Incision and drainage	ITP	Idiopathic thrombocytopenic purpura
I or I_2	Iodine		
IADLs	Instrumental activities of daily living		
		IU	International units
IBD	Inflammatory bowel disease	IUD	Intrauterine device
		IUGR	Intrauterine growth retardation
ICP	Intracranial pressure		
ICU	Intensive care unit	IUP	Intrauterine pregnancy
ID	Infectious disease	iv	Intravenous
IDDM	Insulin-dependent diabetes mellitus	IVC	Inferior vena cava
		IVF	Intravenous fluid
ie	in other words	IVP	Intravenous pyelogram
IEP	Immunoelectrophoresis	IWMI	Inferior wall myocardial infarction
IF	Intrinsic factor		

J	Joule	LMA	Laryngeal mask airway
JODM	Juvenile-onset diabetes mellitus	LMW	Low molecular weight
		LMWH	Low molecular weight heparin
JRA	Juvenile rheumatoid arthritis	LP	Lumbar puncture
JVD	Jugular venous distension	LR	Lactated Ringer's
JVP	Jugular venous pressure/ pulse	LS	Lumbosacral
		LSD	Lysergic diethylamide
		LV	Left ventricle
K	Potassium	LVEDP	Left ventricular end-diastolic pressure
KCl	Potassium chloride		
kg	Kilogram	LVH	Left ventricular hypertrophy
KOH	Potassium hydroxide		
KUB	Abdominal x-ray ("kidneys, ureters, bladder")	lytes	Electrolytes
		M	Male
		m	Meter(s)
L	Liter; or left	M/F	Male/Female
LA	Left atrium; long acting	MAI	*Mycobacterium avium-intracellulare*
Lab	Laboratory tests		
LAD	Left anterior descending	MAO	Monoamine oxidase
LAP	Leukocyte alkaline phosphatase	MAOI	Monoamine oxidase inhibitor
LATS	Long-acting thyroid-stimulating protein	MAP	Mean arterial pressure
		MAT	Multifocal atrial tachycardia
lb	Pound	MAZE	A cardiac procedure creating a surgical maze to treat atrial fibrillation
Lb	Lead		
LBBB	Left bundle branch block		
LDH	Lactate dehydrogenase		
LDL	Low-density lipoproteins		
LES	Lower esophageal sphincter	MB	Isoform 2 of CPK, mainly found in heart
LFTs	Liver function tests	mcg	Microgram
LH	Luteinizing hormone	mcp	Metacarpal-phalangeal joint(s)
LHRH	LH-releasing hormone		
LLQ	Left lower quadrant	MCV	Mean corpuscular volume

MD	Muscular dystrophy; or physician	MRA	Magnetic resonance angiography
MDA	Methylenedioxy-amphetamine	MRFIT	Multiple risk factor intervention trial
MDI	Metered-dose inhaler	MRI	Magnetic resonance imaging
MDMA	3,4-methylene dioxymethamphetamine	MS	Multiple sclerosis; or mitral stenosis
meds	Medications	MSA	Multisystem atrophy
MEN	Multiple endocrine neoplasias	MSE	Mental status examination
mEq	Milliequivalent	MSH	Melanocyte-stimulating hormone
METs	Metabolic equivalents	mtx	Methotrexate
mets	Metastases	Multip	Multiparous patient
Mg	Magnesium	MVP	Mitral valve prolapse
mg	Milligram	MZ	Monozygotic
MHPH	Methoxydydroxy-phenylglycol		
MI	Myocardial infarction; or mitral insufficiency	NA	Narcotics Anonymous
		Na	Sodium
MIC	Minimum inhibitory concentration	NaCl	Sodium chloride
		NAD	Nicotinamide adenine dinucleotide
min	Minute(s)		
mL	Milliliter	NADH	Reduced form of NAD
MM	Isoform 3 of CPK, mainly in skeletal muscle	nbM	Nucleus basalis of Mayner
		NC	Noncontributory
mmHg	Millimeters of mercury	NCI	National Cancer Institute
MMR	Measles, mumps, rubella	ncnc	normochromic normocytic
MMSE	Mini-Mental State Exam	NCV	Nerve conduction velocities
mon	Month	neb	Nebulizer
MOM	Milk of magnesia	neg	Negative
mOsm	Milliosmole(s)	NG	Nasogastric
mp	Metocarpal phalangeal	NGT	Nasogastric tube
MPE	Monophasic equivalents	NH	Nursing home
MPTP	1-methyl-4-phenyl-1,2,3,6-tetrahydropyridine	NH_3	Ammonia
		NICU	Newborn intensive care unit
MR	Mitral regurgitation		

NIDDM	Non-insulin-dependent diabetes mellitus	OM	Otitis media
		OMC	Ostiomeatal complex
NIHSS	National Institutes of Health Scoring System	op	Operative
		OPA	Oral pharyngeal airway
NIX	Permethrin	OPD	Outpatient department
nl	Normal	OPV	Oral polio vaccine
NMDA	N-methyl-D-aspartate	ORS	Oral rehydration solution
NMRI	Nuclear magnetic resonance imaging	ORT	Oral rehydration therapy
		OS	Left eye
NMS	Neuroleptic Malignant Syndrome	osm	Osmoles
		OTC	Over the counter
NNT	Number needed to treat	OU	Both eyes
noninv	Noninvasive	oz	Ounce
NPA	Nasopharyngeal airway		
NPH	Normal-pressure hydrocephalus	P	Pulse
		P_2	Pulmonary (2nd) component of S_2
npo	Nothing by mouth		
NREM	Non-REM	PA	Pernicious anemia; or pulmonary artery
NS	Normal saline		
NSAID	Nonsteroidal anti-inflammatory drug	PABA	Paraminobenzoic acid
		PAC	Premature atrial contraction
NSR	Normal sinus rhythm		
NST	Nonstress test	PAF	Paroxysmal atrial fibrillation
Nullip	Nulliparous patient		
NV + D	Nausea, vomiting, and diarrhea	PAN	Polyarteritis nodosa
		Pap	Papanicolaou
		PAP	Pulmonary artery pressure
O + P	Ova and parasites	PAPP-A	Pregnancy associated plasma protein A
O_2	Oxygen		
OB	Obstetrics	par	Parenteral
OCD	Obsessive Compulsive Disorder	PAS	p-Aminosalicylic acid
		PAT	Paroxysmal atrial tachycardia
OD	Overdose; or right eye		
OGIT	Oral glucose tolerance test	patho-phys	Pathophysiology
OH	Hydroxy-	Pb	Lead
OI	Ostogenesis imperfecta	PBG	Phorphobilinogen

pc	After meals	pheo	Pheochromocytoma
PCI	Percutaneous coronary intervention	PHLA	Post-heparin lipolytic activity
PCN VK	Penicillin	phos	Phosphatase
PCP	*Pneumocystis carinii* pneumonia	PI	Pulmonic insufficiency
		PID	Pelvic inflammatory disease
PCR	Polymerase chain reaction		
PCTA	Percutaneous transluminal angioplasty	PIH	Pregnancy-induced hypertension
PCWP	Pulmonary capillary wedge pressure	pip	Proximal interphalangeal joint
PDA	Patent ductus arteriosus	PJRT	Paroxysmal junctional re-entry tachycardia
PDE	Phosphodiesterase	PMH	Past medical history
PE	Pulmonary embolism or Physical examination	PMI	Point of maximal impulse of heart
PEA	Pulseless Electrical Activity	PMN	Polymorphonuclear neutrophils
Peds	Pediatrics	PMNLs	Polymorphonuclear leukocytes
PEEP	Positive end-expiratory pressure		
		PMR	Polymyalgia rheumatica
PEG	Percutaneous endoscopic gastrostomy	PND	Paroxysmal nocturnal dyspnea
PEP	Protein electrophoresis	PNH	Paroxysmal hemoglobinuria
PERRLA	Pupils equal round reactive to light and accommodation	po	By mouth
		PO_4	Phosphate
PET	Positron emission tomography	polys	Polymorphonuclear leukocytes
PFAPA	Periodic fever, aphthous stomatis, pharyngitis, adenopathy	pos	Positive
		PP	Protoporphyrin
PFTs	Pulmonary function tests	ppd	Pack per day
Pg	Picogram	PPD	Tuberculin skin test
PG	Prostaglandin	PPG	Protoporphyrinogen
PGB	Phorphobilinogen	PPI	Proton pump inhibitor
PGE	Prostaglandin E	pr	Per rectum
PGF	Prostaglandin F	PR	PR interval on EKG

pRBBB	Partial right bundle branch block	RAST	Radioallergosorbent test
PRBC	Packed red blood cells	RBBB	Right bundle branch block
pre-op	Pre-operative	rbc	Red blood cell
prep	Preparation	RCT	Randomized controlled trial
primip	Primiparous patient	RDS	Respiratory distress syndrome
prn	As needed	re	About
PROM	Premature rupture of membranes	rehab	Rehabilitation
PS	Pulmonic stenosis	REM	Rapid eye movement
PSA	Prostate-specific antigen	RES	Reticuloendothelial system
PSVT	Paroxysmal supraventricular tachycardia	retic	Reticulocyte(s)
PT	Prothrombin time	RF	Rheumatoid factor
pt(s)	Patient(s)	Rh	Rhesus factor
PTH	Parathormone	RHD	Rheumatic heart disease
PTSD	Post-traumatic stress disorder	RIA	Radioimmunoassay
		RIND	Reversible ischemic neurologic deficit
PTT	Partial thromboplastin time	RLQ	Right lower quadrant
PTU	Propylthiouracil	RMSF	Rocky Mountain spotted fever
PUD	Peptic ulcer disease		
PUVA	Psoralen + UVA light	RNA	Ribonucleic acid
PVC	Premature ventricular tachycardia	RNP	Ribonucleoprotein
		ROM	Range of motion
		ROS	Review of systems
q	Every	RPR	Rapid plasma reagin
qd	Daily	RR	Respiratory rate
qi	4 times a day	RSI	Rapid sequence intubation
qod	Every other day	RSV	Respiratory syncytial virus
QRS	QRS wave form on EKG	RTA	Renal tubular acidosis
qt	Quart	RUQ	Right upper quadrant
		rv	Review
R	Right; or respirations	RV	Right ventricle
r/o	Rule out	RVH	Right ventricular hypertrophy
RA	Rheumatoid arthritis		
RAIU	Radioactive iodine uptake	rx	Treatment

s/p	Status post	SKSD	Streptokinase, streptodornase
S_1	First heart sound		
S_2	Second heart sound	sl	Sublingual
S_3	Third heart sound, gallop	SLE	Systemic lupus erythematosis
S_4	Fourth heart sound, gallop		
SAB	Spontaneous abortion	SMA	Superior mesenteric artery
SAH	Subarachnoid hemorrhage	SMX	Sulfamethexasole
sat	Saturation	SNF	Skilled nursing facility
Sb	Antimony	soln	Solution
SBE	Subacure bacterial endocarditis	SP	Spontaneous pneumothorax
		specif	Specificity
SBFT	Small bowel follow through	SPECT	Single-photon emission computed tomography
SBP	Spontaneous bacterial peritonitis	SPEP	Serum protein electrophoresis
sc	Subcutaneous	SR	Slow release
SCD	Sickle cell disease	SRS	Slow-reacting substance
SCFE	Slipped capital femoral epiphysis	SS	Sickle cell disease
		SSKI	Saturated solution of potassium iodide
SD	Standard deviation		
sec	Second	SSRI	Selective serotonin reuptake inhibitor
sens	Sensitivity		
serol	Serology(ies)	SSS	Sick sinus syndrome
SFMS	Stroma-free methemoglobin solution	ST	ST segment of EKG
		Staph	Staphylococcus
SGA	Small for gestational age	STD	Sexually transmitted disease
SGGT	Serum gamma-glutamyl-transaminase		
		STEMI	ST elevation myocardial infarction
SGPT	Serum glutanic-pyruvic transminase	STP	2,5-dimethoxy-4-methylamphetamine
SH	Salter-Harris		
SI	Sacroiliac	STS	Serologic test for syphillis
si	Sign(s)	SVC	Superior vena cava
SIADH	Syndrome of inappropriate ADH	SVR	Systemic vascular resistance
SIDS	Sudden infant death syndrome	SVT	Supraventricular tachycardia

sx	Symptom(s)	Tm	Trimethoprim
sys	Systolic	TMP/ SMX	Trimethorprim/ sulfamethoxazole
T + A	Tonsillectomy and adenoidectomy	TNF	Tumor necrosis factor
		TNG	Nitroglycerine
T°	Fever/temperature	TNM	Tumor, nodes, metastases
T_3	Triiodothyronine	TPA	Tissue plasminogen activator
T_4	Thyroxine		
T7	Free thyroxine index	TPN	Total parenteral nutrition
tab	Tablet	TPNH	Triphosphopyridine reduced
TAH	Total abdominal hysterectomy		
		TRH	Thyroid-releasing hormone
TB	Tuberculosis		
TBG	Thyroid-binding globulin	TS	Tricuspid stenosis
TBSA	Total body surface area	TSH	Thyroid-stimulating hormone
TCA	Tricyclic antidepressant		
tcn	Tetracycline	tsp	Teaspoon
Td	Tetanus/diphtheria, adult type	TTE	Transthoracic echocardiogram
TDF	Tenofovir	TTP	Thrombotic thrombocytopenic purpura
TEE	Transesophageal echocardiogram		
TENS	Transcutaneous electrical nerve stimulation	TURP	Transurethral resection of prostate
TFT	Thyroid function test	TWAR	Chlamydia pneumoniae species with subtypes TW-183 and AR-39
TFV	Tenofovir		
TG	Triglycerides		
TGA	Transient global amnesia		
THC	Tetrahydrocannabinol	U	Units
TI	Tricuspid insufficiency	UA	Urinalysis
TIA	Transient ischemic attack	UCSF	University of California, San Francisco
TIBC	Total iron-binding capacity		
		UGI	Upper gastrointestinal
tid	Three times a day	UGIS	Upper gi series
TIMI	Thrombolysis in myocardial infarction	URI	Upper respiratory illness
		U.S.	United States
TM	Tympanic membrane	US	Ultrasound

USPTF	U.S. Preventive Task Force	VT/ Vtach	Ventricular tachycardia
UTI	Urinary tract infection	VZIG	Varicella-zoster immune globulin
UTS	Urine toxicologic screen		
UUB	Urine urobilinogen		
UV	Ultraviolet	w	with
UVA	Ultraviolet A	W/s	Watt/second
UVB	Ultraviolet B	w/u	Work up
		WAP	Wandering atrial pacemaker
V/Q	Ventilation/perfusion		
vag	Vaginally	wbc	White blood cells; or white blood count
val	Valine		
VCUG	Voiding Cystourethrogram	wk	Weeks(s)
VDRL	Venereal Disease Research Lab	WNL	Withing normal limits
		WPW	Wolff-Parkinson-White syndrome
VF/Vfib	Ventricular fibrillation		
VIP	Vasoactive intestinal peptide	wt	Weight
vit	Vitamin	xmatch	Cross-match
VLDL	Very-low density lipoprotein		
		yr	Year(s)
VMA	Vanillymandelic acid		
vol	Volume	ZE	Zollinger-Ellison syndrome
vs	Versus		
VSD	Ventricular septal defect	Zn	Zinc

Journal and Reference Abbreviations

Acad Emerg Med	Academic Emergency Medicine
ACP J Club	American College of Physicians Journal Club (supplement to Annals of Internal Medicine)
Acta Anaesthesiol Scand	ACTA Anaesthesiologica Scandinavica (Copenhagen)
Acta Belg Med Phys	ACTA Belgica Medica Physiologica
Acta Derm Venereol	ACTA Dermato-Venereolgica
Acta Med Scand	ACTA Medica Scandiavica
Acta Neurochir	ACTA Neurochirurgica
Acta Obgyn	ACTA Obstetricia et Gynecologica Scandinavica
Acta Ophthalm Scand	ACTA Ophthalmologica Scandinavica
Acta Otolaryngol	ACTA Oto-laryngologica
Acta Paediatr	ACTA Paediatrica
Acta Paediatr Scand	ACTA Paediatrica Scandinavica
Acta Urol Belg	ACTA Urologica Belgica
Adv Exp Med Biol	Advances in Experimental Medicine and Biology
Adv IM	Advances in Immunology
Adv Neurol	Advances in Neurology
Adv Pharmacol	Advances in Pharmacology
Age Aging	Age and Aging
AIDS	AIDS
AIDS Read	AIDS Reader
Alcohol	Alcohol
Aliment Pharmacol Ther	Alimentary Pharmacology and Therapeutics
Allergy	Allergy

Allergy Asthma Proc	Allergy and Asthma Proceedings
Allergy Clin Immunol	Allergy and Clinical Immunology
Am Fam Phys	American Family Physician
Am Hrt J	American Heart Journal
Am J Cardiol	American Journal of Cardiology
Am J Clin Path	American Journal of Clinical Pathology
Am J Dis Child	American Journal of Diseases of Childhood
Am J Emerg Med	American Journal of Emergency Medicine
Am J Epidem	American Journal of Epidemiology
Am J Gastroenterol	American Journal of Gastroenterology
Am J Hematol	American Journal of Hematology
Am J Hlth Sys Pharm	American Journal of Health-System Pharmacy
Am J Hosp Pharm	American Journal of Hospital Pharmacy
Am J Infect Control	American Journal of Infection Control
Am J Kidney Dis	American Journal of Kidney Diseases
Am J Med	American Journal of Medicine
Am J Med Sci	American Journal of the Medical Sciences
Am J Neuroradiol	American Journal of Neuroradiology
Am J Obgyn	American Journal of Obstetrics and Gynecology
Am J Ophthalm	American Journal of Ophthalmology
Am J Orthop	American Journal of Orthopedics
Am J Otol	American Journal of Otology
Am J Otolaryngol	American Journal of Otolaryngology
Am J Perinatol	American Journal of Perinatology

Am J Phys Med Rehabil	American Journal of Physical Medicine and Rehabilitation
Am J Psych	American Journal of Psychiatry
Am J Pub Hlth	American Journal of Public Health
Am J Respir Crit Care Med	American Journal of Respiratory and Critical Care Medicine
Am J Respir Med	American Journal of Respiratory Medicine
Am J Roentgenol	American Journal of Roentgenology
Am J Roentgenol Radium Ther Nucl Med	American Journal of Roentgenology Radium Therapy and Nuclear Medicine
Am J Surg	American Journal of Surgery
Am J Ther	American Journal of Therapy
Am Rv Respir Dis	American Review of Respiratory Disease
Am Surg	American Surgeon
Anaesth Intensive Care	Anaesthesia and Intensive Care
Anaesthesia	Anaesthesia
Anaesthesist	Anaesthetist
Anesth Analg	Anesthesia and Analgesia
Anesthesiology	Anesthesiology
Ann Allergy	Annals of Allergy
Ann Chir Gynaecol Fenn	Annales Chirurgiae et Gynaecologiae
Ann Clin Biochem	Annals of Clinical Biochemistry
Ann EM	Annals of Emergency Medicine
Ann Fam Med	Annals of Family Medicine
Ann IM	Annals of Internal Medicine
Ann Med Interne (Paris)	Annales de Medecine Interne (Paris)
Ann N Y Acad Sci	Annals of New York Academy of Sciences
Ann Neurol	Annals of Neurology
Ann Ophthalm	Annals of Ophthalmology

Ann Otol Rhinol Laryngol	Annals of Otology, Rhinology and Laryngology
Ann Pharmacother	The Annals of Pharmacotherapy
Ann Plast Surg	Annals of Plastic Surgery
Ann R Coll Surg Engl	Annals of the Royal College of Surgeons of England
Ann Rv Public Health	Annual Review of Public Health
Ann Surg	Annals of Surgery
Ann Thorac Surg	Annals of Thoracic Surgery
Antimicrob Agents Chemother	Antimicrobial Agents and Chemotherapy
Arch Derm	Archives of Dermatology
Arch Dis Child	Archives of Disease in Childhood
Arch EM	Archives of Emergency Medicine
Arch Environ Contam Toxicol	Archives of Environmental Contamination and Toxicology
Arch Environ Hlth	Archives of Environmental Health
Arch Gen Psychiatry	Archives of General Psychiatry
Arch IM	Archives of Internal Medicine
Arch Neurol	Archives of Neurology
Arch Ophthalm	Archives of Ophthalmology
Arch Otolaryngol Head Neck Surg	Archives of Otolaryngology— Head and Neck Surgery
Arch Otorhinolaryngol	Archives of Oto-Rhino-Laryngology
Arch Ped Adolesc Med	Archives of Pediatrics and Adolescent Medicine
Arch Phys Med Rehab	Archives of Physical Medicine and Rehabilitation
Arch Surg	Archives of Surgery
Arthritis Rheum	Arthritis and Rheumatism
Asia Oceania J Obgyn	Asia-Oceania Journal of Obstetrics and Gynaecology
Aust N Z J Ophthalm	Australian and New Zealand Journal of Ophthalmology

Aust N Z J Surg	Australian and New Zealand Journal of Surgery
Aviat Space Environ Med	Aviation Space and Environmental Medicine
Biol Psych	Biological Psychiatry
Blood	Blood
BMJ	British Medical Journal
Brain	Brain
Brain Inj	Brain Injury
Brain Res	Brain Research
Brit Hrt J	British Heart Journal
Brit J Addict	British Journal of Addiction
Brit J Anaesth	British Journal of Anaesthesia
Brit J Clin Pharmacol	British Journal of Clinical Pharmacology
Brit J Dermatol	British Journal of Dermatology
Brit J Gen Pract	British Journal of General Practice
Brit J Haematol	British Journal of Haematology
Brit J Neurosurg	British Journal of Neurosurgery
Brit J Obgyn	British Journal of Obstetrics and Gynaecology
Brit J Opthalm	British Journal of Ophthalmology
Brit J Pharmacol	British Journal of Pharmacology
Brit J Plast Surg	British Journal of Plastic Surgery
Brit J Psych	British Journal of Psychiatry
Brit J Radiol	British Journal of Radiology
Brit J Rheum	British Journal of Rheumatology
Brit J Sports Med	British Journal of Sports Medicine
Brit J Surg	British Journal of Surgery
Brit J Urol	British Journal of Urology
Brit J Vener Dis	British Journal of Venereal Diseases
Bull Am Coll Surg	Bulletin of the American College of Surgeons
Bull Rheum Dis	Bulletin of Rheumatic Diseases
Bull World Hlth Organ	Bulletin of the World Health Organization
Burns	Burns

Can Assoc Radiol J	Canadian Association of Radiologists Journal
Can J Cardiol	Canadian Journal of Cardiology
Can J Ophthalm	Canadian Journal of Ophthalmology
Can J Psychiatr	Canadian Journal of Psychiatry
Can J Surg	Canadian Journal of Surgery
Can J Urol	Canadian Journal of Urology
Can Med Assoc J	Canadian Medical Association Journal
Cancer Control	Cancer Control
Cancer Epidem Biomarkers Prev	Cancer Epidemiology, Biomarkers & Prevention
Cardiol Clin	Cardiology Clinics
Cardiol Rev	Cardiology in Review
Cardiologia	Cardiologia
Cardiology	Cardiology
Cardiovasc Clin	Cardiovascular Clinics
Cardiovasc Drugs Ther	Cardiovascular Drugs and Therapy
Cardiovasc Surg	Cardiovascular Surgery
Cathet Cardiovasc Diagn	Catheterization and Cardiovascular Diagnosis
Cephalalgia	Cephalgia
Cerebrovasc Dis	Cerebrovascular Diseases
Chest	Chest
Child Abuse Negl	Child Abuse and Neglect
Child Nephrol Urol	Child Nephrology and Urology
Chin Med J	Chinese Medical Journal
Circ Res	Circulation Research
Circ	Circulation
Clao J	Clao Journal
Cleve Clin J Med	Cleveland Clinic Journal of Medicine
Clin Cardiol	Clinical Cardiology
Clin Chem	Clinical Chemistry
Clin Chest Med	Clinics in Chest Medicine
Clin Chim Acta	Clinica Chimica ACTA

Clin Cornerstone	Clinical Cornerstone
Clin Electroencephalogr	Clinical Electroencephalography
Clin Exp Allergy	Clinical and Experimental Allergy
Clin Exp Dermatol	Clinical and Experimental Dermatology
Clin Exp Hypertens	Clinical and Experimental Hypertension
Clin Exp Immunol	Clinical and Experimental Immunology
Clin Exp Neurol	Clinical and Experimental Neurology
Clin Exp Rheum	Clinical and Experimental Rheumatology
Clin Ger Med	Clinics in Geriatric Medicine
Clin Imaging	Clinical Imaging
Clin Immunol Immunopathol	Clinical Immunology and Immunopathology
Clin Infect Dis	Clinical Infectious Diseases
Clin J Sport Med	Clinical Journal of Sports Medicine
Clin Lab Haematol	Clinical and Laboratory Haematology
Clin Lab Med	Clinics in Laboratory Medicine
Clin Microbiol Rv	Clinical Microbiology Reviews
Clin Nephrol	Clinical Nephrology
Clin Neurol Neurosurg	Clinical Neurology and Neurosurgery
Clin Neuropathol	Clinical Neuropathology
Clin Obgyn	Clinical Obstetrics and Gynecology
Clin Orthop	Clinical Orthopedics and Related Research
Clin Perinatol	Clinical Perinatology
Clin Pharm	Clinical Pharmacy
Clin Pharmacokinet	Clinical Pharmocokinetics
Clin Pharmacol Ther	Clinical Pharmacology and Therapeutics
Clin Physiol Biochem	Clinical Physiology and Biochemistry

Clin Physiol Funct Imaging	Clinical Physiology and Functional Imaging
Clin Plast Surg	Clinics in Plastic Surgery
Clin Radiol	Clinical Radiology
Clin Rheumatol	Clinical Rheumatology
Cochrane Database Sys Rv	Cochrane Database Sys
Conn Med	Connecticut Medicine
Contraception	Contraception
Contraceptive Tech	Contraceptive Technology
Contrib Nephrol	Contributions to Nephrology
Crit Care	Critical Care
Crit Care Clin	Critical Care Clinics
Crit Care Med	Critical Care Medicine
Crit Rev Toxicol	Critical Reviews in Toxicology
Curr Clin Top Infect Dis	Current Clinical Topics in Infectious Disease
Curr Concepts Cerebro Dis	Current Concepts of Cerebrovascular Disease
Curr Drug Targets	Current Drug Targets
Curr Med Res Opin	Current Medical Research and Opinion
Curr Opin Cardiol	Current Opinion in Cardiology
Curr Opin Obgyn	Current Opinion in Obstetrics and Gynecology
Curr Opin Ophthalmol	Current Opinion in Ophthalmology
Curr Opin Peds	Current Opinion in Pediatrics
Curr Opin Rheumatol	Current Opinion in Rheumatology
Curr Ther Res Clin Exp	Current Therapeutic Research-Clinical and Experimental
Cutis	Cutis
Dement Geriatr Cogn Disord	Dementia and Geriatric Cognitive Disorders
Diab Care	Diabetes Care
Diab Res Clin Pract	Diabetes Research and Clinical Practice

Diabetes	Diabetes
Dig Dis	Digestive Diseases
Dig Dis Sci	Digestive Diseases and Sciences
Dis Chest	Diseases of the Chest
Dis Colon Rectum	Diseases of the Colon and Rectum
Drug Alcohol Depend	Drug and Alcohol Dependence
Drug Saf	Drug Safety
Drugs	Drugs
Ear Nose Throat J	Ear, Nose and Throat Journal
Eff Clin Prac	Effective Clinical Practice
EM Australas	Emergency Medicine Australasia
Emerg Infect Dis	Emerging Infectious Diseases
Emerg Med Clin N Am	Emergency Medical Clinics of North America
Emerg Radiol	Emergency Radiology
EMJ	Emergency Medicine Journal
Endocrinol Metab Clin N Am	Endocrinology and Metabolism Clinics of North America
Endoscopy	Endoscopy
Environ Hlth Perspect	Environmental Health Perspectives
Epidem Rev	Epidemiology Review
Epidemiology	Epidemiology
Epilepsia	Epilepsia
Eur Hrt J	European Heart Journal
Eur J Cancer	European Journal of Cancer
Eur J Cardiol	European Journal of Cardiology
Eur J Clin Invest	European Journal of Clinical Investigation
Eur J Clin Microbiol Infect Dis	European Journal of Clinical Microbiology and Infectious Diseases
Eur J Clin Pharmacol	European Journal of Clinical Pharmacology
Eur J Emerg Med	European Journal of Emergency Medicine

Eur J Ped Surg	European Journal of Pediatric Surgery
Eur J Peds	European Journal of Pediatrics
Eur Respir J	European Respiratory Journal
Eur Urol	European Urology
Eye	Eye
Eye Ear Nose Throat Mon	Eye, Ear, Nose and Throat Monthly
Fam Med	Family Medicine
Fam Pract Recert	Family Practice Recertification
Fam Pract Survey	Family Practice Survey
FDA Bul	Federal Drug Administration Bulletin
Fertil Steril	Fertility and Sterility
Foot Ankle Int	Foot & Ankle International
Fortschr Ophthalm	Fortschritte der Ophthalmologie
Fundam Clin Pharmacol	Fundamental and Clinical Pharmacology
Gastrointest Endosc	Gastrointestinal Endoscopy
GE	Gastroenterology
Gen Dent	General Dentistry
Genitourin Med	Genitourinary Medicine
Ger Med Mon	German Medical Monthly
Ger Med Today	Geriatric Medicine Today
Ger Rv Syllabus	Geriatric Review Syllabus
Geriatrics	Geriatrics
Gerontol	Gerontologist
Graefes Arch Clin Exp Ophthalm	Graefes Archive for Clinical and Experimental Ophthalmology
Gut	Gut
Haematologica	Haematologica
Haemostasis	Haemostasis
Hand Clin	Hand Clinics
Hawaii Med J	Hawaii Medical Journal

Head Neck Surg	Head and Neck Surgery
Headache	Headache
Heart	Heart
Heart Lung	Heart and Lung
HEC Forum	Healthcare Ethics Committee Forum
Hepatology	Hepatology
Hlth Technol Assess	Health Technology Assessment Reports
Hosp Community Psychiatry	Hospital and Community Psychiatry
HT	Hypertension
Hum Exp Toxicol	Human and Experimental Toxicology
Hum Pathol	Human Pathology
Hum Reprod	Human Reproduction
Hum Toxicol	Human Toxicology
Immunodefic Rev	Immunodeficiency Reviews
Immunopharmacol	Immunopharmacology
Indian J Peds	Indian Journal of Pediatrics
Inf Contr Hosp Epidem	Infection Control and Hospital Epidemiology
Inf Dis Clin North Am	Infectious Disease Clinics of North America
Inf Dis Ob/Gyn	Infectious Diseases in Obstetrics and Gynecology
Infection	Infection
Injury	Injury
Instr Course Lect	Instructional Course Lectures
Int Angiol	International Angiology
Int J Antimicrob Agents	International Journal of Antimicrobial Agents
Int J Cardiol	International Journal of Cardiology
Int J Dermatol	International Journal of Dermatology

Int J Dev Neurosci	International Journal of Developmental Neuroscience
Int J Gynaecol Obstet	International Journal of Gynaecology and Obstetrics
Int J Hyg Environ Hlth	International Journal of Hygiene and Environmental Health
Int J Oncol	International Journal of Oncology
Int J Oral Surg	International Journal of Oral Surgery
Int J Radiat Oncol Biol Phys	International Journal of Radiation Oncology, Biology, Physics
Int Ophthalm Clin	International Ophthalmology Clinics
Intensive Care Med	Intensive Care Medicine
Intern Med	Internal Medicine
Ir Med J	Irish Medical Journal
J Accid Emerg Med	Journal of Accident and Emergency Medicine
J Acquir Immune Defic Syndr	Journal of Acquired Immune Deficiency Syndromes
J Allergy Clin Immunol	Journal of Allergy and Clinical Immunology
J Am Acad Derm	Journal of the American Academy of Dermatology
J Am Acad Orthop Surg	Journal of the American Academy of Orthopedic Surgery
J Am Board Fam Pract	Journal of the American Board of Family Practice
J Am Coll Cardiol	Journal of the American College of Cardiology
J Am Coll Surg	Journal of the American College of Surgery
J Am Ger Soc	Journal of the American Geriatric Association
J Am Mosq Control Assoc	Journal of the American Mosquito Control Association

J Am Soc Nephrol	Journal of the American Society of Nephrology
J Anal Toxicol	Journal of Analytical Toxicology
J Antimicrob Chemother	Journal of Antimicrobial Chemotherapy
J Appl Bacteriol	Journal of Applied Bacteriology
J Appl Physiol	Journal of Applied Physiology
J Assoc Physicians India	Journal of the Association of Physicians of India
J Asthma	Journal of Asthma
J Biol Chem	Journal of Biological Chemistry
J Bone Joint Surg	Journal of Bone and Joint Surgery
J Burn Care Rehab	Journal of Burn Care and Rehabilitation
J Card Fail	Journal of Cardiac Failure
J Card Surg	Journal of Cardiac Surgery
J Cardiovasc Pharmacol	Journal of Cardiovascular Pharmacology
J Cardiovasc Pharmacol Ther	Journal of Cardiovascular Pharmacology Therapy
J Cardiovasc Risk	Journal of Cardiovascular Risk
J Cataract Refract Surg	Journal of Cataract and Refractive Surgery
J Child Neurol	Journal of Child Neurology
J Child Psychol Psychiatry	Journal of Child Psychology and Psychiatry and Allied Disciplines
J Chronic Dis	Journal of Chronic Disease
J Clin Anesth	Journal of Clinical Anesthesia
J Clin Endocrinol Metab	Journal of Clinical Endocrinology and Metabolism
J Clin Epidem	Journal of Clinical Epidemiology
J Clin Immunol	Journal of Clinical Immunology
J Clin Microbiol	Journal of Clinical Microbiology
J Clin Oncol	Journal of Clinical Oncology
J Clin Pharmacol J New Drugs	Journal of Clinical Pharmacology/Journal of New Drugs

J Clin Psych	Journal of Clinical Psychiatry
J Clin Psychopharmacol	Journal of Clinical Psychopharmacology
J Clin Ultrasound	Journal of Clinical Ultrasound
J Clin Virol	Journal of Clinical Virology
J Crit Illn	Journal of Critical Illness
J Cutan Med Surg	Journal of Cutaneous Medicine and Surgery
J Dermatol	Journal of Dermatology
J Dermatol Surg Oncol	Journal of Dermatologic Surgery and Oncology
J Electrocardiol	Journal of Electrocardiology
J Emerg Med	Journal of Emergency Medicine
J Epidem Community Hlth	Journal of Epidemiology and Community Health
J Eur Acad Dermatol Venereol	Journal of the European Academy of Dermatology and Venereology
J Fam Pract	Journal of Family Practice
J Foot Ankle Surg	Journal of Foot and Ankle Surgery
J Forensic Sci	Journal of Forensic Sciences
J Gastroenterol Hepatol	Journal of Gastroenterology and Hepatology
J Gen Intern Med	Journal of General Internal Medicine
J Ger Psych Neurol	Journal of Geriatric Psychiatry and Neurology
J Gerontol	Journal of Gerontology
J Gerontol A Biol Sci Med Sci	Journals of Gerontology Series A: Biological Sciences and Medical Sciences
J Hand Surg [Am]	Journal of Hand Surgery [American Volume]
J Hand Surg [Br]	Journal of Hand Surgery [British Volume]
J Hrt Lung Transplant	Journal of Heart and Lung Transplantation

J Hum Hypertens	Journal of Human Hypertension
J Hyg	Journal of Hygiene
J Infect	Journal of Infection
J Infect Dis	Journal of Infectious Disease
J Inherit Metab Dis	Journal of Inherited Metabolic Disease
J Intern Med	Journal of Internal Medicine
J Invasive Cardiol	Journal of Invasive Cardiology
J Investig Derm	Journal of Investigative Dermatology
J Lab Clin Med	Journal of Laboratory and Clinical Medicine
J Laryngol Otol	Journal of Laryngology and Otology
J Med Assoc Ga	Journal of the Medical Association of Georgia
J Med Virol	Journal of Medical Virology
J Nat Prod	Journal of Natural Products
J Natl Cancer Inst	Journal of the National Cancer Institute
J Neurol	Journal of Neurology
J Neurol Neurosurg Psychiatry	Journal of Neurology, Neurosurgery and Psychiatry
J Neurol Sci	Journal of the Neurological Sciences
J Neuroophthalmol	Journal of Neuro-Ophthalmology
J Neurosurg Anesthesiol	Journal of Neurosurgical Anesthesiology
J Neurosurg	Journal of Neurosurgery
J Neurotrauma	Journal of Neurotrauma
J Neurovirol	Journal of Neurovirology
J Nucl Cardiol	Journal of Nuclear Cardiology
J Nucl Med	Journal of Nuclear Medicine
J Nurs Adm	Journal of Nursing Administration
J Nutr	Journal of Nutrition
J Oral Maxillofac Surg	Journal of Oral and Maxillofacial Surgery

J Orthop Res	Journal of Orthopedic Research
J Oslo City Hosp	Journal of the Oslo City Hospitals
J Otolaryngol	Journal of Otolaryngology
J Paediatr Child Health	Journal of Paediatrics & Child Health
J Ped Gastroenterol Nutr	Journal of Pediatric Gastroenterology and Nutrition
J Ped Orthop	Journal of Pediatric Orthopaedics
J Ped Surg	Journal of Pediatric Surgery
J Peds	Journal of Pediatrics
J Perinat Med	Journal of Perinatal Medicine
J Perinatol	Journal of Perinatology
J Pharm Experim Ther	Journal of Pharmacology and Experimental Therapeutics
J Postgrad Med	Journal of Postgraduate Medicine
J Psychoactive Drugs	Journal of Psychoactive Drugs
J Psychopharm	Journal of Psychopharmacology
J Refract Corneal Surg	Journal of Refractive and Corneal Surgery
J Reproduct Med	Journal of Reproductive Medicine
J Rheumatol	Journal of Rheumatology
J Spinal Disord	Journal of Spinal Disorders
J Surg Oncol	Journal of Surgical Oncology
J Thromb Thrombolysis	Journal of Thrombosis and Thrombolysis
J Toxicol Clin Toxicol	Journal of Toxicology—Clinical Toxicology
J Trauma	Journal of Trauma—Injury, Infection and Critical Care
J Ultrasound Med	Journal of Ultrasound in Medicine
J Urol	Journal of Urology
J Vasc Surg	Journal of Vascular Surgery
J Water Health	Journal of Water and Health
J Wildl Dis	Journal of Wildlife Diseases
Jama	Journal of the American Medical Association
Joint Bone Spine	Joint Bone Spine

Jpn Circ J	Japanese Circulation Journal—English Edition
Jpn J Surg	Japanese Journal of Surgery
JR Coll Physicians Lond	Journal of the Royal College of Physicians of London
JR Coll Surg Edinb	Journal of the Royal College of Surgeons of Edinburgh
JR Soc Med	Journal of the Royal Society of Medicine
Kidney Int	Kidney International
Lab Anim	Lab Animal
Lancet	Lancet
Laryngoscope	Laryngoscope
Leuk Lymphoma	Leukemia & Lymphoma
Leukemia	Leukemia
Life Sci	Life Sciences
Lik Sprava	Likars'ka Sprava
Lupus	Lupus
Mccvd	Modern Concepts of Cardiovascular Disease
Md State Med Assoc J	Maryland State Medical Association Journal
Med	Medicine
Med Care	Medical Care
Med Clin N Am	Medical Clinics of North America
Med Decis Making	Medical Decision Making
Med Hypotheses	Medical Hypotheses
Med J Aust	Medical Journal of Australia
Med Lett Drugs Ther	Medical Letter of Drugs and Therapeutics
Med Sci Sports Exerc	Medicine and Science in Sports and Exercise
Med Toxicol	Medical Toxicology

Metabolism	Metabolism—Clinical and Experimental
Mil Med	Military Medicine
Millbank Q	Millbank Quarterly
Mmwr	CDC Morbidity and Mortality Weekly Review
Mod Med	Modern Medicine
Nejm	New England Journal of Medicine
Nephrol Dial Transplant	Nephrology Dialysis Transplantation
Nephron	Nephron
Neuroimaging Clin N Am	Neuroimaging Clinics of North America
Neurol Clin	Neurologic Clinics
Neurol Res	Neurological Research
Neurol	Neurology
Neurosurgery	Neurosurgery
Obgyn Cl N Am	Obstetrics and Gynecology Clinics of North America
Obgyn	Obstetrics and Gynecology
Occup Med	Occupational Medicine—State of the Art Reviews
Ophthalm	Ophthalmology
Ophthalmic Res	Ophthalmic Research
Ophthalmic Surg	Ophthalmic Surgery
Ophthalmologica	Ophthalmologica
Optom Clin	Optometry Clinics
Optom Vis Sci	Optometry and Vision Science
Oral Dis	Oral Diseases
Orthop Clin N Am	Orthopedic Clinics of North America
Orthop Rev	Orthopaedic Review
Otolaryngol Clin N Am	Otolaryngologic Clinics of North America

Otolaryngol Head Neck Surg	Otolaryngology-Head and Neck Surgery
Pacing Clin Electrophysiol	Pacing and Clinical Electrophysiology
Paediatrician	Paediatrician
Pain	Pain
Paraplegia	Paraplegia
Ped Anaesth	Paediatric Anaesthesia
Ped Ann	Pediatric Annals
Ped Cardiol	Pediatric Cardiology
Ped Clin N Am	Pediatric Clinics of North America
Ped Dent	Pediatric Dentistry
Ped Derm	Pediatric Dermatology
Ped Emerg Care	Pediatric Emergency Care
Ped Hematol Oncol	Pediatric Hematology and Oncology
Ped Infect Dis J	Pediatric Infectious Disease Journal
Ped Nephrol	Pediatric Nephrology
Ped Neurol	Pediatric Neurology
Ped Pulmonol	Pediatric Pulmonology
Ped Radiol	Pediatric Radiology
Ped Rv	Pediatric Review
Peds	Pediatrics
Peds Int	Pediatrics International
Perit Dial Int	Peritoneal Dialysis International
Pharmacoeconomics	Pharmacoeconomics
Pharmacol	Pharmacology
Pharmacotherapy	Pharmacotherapy
Phys Ther	Physical Therapy
Physiol Rev	Physiological Reviews
Plast Reconstr Surg	Plastic and Reconstructive Surgery
Post Grad Med J	Postgraduate Medicine Journal
Practitioner	Practitioner
Prehosp Diaster Med	Prehospital and Disaster Medicine

Prehosp Emerg Care	Prehospital Emergency Care
Prev Med	Preventive Medicine
Proc Natl Acad Sci USA	Proceedings of the National Academy of Sciences of the United States of America
Proc Soc Exp Biol Med	Proceedings of the Society for Experimental Biology and Medicine
Prog Cardiovasc Dis	Progress in Cardiovascular Diseases
Prostate	Prostate
Psychiat Ann	Psychiatric Annals
Psychiatry Res	Psychiatry Research
Psychol Rep	Psychological Reports
Psychosomatics	Psychosomatics
Public Hlth Rep	Public Health Reports
Qjm	Quarterly Journal of Medicine
Radiol Clin N Am	Radiologic Clinics of North America
Radiology	Radiology
Recenti Prog Med	Recenti Progressi in Medicina
Ren Fail	Renal Failure
Respir Med	Respiratory Medicine
Respiration	Respiration
Resuscitation	Resuscitation
Rev Cardiovasc Med	Reviews in Cardiovascular Medicine
Rev Inf Dis	Review of Infectious Disease
Rev Rhum Ed Fr	Revue du Rhumatisme. Edition Francaise
Rheum Dis Clin N Am	Rheumatic Disease Clinics of North America
Rheumatology	Rheumatology
Sarcoidosis Vasc Diffuse Lung Dis	Sarcoidosis Vasculitis and Diffuse Lung Diseases

Scand J Clin Lab	Scandinavian Journal of Clinical Laboratory
Scand J Clin Lab Invest	Scandinavian Journal of Clinical & Laboratory Investigation
Scand J Gastroenterol	Scandinavian Journal of Gastroenterology
Scand J Infect Dis	Scandinavian Journal of Infectious Diseases
Scand J Rheumatol	Scandinavian Journal of Rheumatology
Scand J Work Environ Hlth	Scandinavian Journal of Work Environment & Health
Schweiz Arch Neurol Psychiatr	Schweizer Archiv fur Neurologie und Psychiatrie
Sci Am Text Med	Scientific American Textbook of Medicine
Science	Science
Semin Arth Rheum	Seminars in Arthritis and Rheumatology
Semin Interv Cardiol	Seminars in Interventional Cardiology
Semin Nephrol	Seminars in Nephrology
Semin Ophthalm	Seminars in Ophthalmology
Semin Ped Surg	Seminars in Pediatric Surgery
Semin Roentgenol	Seminars in Roentgenology
Semin Thorac Cardiovasc Surg	Seminars in Thoracic and Cardiovascular Surgery
Sex Transm Dis	Sexually Transmitted Diseases
South Med J	Southern Medical Journal
Spinal Cord	Spinal Cord
Spine	Spine
Sports Med	Sports Medicine
Stroke	Stroke
Surg Forum	Surgical Forum
Surg Gynecol Obstet	Surgery Gynecology & Obstetrics

Surg Neurol	Surgical Neurology
Surgery	Surgery
Thorax	Thorax
Thromb Haemost	Thrombosis and Haemostasis
Thromb Res	Thrombosis Research
Toxicol Lett	Toxicology Letters
Toxicol Sci	Toxicological Sciences
Toxicology	Toxicology
Transfuse Med	Transfusion Medicine
Undersea Hyperb Med	Undersea & Hyperbaric Medicine
Urol Radiol	Urologic Radiology
Urology	Urology
Vet Hum Toxicol	Veterinary and Human Toxicology
Vet Surg	Veterinary Surgery
West J Med	Western Journal of Medicine
Wis Med J	Wisconsin Medical Journal
World J Surg	World Journal of Surgery
Yale J Biol Med	Yale Journal of Biology and Medicine

Notice

We have made every attempt to summarize accurately and concisely a multitude of references. However the reader is reminded that times and medical knowledge change, transcription or understanding error is always possible, and crucial details are omitted whenever such a comprehensive distillation as this is attempted in limited space. And the primary purpose of this compilation is to cite literature on various sides of controversial issues; knowing where "truth" lies is usually difficult. We cannot, therefore, guarantee that every bit of information is absolutely accurate or complete. The reader should affirm that cited recommendations are reasonable still, by reading the original articles and checking other sources, including local consultants as well as recent literature, before applying them.

Drugs and medical devices are discussed that may have limited availability controlled by the Food and Drug Administration (FDA) for use only in research study or clinical trial. The drug information presented has been derived from reference sources, recently published data, and pharmaceutical tests. Research, clinical practice, and government regulations often change the accepted standard in this field. When consideration is being given to use of any drug in the clinical setting, the clinician or reader is responsible for determining FDA status of the drug, reading the package insert, and prescribing information for the most up-to-date recommendations on dose, precautions, and contraindications and determining the appropriate usage for the product. This is especially important in the case of drugs that are new or seldom used.

Chapter 1

Allergy

1.1 Anaphylaxis

Med Clin N Am 1992;76:841; Ann Allergy 1992;69:87

Cause: Aspiration, ingestion and/or parenteral use of drugs or other haptens including foreign antigens (insect stings), desensitization shots, semen, or polysaccharides.

Epidem: True anaphylaxis not common; the statistics are not well elucidated because this dx is too broad. Of note, no real cross-reactivity between sulfonamide antibiotics and sulfonamide non-antibiotics (Nejm 2003;349:1628).

Pathophys: Respiratory distress due to both upper tract edema and lower tract bronchospasm, consider leukotrienes, also known as slow-reacting substance. Histamine release causes hypotension. Diarrhea and gi symptoms due to serotonin. Some reactions not IgE mediated, which is probably a function of clinical inclusion criteria being too broad.

Sx: Dizziness, dyspnea, pruritus, nausea, vomiting, diarrhea.

Si: Diffuse erythema (lobster red skin), tachypnea, decreased breath sounds, hypotension, altered mental status.

Crs: Onset in ½-3 min, death usually in 15-120 min; recurs in 28% if re-challenged.

Cmplc: Respiratory or vascular collapse, death.

Diff Dx: Differentiate from other forms of shock that include cardio-vascular, septic, or neurogenic; and differentiate from other causes of airway compromise that include asthma, COPD, airway foreign body, aspiration, near drowning, or pneumothorax.

Lab: Check for other reasons for respiratory and/or vascular collapse, and monitor vital functions—CBC with diff, ABG, serum tryptase level (Lik Sprava 1992:76) increases and helps distinguish from other forms of shock, EKG, pan culture, metabolic profile, CXR, ethanol level, urine toxic screen, O_2 sat.

Emergency Management:

- Secure airway, O_2
- Epinephrine 0.5-1.0 mg iv or im; peds dose 0.01 cc/kg of 1:1000 im (Ann EM 1995;25:785); Not sc (J Allergy Clin Immunol 1998;101:33). Despite prompt epinephrine treatment, some will still succumb to anaphylaxis and there will be the rare death from MI in those without true anaphylaxis—previous history of severe allergic reaction is not a good prognosticator for those who need home epinephrine kits (Clin Exp Allergy 2000;30:1144).
- Iv access (Crit Care Clin 1993;9:313) with NS wide open treat for shock.
- Trendelenburg if hypotensive, short term (J Trauma 1986;26: 718) with potentially minimal effects (Ann EM 1985;14:641; Crit Care Med 1979;7:218).
- Diphenhydramine 25-50 mg iv (peds 1 mg/kg) (J Appl Physiol 1988;64:210; J Allergy Clin Immunol 1990;86:684).
- Methylprednisolone 125 mg iv (peds 2 mg/kg) (Ann Allergy 1989;62:201).
- Nebs [β-agonists with equivocal data—patient pool with multiple diagnoses (Prehosp Emerg Care 2004;8:34), ipratropium].
- Selective H_2 blockers controversial, but may dose cimetidine 300 mg iv (Ann Allergy 1987;58:447).
- Aminophylline controversial (9 mg/kg load, 0.7 mg/kg/hr) (Brit J Pharmacol 1980;69:467).

1.2 Angioedema

J Am Acad Derm 1991;25:146; Ped Rv 1992;13:387

Cause: Genetic, autosomal dominant type (Clin Immunol Immunopathol 1991;61:S78); medications—eg, ACEIs; foods—eg, beer; environmental challenges; bacteria or viruses—eg, hep C, not *H. pylori;* drugs of abuse—eg, cocaine.

Epidem: Most Western races.

Pathophys: Deficiency of inhibitor of complement C'1a esterase, which also inactivates clotting factors XII and XI; the latter build up and release kallikreins/kinins causing pain, shock, etc. (Blood 1991;77:2660).

Sx: Frequently precipitated by trauma, psychological stress; pharyngitis; abdominal pain

Si: Edema of skin, upper gi tract, and respiratory tracts, recurrent, acute, nonpitting, nonpruritic, circumscribed, transient, involves localized areas, edema of uvula. [Quincke's edema (Arch Otolaryngol Head Neck Surg 1991;117:100)].

Crs: Onset not until 20-50 yr of age.

Cmplc: Laryngeal edema causing asphyxia (26% of patients die this way), r/o
- Acquired angioedema—common, benign—treat with prednisone plus hydroxyzine
- "Pseudo-angioedema" associated with lymphoma and colon Ca
- Uvular edema of Franklin's disease (Nejm 1993;329:1389)—a B-cell lymphoma with uvular edema as a prominent si/sx
- ACEI angioedema (Immunopharmacol 1999;44:21)

Lab: Assess for other reasons and severity of airway compromise—CBC with diff, ABG, carbon monoxide level, urine tox screen.

Emergency Management:
- See Anaphylaxis, p1.
- Airway management in these cases may include nasal trumpet as most efficacious; most cases with anterior airway edema sparing the pharynx. More aggressive cases may require naso-tracheal intubation.
- C'1a inhibitor form vapor-heated pooled plasma concentrate.
- Consider injection of unfractionated heparin at base of tongue—heparin is anti-inflammatory (Adv Pharmacol 1999;46:151; Ann Pharmacother 2001;35:1161) but its exact role in this condition has not been elucidated.

1.3 Urticaria

Am Fam Phys 2004;69:1123; Clin Exp Allergy 1999;29:31; Clin Exp Dermatol 1999;24:424

Cause: 80% idiopathic, and see Pathophys.

Epidem: 25% of adult population has had chronic urticaria (including mild form)

Pathophys: Direct histamine release by opiates, NSAIDs, IVP dye, thiamine, curare, dextrans, and some antibiotics; ubiquitous involvement of cytokines (J Allergy Clin Immunol 1999;103:307).

Immunologic is one of five etiologies:
- C' activation by cryoglobulins (IgG or cold agglutinins produced by tumors, multiple myeloma, SLE, arteritis, etc) or by B1C globulin damage (snake venom, DIC). Angioneurotic edema is C' mediated, but not urticaria.
- Antibodies vs mast cells: or, in chronic urticaria, their IgE receptors.
- Mast cells as "innocent bystanders," eg, SLE, serum sickness, antigens in all lesions, leukemias, and other malignancies,

drugs, parasites, hepatitis B, perhaps mononucleosis plus ampicillin; nearly all recurrent erythema multiforme and most primary episodes are due to HSV, but a few of the latter are due to mycoplasma and drugs.

- Mast cell fixed antibody (IgE), eg, to fish, bee sting, PCN.
- Type IV (DHS) immune reaction leads to vasculitis.
    Physical/"neurogenic" is one of six categories:
- Cold urticaria (test with ice cube), perhaps IgE attaches to a cold-dependent skin antigen and releases platelet-activating factor (Nejm 1985;313:405).
- Local heat urticaria.
- Systemic heat urticaria, cholinergic; seen when core body temperature is elevated, starts around hair follicles; seen in runners, tennis players, etc.
- Light/solar
- Stress
- Dermatographia
    Associated diseases: urticaria pigmentosa occasionally and anaphylaxis

Sx: Itching, mucosal swelling (with all but physical types), and abdominal pain.

Si: Target skin lesion of erythema multiforme, raised urticarial lesions; bilateral symmetry always suggests drug-induced first.

Crs: Most lesions last < 24 hr, except in vasculitis, immunologic, and physical types.

Cmplc: Epidermal detachment of mucous membranes, locally in Stevens-Johnson Syndrome with 5% mortality or extensively in toxic epidermal necrolysis with 30% mortality.

Lab: Consider r/o of toxic shock and vasculitis: CBC with diff, liver profile, metabolic profile, ESR, UA. Skin biopsy at time or urticaria to also r/o vasculitis.

Emergency Management: Acute rx: See Anaphylaxis p 1.

- 2% ephedrine spray for angioedema; H_1 receptor antagonist antihistamines, like loratadine 10 mg po qd (Drugs 1999; 57:31); H_2 blockers, like cimetidine with equivocal efficacy (J Allergy Clin Immunol 1995;95:685).

Chronic: Avoid ACEIs and NSAIDs; hydroxyzine 25 mg po three to four times a day, or diphenhydramine 25-50 mg qd 4-6 hr; cetirizine 10 mg po qd (Ann Pharmacother 1996;30:1075); or terfenadine 60 mg po bid (Ann Allergy 1989;63:616).

If these do not work, second line may warrant fexofenadine 180 mg qd or 60 mg tid, or desloratdatine 5 mg qd, or loratadine 10 mg qd.

If second line does not work, may try ranitidine 150 mg bid, or doxepin 10-25 mg bid, or cimetidine 400 mg tid.

If third line does not work, may elect to try montelukast 10 mg qd or zafirlukast 20 mg bid.

N.B. The above mentioned selective H_1-antihistamines, which include loratadine, terfenadine, and cetirizine, have not been optimally studied (Nejm 2004;351:2203) and much of this empiric practice is just better than anecdotal.

- Cold urticaria: Cyproheptadine at 4 mg up to tid a day is best (Arch Derm 1977;113:1375); doxepin 10-25 mg po bid (J Am Acad Derm 1984;11:483).
- Heat (cholinergic) type: hydroxyzine.
- Vasculitis: Steroids, may elect short course of prednisone 40 mg qd for 1 wk.
- Mast Cell Types: Ketotifen 2 mg po bid, stabilizes mast cells (Ann Allergy 1989;62:322); Acyclovir for, at least, recurrent erythema multiforme.
- Consider consult to allergist, dermatologist, or immunologist.

Chapter 2

Cardiovascular

2.1 Acute Coronary Syndrome

Int J Cardiol 1995;49:S3; J Thromb Thrombolysis 1999;8:113; Ann EM 2001;38:229

Events that have sudden onset and could lead to significant morbidity or mortality if not recognized include myocardial infarction, which includes ST-elevation MI (STEMI), myocardial stunning, coronary artery vasospasm, or unstable angina.

Cause: Atherosclerosis (85%), including spasm with superimposed thrombus in 90% of those; emboli (15%) and may also be due to cocaine-induced spasm when cocaine is used as anesthesia or a recreational drug.

Epidem: Increased incidence with h/o the following:
- Carbon monoxide acute exposures, eg, firefighters; and chronic carbon disulfide exposures, eg, disulfiram use, rayon manufacturing (Arch Environ Hlth 1989;44:361; Nejm 1989; 321:1426).
- Cholesterol elevations of total and/or LDL (Jama 1998;279: 445). Consider with cholecystitis history, presence of an arcus senilis (Am Hrt J 1965;70:838; Brit Hrt J 1970;32:449).
- Cocaine use or withdrawal (J Am Coll Cardiol 1990;16:74; Nejm 2001;345:351).
- Postmenopausal hormone therapy was thought to be cardioprotective until contrary data published at the end of the twentieth century (Jama 1998;280:605; 2002;288:49)—

CARDIOVASCULAR

current trends show more women discontinuing or tapering their doses in response to the potential harm of this therapy (Jama 2004;291:47).

- Coffee data equivocal (J Epidem Community Hlth 1999; 53:481).
- Exercise test showing ischemia; limited in asymptomatic individuals (Aviat Space Environ Med 1982;53:379), and most sensitive is MIBI-SPECT with dobutamine infusion and most specific is stress echocardiography (Heart 1998;80:370).
- Family history of MIs prematurely (age < 55 years males, < 65 years females)(Prev Med 1980;9:773; Am J Cardiol 1988;62:708; Brit Hrt J 1982;47:78; Nejm 1994;330:1041).
- Variant 5-lipoxygenase genotypes (5-lipoxygenase gives rise to leukotrienes from arachidonic acid) with increased atherosclerosis, and this atherosclerotic effect is worsened by n-6 polyunsaturated fatty (arachidonic) acids and improved by marine n-3 fatty acids (Nejm 2004;350:29).
- Homocysteine levels > 15 μM/L correlate with worse prognosis, data equivocal (Semin Interv Cardiol 1999;4:121; Circ 1998;98:204).
- Hypertension (Am Hrt J 1988;116:1713; Nejm 2001;345: 1291).
- Diabetes Mellitus (Am Hrt J 1988;116:1713); a corollary of this would be women with polycystic ovarian syndrome (Nejm 2005;352:1223).
- Lysosomal storage diseases such as α-galactosidese A deficiency (Fabry disease) which can be now treated with agalsidase beta (Fabrazyme) (Med Lett Drugs Ther 2003;45:74).
- Estrogen receptor gene variation: ESR1 c.454-397CC (Jama 2003;290:2263).
- Sedentary work or lifestyle (Scand J Work Environ Hlth 1979;5:100).

- Sexual activity can induce myocardial ischemia, silent or symptomatic (Am J Cardiol 1995;75:835).
- Smoking increases risk times 3, but risk decreases to normal over 2 yr after cessation; increases risk 5 times if > 1 ppd, 2 times if 1-4 cigarettes qd in women; also passive smoking (Nejm 1999;340:920). Smokers usually have thrombogenic MI rather than diffuse vessel disease, and the mortality/morbidity benefits seen from smoking are due to lack of other risk factors and relative youth of this population—NOT a protective effect of smoking (J Cardiovasc Risk 1999;6:307). This effect of thrombogenesis with tobacco use is increased with concomitant use of bcp's and uncontrolled (unscreened) HT—bcp's alone have small risk for MI (Lancet 1997;349:1202).
- Any renal disease (including mild) is a risk for worse morbidity/mortality after an MI. In other words, decreased GFR with increased risk of poor outcome (Nejm 2004; 351:1285; 2004;351:1296).
- Stress, day-to-day, but not type A nor distressed personality; possibly hostility—(Psychol Rep 1999;85:505) vs (Nejm 2000;343:1298).
- Viral URI in past 2 wk; or chronic *Chlamydia pneumoniae* infections, although a 3-mon empiric trial of Azithromycin in those with *C. pneumoniae* exposure made no difference on morbidity or mortality in regards to cardiac disease (Jama 2003;290:1459)—(Ann IM 1992;116:273; J Am Coll Cardiol 1998;31:827) vs (Clin Cardiol 1999;22:85). Perhaps chronic *H. pylori* infection, as well (BMJ 1995;311:711).
- Peri-operative without β-blockade (Nejm 1996;335:1713; 1999;341:1789).
- Mercury exposure may convey some risk for CAD (Nejm 2002;347:1747; 2002;347:1755).

- Ephedra alkaloids (dietary supplement aka ma huang) (Nejm 2000;343:1833).
- Decreased activity level of red-cell glutathione peroxidase 1, this is measured in U/g of Hgb (Nejm 2003;349:1605).
- Rare instance of Raynaud's type phenomenon in those with progressive systemic sclerosis having coronary vasospasm and MI (Am Hrt J 1978;95:563).
- Systemic respiratory infections associated with an increase in vascular events in the first 3 d of illness—this is not seen with immunizations (Nejm 2004;351:2611).

Decreased incidence with:
- Exercise, walking or vigorous exercise 3-4 times per wk (Nejm 1999;341:650).
- Fish intake 1-4 times/mon (Nejm 1985;312:1205; Jama 2002;287:1815); also lowers risk of sudden death (Nejm 2002;346:1113) and healthy diet (optional) (Jama 2002;288:2569). Following the Mediterranean diet, imbibing in moderate alcohol consumption, and at least 30 min of physical activity per day is associated with a lower mortality rate from coronary artery disease and is associated with a 50% lower rate of all-cause and cause-specific (coronary heart disease, cardiovascular diseases, cancer, and other causes) mortality (Jama 2004;292:1433).
- Daily ASA 325 mg po qod (Nejm 1989;321:129); even helpful post CABG (Nejm 2002;347:1309); avoid Ibuprofen for this to work (Nejm 2001;345:1809); not as effective in women (Nejm 2005;352:1293).
- Plasma homocysteine level < 9 μmol/L, and if hyperhomocysteinemia is a problem, use folate (Nejm 2001;345:1593).
- Ethanol 2-3 drinks qd in men vs 2-3/wk in women (BMJ 1999;319:1523); or 3-7 drinks per wk in men with decreased

risk of MI (Nejm 2003;348:109); better still if alcohol dehydrogenase type 3 with γ_2 homozygous (Nejm 2001;344:549).

- Better control of HT, cholesterol [statin therapy specifically (Nejm 2005;352:29)] (Nejm 2001;345:1583), etc in U.S. (Nejm 1999;340:1994; 1999;341:410) and this may extend to giving antihypertensives to those with CAD and normal blood pressure (Jama 2004;292:2217).
- High plasma adiponectin levels—those in highest quintile fared healthier than those in lowest quintile (Jama 2004;291:1730).
- Possibly decreased risk of CAD and Type II DM with increased dairy consumption (Jama 2002;287:2081).
- Antioxidant data equivocal (Nejm 2001;345:1583) including vit E (Jama 2005;293:1338).

Pathophys: Platelet aggregations and thrombi on plaque fissures cause thrombosis with or without spasm (Intern Med 2000;39:333); or paradoxical vasoconstriction with stress because plaque prevents normal endothelial cell induction of coronary dilatation.

Sx: Chest pain, substernal, in "distribution of a tree," worse supine: diaphoresis, dyspnea; associated with heavy exertion 5-40 times more frequently depending on conditioning state; atypical presentations in women; CNS symptoms are the presenting symptoms in 50% of patients > 60 yr and 31% with cardiac syncope have syncope due to ischemia or infarction (Nejm 2002;347:878)

Si: Pericardial rub on day 2+, usually without ST changes; S_3 gallop or S_4 gallop; fever < 103°F (39.4°C); transient S_2 paradoxical split. Chest wall tenderness does not exclude ischemic or infarcting myocardium (Arch IM 1985;145:65). Rectal exam for guaiac.

Crs:

- 25% are unrecognized and half are asymptomatic—yet prognosis is just as bad (Nejm 1984;311:1144); 15% in-hospital mortality before thrombolytics, now 7-10%; 10% of survivors get severe pump failure, another 10% get persistent angina, 10% "flunk" discharge mini-ETT, another 10% "flunk" maximal ETT at 6 wk follow-up; remaining 50% do fine (J Cardiovasc Risk 1999;6:69); frequent PVCs ($>$ 7/min) post test predictive of increased risk of death (5-yr death rate 11%) (Nejm 2003;348:781).
- Age-adjusted survival for women may be worse when compared to men, but studies have yet to prove (Am J Cardiol 2000;85:147)—treatment should be gender-blind.
- Cardiac arrest survival is 3.5% in out-of-hospital CPR, 8.8% if VF/VT; more survivors if bystander CPR initiated (Ann EM 1999;33:44).
- In the very elderly, aggressive invasive study and treatment do not improve mortality (Jama 2005;293:1329).

Cmplc:

- Altered binding proteins change meaning of measured levels of quinidine, cholesterol, etc.
- Aneurysm of left ventricle occurs in 40% of those with anterior MI and 13.5 % overall, develops in first 48 hr, leads to emboli, CHF, PVCs, 75% 5-yr mortality (Eur Hrt J 1990; 11:441).
- Arrhythmias (Physiol Rev 1999;79:917; Eur Hrt J 1999; 20:748); Afib is a risk factor for worse outcome (J Am Coll Cardiol 1997;30:406).
- Dressler syndrome (Cardiol Clin 1990;8:601), which may be on a continuum of pericarditis of AMI; this may lead to pericardial tamponade from inflammation (r/o RV infarct) since both functionally acutely constrict pericardial space by fluid or dilated RV.

- Heart block occurs in 5% of inferior MIs, 3% of anterior MIs, and in 100% with anterior MI + RBBB causing a 75% mortality (Chest 1976;69:599; Am J Cardiol 1992;69:1135)
- Mural thrombi without aneurysm in 11% of acute MIs, 2% of others.
- Papillary muscle rupture causes CHF with a normal-sized left atrium by TEE, occurs most often with inferior MIs, and surgery.
- Rupture of septal wall to create a VSD or rupture into pericardial sac causing tamponade.
- Syncope associated with 60% 5-yr survival (Nejm 2002; 347:878).
- Non-hemorrhagic stroke, especially if EF <28% post MI, older age, h/o hypertension or other common stroke risk factors—prevent with warfarin anticoagulation (Circ 1998;97:757).
- Anxiety neurosis, impotence.

Diff Dx:
- Of chest pain: pulmonary embolus, aortic dissection, pneumonia, rib fracture, GERD, cholecystitis.
- Of ST elevation (Nejm 2003;349:2128): pericarditis, myocarditis, hyperkalemia, LBBB, pulmonary embolus, early repolarization (see discussion under "EKG" for Brugada syndrome).

Scoring System:
- TIMI Risk Score for complications in non-ST Elevation MI or Unstable angina: (1) age > 65 yr; (2) at least 3 risk factors for CAD; (3) prior coronary stenosis of 50% or more; (4) ST segment deviation on EKG; (5) at least 2 anginal events in the prior 24 hr; (6) use of ASA in the prior 7 d; and (7) elevated serum cardiac markers (Jama 2000;284:835). Increased risk of complications with increasing score.

- Killip classification (Am J Cardiol 1967;20:457; Jama 2003;290:2174) with findings for risk of arrhythmia, cardiac arrest or death (CHF defined as rales, S_3 gallop, and venous HT; Pulmonary edema defined as severe CHF; and shock is cardiogenic shock). See Table 2.1.

Table 2.1 Killip Classification

Condition	Life-threatening Arrhythmia	Cardiac Arrest	Death
No CHF	36%	5%	6%
CHF	46%	15%	17%
Pulm Edema	73%	46%	38%
Shock	94%	77%	81%

Lab:

Chem Markers: (J Am Coll Cardiol 1999;34:739; Scand J Clin Lab Invest suppl 1999;230:103) These results may alter hospital course, but should not be the determining factors for those who need admission for cardiac evaluation (Heart 1999;82:614). CPK and Troponin may be "erroneously" elevated in those with renal failure (Nephrol Dial Transplant 1999;14:1489). Serial evaluation in ER may increase yield for those having acute MIs (Acad Emerg Med 1997;4:869). Hospital laboratories will determine the parameters that they find useful in determining abnormal marker values based on their specific test and QI testing.

CPK and fractions up in 12 hr, peak at 2 d and last 4 d, CPK-MB subfractions MB2 and MB1 rise in first 6 hr after onset of pain and have 95% sensitivity and specificity; total CPK correlates with MI size; may double in MI, but still be less than upper limit of normal; MB band is increased also by increased death and regeneration of skeletal muscle, and by decreased clearance in myxedema; MM is increased by hypothyroidism, myopathy; BB band is increased by CNS and/or smooth muscle damage.

Cardiac troponin I and T levels elevate in 4-6 hr and are specific to myocardium (Am Hrt J 1999;137:1137); 95-100% sensitivity, 22-33% specific for infarction but "false positives" really represent ischemia (unstable angina) (Clin Chim Acta 1999; 284:161) with suggestive hx—other etiologies are possible such as sepsis, endocrine disorders, rheumatologic disorders, myocarditis, pericarditis, COPD (EM Australas 2004;16:212), pulmonary embolus, cardiomyopathy, renal failure, in those receiving monoclonal antibodies, those receiving cancer therapy, those on anticoagulation and other chronic diseases (Chest 2004;125:1877; Am J Emerg Med 1999;17:225); higher levels correlate with worse outcomes (Am J Cardiol 1999;84:1281); also used perioperatively when surgery may increase CPK; Troponin T levels predictive of ACS even in the setting of abnormal renal function (Nejm 2002;346:2047).

Myoglobin peaks early (2 hr) and is sensitive, but not specific (Ann EM 1987;16:851).

LDH and fractions: isoenzymes 4 and 5 (rapidly migrating) increased, r/o renal and red cell source.

AST (SGOT) up in 24 hr, peaks at 2-4 d, lasts up to 7 d.

Increase in myeloperoxidase level prognostic for MI, and 30-day and 6-mon adverse cardiac events—exact level to be elucidated (Nejm 2003;349:1595).

Acute phase reactants [C-reactive protein (Nejm 2004; 350:1387; 2004;351:2599), fibrinogen] and Troponin T may have prognostic value if they are elevated (Nejm 2000;343:1139); Phospholipase A2 predictive for CAD (Nejm 2000;343:1148).

B-type natriuretic peptide, predictive of ongoing cardiac risk (Nejm 2001;345:1014) or other risk for mortality (Nejm 2004;

CARDIOVASCULAR

350:655); useful as ER test, if rapid assay available to help in diagnosis of CHF.

The N-terminal fragment produced by the cleavage of the precursor to BNP is called pro-BNP (the other product is BNP). This is being studied for utility in diagnosis of CHF and long-term mortality in those with CAD (Nejm 2005;352:666).

Pregnancy-associated plasma protein A (PAPP-A): increased level with placque rupture—needs more study (Nejm 2001;345:1022).

Non-invasive lab: ECHO for mitral regurgitation, aneurysm, ejection fraction estimation, and mural thrombi with 77% sensitivity and 93% specificity. Also looking for wall motion abnormalities, although the ECHO exam may not determine the onset of any abnormalities.

Field EKG with telemetry to ER does help (Am Hrt J 1992;123:835). EKG (Nejm 2003;348:933) may show ST eleva-tion (50% sensitivity), duration of elevation correlates with extent of injury, height of at least 1 mm in limb leads and 2 mm in precordial leads; sum of elevation correlates directly with severity of injury (and thus prognosis) (Jama 1998;279:387); T wave inversions (r/o acute cholecystitis). Persistent ST eleva-tion anteriorly has low association with LV aneurysm (Am J Cardiol 1984:84; Eur Hrt J 1994:1500). New LBBB extremely compelling (Ann EM 2000;36:561) and should be treated as acute injury. New RBBB indicates occlusion of anterior descending proximal to first septal branch, new complete RBBB or LBBB denotes higher mortality (J Am Coll Cardiol 1998;31:105). LBBB to be treated as ST elevation even in patient with ASHD, old LBBB, and an H & P consistent with acute infarct—ie, thrombolytic candidate per protocol; may also apply the Sgarbossa criteria for those with old LBBB: (1) ST ele-vation ≥ 1 mm concordant with QRS complex, (2) ST elevation > 5 mm if discordant with QRS complex, and (3) ST depression in leads V1 thru V3. The Sgarbossa criteria cannot be used to rule out the possibility of MI (Ann EM 2000;36:561) but rather should be used to identify those who qualify for thrombolytic or invasive therapy (Ann EM 2000;36:566).

Serial EKGs in ER are less helpful than serial serum markers (Ann EM 1992;21:1445), but repeating the EKG in 30-60 min can help determine whether a patient has dynamic changes on the EKG—in other words, not just looking for STEMI. Ideally, look at the ST segment 0.08 sec (2 small boxes) after the J-point to read changes from baseline.

Coronary MRA for screening (Nejm 2001;345:1863)

ETT: May be useful if done from ER in patients who do not have known CAD, an evolving MI, or unstable angina based on EKG and serial markers, yet they are stable and no plausible explanation for their symptoms; heart rate recovery in 1st min is predictive (Nejm 1999;341:1351) and decreased exercise capacity prognostic for mortality (Nejm 2002;346:793).

Radiology: Ventriculogram with technetium scan; ejection fraction, if < 40%, 1-yr mortality climbs steeply from 5%; sestamibi perfusion imaging at rest in those with high suspicion and normal or non-diagnostic EKG (Jama 2002;288:2693)

Other reasons: Abnormal EKG or cardiac injury may be found through the following tests: CBC with diff, metabolic profile, CXR, drug/toxin screens.

Emergency Management for ST Elevation MI: [better patient outcomes with use of clinical pathways (Jama 2002;287:1269)]: (Nejm 1997;336:847)

Drugs:
- O$_2$ (Acta Anaesthesiol Scand 1981;25:303)
- ASA 81 mg, 2-4 tabs po immediately; no difference in regular vs prostacyclin-sparing ASA (Eur Hrt J 1994;15:1196); clopidogrel 300 mg po (a thienopyridine derivative) with ASA

decreases death or other primary complications of atherosclerotic disease, but increased risk of bleeding, would consider in non-ST elevation MI (Nejm 2001;345:494); the effect of ASA is blocked by COX-2 medications, especially if they are very COX-2 selective (Lancet 2005;365:475).

- TNG, as sl or iv (Scand J Clin Lab Invest suppl 1984;173:27) if BP OK, especially if continued pain, perhaps even if no pain; especially helpful if any element of CHF or if large anterior MI—Avoid if sildenafil or other drugs for erectile dysfunction, and time of avoidance is specific to the medication—sildenafil needs a 24-hr free window to consider TNG use, and other drugs in this class require longer waiting periods!
- Narcotic analgesia and/or anxiolysis.
- Heparin: Unfractionated vs LMWH (J Am Coll Cardiol 2000;35:1699) (Jama 2004;292:55); at least with enoxaparin, no difference for those with early invasive strategy, as well (Jama 2004;292:45)—this was an open label study.
- Thrombolysis with streptokinase, TPA, Retavase, etc—TPA the standard (Nejm 1993;329:673):
    i) Helps all patients including those > 75 yr.
    ii) If systolic BP ≥ 175 or diastolic ≥ 100, bleeding risk is double.
    iii) Use if pain is < 6 hr duration, or if 6-12 hr and STs still elevated, or LBBB and good story.
    iv) More effective re: mortality if used in smokers (Qjm 1999;92:327).
    v) Potential complications include bleeding, such as intracranial, cardiac rupture (J Am Coll Cardiol 1999;33:479), or intra-abdominal; intracranial associated with older age and hypertension (Am J Cardiol 1991;68:166).
    vi) Contraindications may include recent stroke, recent major surgery, recent major dental work, trauma, hemop-

tysis, hematemesis, melena, hematochezia, hematuria, cancer, new headaches, bleeding diathesis, or h/o aneurysms.
vii) Not for ST depression, even if markers positive.
viii) Prehospital thrombolytics have not been shown to improve outcome and will probably have high skill attrition secondary to paucity of use (Am Hrt J 1991;121:1), unless in areas where transport times are consistently $> 1^1/_2$ hr. With the advent of aeromedical care, transport to a primary catheterization center without thrombolysis may make more sense. In Donegal, Ireland, patients with extended transport times have shown improvement with prehospital thrombolysis, but this is in a setting where a physician responds to the prehospital scene and thrombolysis is given in consult with a cardiologist (Ir Med J 2003;96:70). Thrombolysis vs primary angioplasty showed a favor toward angioplasty for the endpoint of reinfarction but not death or stroke if the procedure could be accomplished within 3 hr (Nejm 2003;349:733) and further analysis shows that a delay of balloon inflation time of > 1 hr compared to the standard time for thrombolysis does not convey a greater benefit when compared to thrombolysis (Am J Cardiol 2003;92:824).

- G IIb/IIIa agents (Drugs 1999;58:609) helpful around time of catheterization (Am J Cardiol 1999;84:779; 2001;88:A6,62), not proven to be helpful otherwise in combination with thrombolytics at this time, ongoing trials to assess whether lower thrombolytic doses could be used if G IIb/IIIa agents given in conjunction (Lancet 2000;355:337). Pro study of abciximab compared to tirofiban in preventing ischemia (Nejm 2001;344:1888; 2002;346:957)

- β-blocker within 24 hr of MI (OK to give in ER and continued indefinitely), helps prevent recurrent MIs and fatal ventricular arrhythmias in all (including the elderly) (Prog Cardiovasc Dis 1993;36:261), increase survival for > 6 yr; one example for loading is metoprolol 5 mg iv over 5 min × 3 and then 50-100 mg po.
- Consider direct thrombin inhibitor such as bivalirudin 0.75 mg/kg iv bolus prior to PCI, followed by 1.75 mg/kg/hr iv infusion per length of procedure for those who are receiving IIb/IIIa agent instead of heparin—preliminary data (Jama 2004;292:696).
- ACEIs within 24 hr of MI and for 6 wk, but continue indefinitely if EF < 40%; may also help with CHF emergently, as long as no AS with captopril 6.25 mg sl; captopril 50 mg tid increases ETT performance and decreases LV size; especially in anterior MIs; prolong life after MI even if no symptoms but not efficacious in those with preserved left ventricular function (Nejm 2004;351:2058).
- Angiotensin-receptor blockers (ARBs) such as valsartan may be as effective as ACEIs, but no value in combining these two therapies—head-to-head study of valsartan with captopril (Nejm 2003;349:1893).
- Eplerenone 25 mg qd for 4 wk and then increased to 50 mg qd to decrease morbidity/mortality after MI in those with EF < 40% (Nejm 2003;348:1309)—this is a selective aldosterone blocker for the mineralcorticoid receptor.
- PRBC if age > 65 yr and Hct < 30% (Nejm 2001; 345:1230); note that transfusion in these patients is associated with higher mortality (Jama 2004;292:1555)
- $MgSO_4$ perhaps, 8 nm bolus over 5 min, then 65 nm over 24 hr; if Mg low, perhaps for all; improves survival in one study from 89% to 92%; but of no help in ISIS-4.
- Historical consideration of insulin iv then sc qid for months in all patients. Diabetics with intensive insulin therapy will have

decreased mortality at 1 yr. Low dose Glucose-Insulin-Potassium (GIK) is not effective (Cardiology 1966;49:239, Cardiovasc Drugs Ther 1999;13:191).

Surgical:
- Angioplasty (PCI) as primary treatment for STEMI if available (J Invasive Cardiol 1999;11:61; Circ 1999;100:14) and < 12 hr of symptoms gives a better outcome when looking at the triple end-point of death, re-infarction, or CVA but no difference when just looking at death (Jama 2002;287:1943). Discussion of regionalization for primary PCI if available at other facility within 2 hr (this is time to balloon open) of original hospital or from prehospital site (Nejm 2003;349:733), 90 min per Nallamothu (Am J Cardiol 2003;92:824), or facilitated PCI which would be after thrombolysis if symptoms or ischemia persist. Aggressive intervention touted as superior to aggressive medical management is challenged when looking at a 7-yr outcome (Jama 2005;293:1329). PCI is preferred if coincident heart failure or cardiogenic shock (J Am Coll Cardiol 1991;18:1077)—thrombolytics of equivocal efficacy in this setting (Eur Hrt J 1999;20:128). PCI as acute treatment has the findings of 90% successful, 3% require emergency CABG, 5% infarct, and 1% mortality.
- CABG after angio if low EF (21-49%) and multivessel disease, or if left main disease; can do it 1 mon post-MI, although better 6-mon survival, if done immediately for cardiogenic shock (Nejm 1999;341:625).
- Atherectomy less good.

2.2 Right Ventricular Infarct

Eur J Cardiol 1976;4:411.

Epidem: Seen with inferior wall MIs (IWMI) and increase the mortality from 6% to 30% (Nejm 1993;328:981); mitral regurgitation, when severe, is associated with a 50% 1-yr mortality despite all interventions; increased risk also seems to be age related (Circ 1998;98:1714).

Pathophys: Right ventricular infarct syndrome—acute inferior MI, Kussmaul's sign (paradoxical increases in jugulovenous pulsation with inspiration), high CVP with low PA pressure and low PCWP so all nearly equal (like pericardial tamponade), low cardiac output; occur in 50% of inferior wall MI patients but clinically significant in 30% and nearly 10% of those with CPK levels > 2000 IU; reversible with reperfusion treatment.

Lab/EKG: ST elevation in RV4; get right-sided EKG in all patients with IWMI.

Rx: Consider increasing preload with saline; use dobutamine, nitroprusside,and sequential pacing as needed; avoid nitrates and diuretics; isoproterenol may unload RV but concerns of increasing mortality. Thrombolytics helpful (Am J Cardiol 1984;54:951), but not as good as for other regions of the heart unless heart block or hypotension (larger infarct) (J Am Coll Cardiol 1998;32:876).

2.3   Unstable Angina/non-Q wave MI

Circ 1994;89:81

Complc: See p 13 for TIMI Risk Score.

EKG: ST depressions or even no acute changes

Rx: Unstable angina may be amenable to medical therapy, and acutely should use ASA, nitroglycerin drip, and heparin—unfractionated vs LMWH is an active area of research (Circ 1999;100:1593). If ischemia or pain cannot be remedied, this should be treated in a similar fashion to post-infarction angina and coronary angiography is indicated—a "cooling off" period with antithrombotics is not helpful (Jama 2003;290:1593). Whether treatment with primary coronary catheterization with G IIb/IIIa therapy is a better treatment is still not fully elucidated (Am J Cardiol 1998; 82:731).

Crs: Prognosis is similar for Q-wave and non-Q-wave infarcts, although non-Q-wave MIs are followed by more infarcts and angina but are associated with less CHF; is not affected by 1st-degree heart block, PVCs, Vtach, or RBBB; better prognosis if preinfarction angina preceded.

2.4   Atrial Fibrillation and Flutter

J Cardiovasc Pharmacol Ther 2000;5:11; Nejm 2001;344:1067; 2004;351:2408.

Cause: Associated with: normal variations, idiopathic, CHF, and RHD, atrial dilatation (eg, in mitral stenosis or regurgitation), pericarditis, COPD especially with hypoxia and bronchodilators, ASHD; with hyperthyroidism especially in the elderly as measured by low TSH, which has a 30% 10-yr incidence in contrast to 10% 10-yr incidence with normal TSH and with toxic multinodular goiter; with alcoholic cardiomyopathy or "holiday heart"; marijuana use (Ped Cardiol 2000;21:284); and Wolff-Parkinson-White (WPW) syndrome (Am J Cardiol 2000;85:1256).

Aflut and multifocal atrial tachycardia often (60%) from pulmonary disease including pulmonary emboli and theophylline use.

Wandering atrial pacemaker (WAP), multifocal atrial tachycardia, and sick sinus syndrome (SSS) are also supraventricular arrhythmias.

Epidem: Common; supraventricular prematures are not associated with ASHD or sudden death; 40-65% incidence after cardiac surgery (Ann Thorac Surg 2000;69:300). Afib is more common with increasing BMI (Jama 2004;292:2471). BMI = Weight in lbs/(height in inches)^2 × 703.

Pathophys: Unknown, hypotheses of conduction problems vs structural problems as primary insult, probably many variables. Whether dilatation of the atrium(a) is cause or effect is debatable, but is associated with Afib. Many different frequencies and duration of Paroxysmal Afib. (Curr Opin Cardiol 2000;15:54).

Sx: Polyuria, palpitations, and faintness; 51% of cardiac syncope due to arrhythmias (Nejm 2002;347:878)

Si: Tachycardia; irregularly, irregular rhythm with Afib.

Crs: Rate control is key to maximize Starling hemodynamics; anticoagulation in chronic/recurrent Afib to prevent thromboembolic sequelae; losing atrial ability to fill the last 10% of ventricular diastolic volume may be an issue with low EF, leading to CHF; 60% 5-yr survival if associated with syncope (Nejm 2002; 347:878).

- A flutter in neonates is of serious consequence (J Am Coll Cardiol 2000;35:771)

Cmplc: Chronic Afib, Aflut, and SSS cause embolic CVA in 20% if recent CHF, HT, or previous embolus but < 1% per yr if none of those and no increase in LA size or LV dyskinesis on ECHO; likewise others find rate only 1.3% after 15 yr where no other disease and > 60 yr of age; embolic CVA increased 5 times in ASHD type compared to age-matched controls, 17 $\times$s in RHD.

- In SSS, 16% per year develop arterial emboli.

Diff Dx: Other SVT.

Lab: CBC with diff; metabolic profile; TSH; consider ethanol level, digoxin level, or theophylline level; experimental—elevated atrial natriuretic peptide (ANP) (J Am Coll Cardiol 2000; 35:1256).

- EKG:
    a) SSS is diagnosed by SVTs alternating with some heart block, and suggested by P < 90 beat/min after 1-2 mg atropine, or asystole $\geq$ 3 sec after carotid sinus massage.

b) MAT, P > 100 beat/min, and > 3 different PR intervals and P-wave morphologies; looks superficially like Afib, but digoxin will not help it; WAP is same thing but rate < 100 beat/min.

- Holter to find when intermittent; event monitor is even better.
- TEE is 99% specific, 100% sensitive for LA thrombus.

Emergency Management:

Afib:

(Curr Opin Cardiol 2000;15:23)

- Perioperative prevention post CABG with amiodarone 30 mg/kg po (Am J Cardiol 2000;85:462).
- Rate control: iv β-blocker, like propranolol or esmolol; iv calcium-channel blocker such as verapamil or diltiazem—may pretreat with 5 cc of iv calcium chloride if no contraindications to prevent calcium-channel blocker induced hypotension although this may be equivocal (J Emerg Med 2004;26:395) and would avoid calcium-channel blockers if any concern of under-lying cardiac ischemia; diltiazem purported to not cause as signifi-cant ionotropic suppression as compared to verapamil (most likely equivocal). If time to conversion not a factor, consider digoxin—rate is easily overridden by catechol/exercise stimulation.
- Conversion: especially if LA size is < 50 mm, significant CHF or ischemia—consider electricity if patient unstable; embolic risk post-conversion in 1st 48 hr ≤ 1%, but if > 48 hr the risk is 5-7%, and thus, should anticoagulate first with short-term anticoagulation, even if TEE is negative while others report no emboli if TEE is negative (Nejm 2001;344:1411).
- Medical conversion with propafenone (Rythmol) 450 mg po if > 70 kg or 600 mg po if < 70 kg; or flecainide 200 mg po for those < 70 kg, or 300 mg po if ≥ 70 kg—may try this as out-patient treament for those with recurrent Afib following these caveats (Nejm 2004;351:2384): age 18 to 75 yr; heart rate

> 70 beat/min; systolic blood pressure > 100 mm Hg; palpitations of abrupt onset that is well-tolerated without dyspnea, syncope, or presyncope; no chest pain; and less than 12 episodes per yr. Propafone 300 mg po converts 75% within 8 hr safely, or may use 2 mg/kg iv over 10 min to convert within 30 min (Am J Cardiol 1999;84:345,A8); or ibutilide (Corvert) 1 mg iv over 10 min, may repeat one time (Clin Cardiol 2000;23:265); or dofetilide 8 μg/kg 15-min infusion (Am J Cardiol 2000;85:1031); or perhaps with procainamide, amiodarone, or clonidine 0.075 mg po repeat in 2 hr by decreasing sympathetic tone; digoxin alone is no better than placebo.

- Electrical cardioversion with synchronized mode if unstable or eventually if meds fail—biphasic OK (Am J Cardiol 2003; 92:810). OK to do even if dig on board as long as levels therapeutic and not toxic, and K^+ OK. Begin with monophasic equivalents (MPE) of 100 J, then 200 J, then 300 J, then 360 J (AHA recommendations)—increase the energy if no conversion.

- Maintenance treatment: β-blockers, amiodarone, verapamil, digoxin, sotalol, or dofetilide (Med Lett Drugs Ther 2000;42:41); quinidine po, which holds in NSR but death rate is 3 times placebo or procainamide.

- Anticoagulate chronic or intermittent Afib if clinically able with warfarin to INR > 2 but < 4—this provides the best risk/benefit balance which reduces the risk of CVA from 7% to 12% at any age especially in SSS variant (Cerebrovasc Dis 2000;10:39). Annual bleeding risk is approximately 2.5%; no need to anticoagulate chronic Afib if age < 60 yr, no h/o TIA, no valve disease, normal ECHO, and no HT (Lancet 2000; 355:956). Use ASA if cannot use warfarin, might help at least under age 75.

- Anticoagulate option with Ximelagatran 36 mg po bid, which is as effective as warfarin, although elevated LFTs are a concern (Jama 2005;293:690).

- Conduction affected by $MgSO_4$ with delay in RR interval, no change with use of glucose, insulin, or potassium (J Electrocardiol 1998;31:281)
- AV nodal ablation, area of active research (Pacing Clin Electrophysiol 2000;23:395), but most are pacemaker dependent afterwards (Am Hrt J 2000;139:122); although in peds, ablation prophylactically in asymptomatic yet high-risk patients reduces the risk of arrhthmia that is life-threatening (Nejm 2004;351:1197); open surgery using the MAZE procedure to let incisions guide impulses from the SA to AV node (Semin Thorac Cardiovasc Surg 2000;12:2)

Aflut: Carotid sinus pressure trial, then treat as Afib above. Electrical cardioversion if needed may begin at 50 J MPE, and then follow the aforementioned increases.

MAT: Treat the primary disease (COPD, sepsis) or theophylline toxicity if appropriate, and may be only treatment necessary; verapamil iv with pretreatment with iv $CaCl_2$ or po for chronic; $MgSO_4$ iv, especially if low serum level; β-blockers OK if no COPD, but may consider carvedilol (Coreg) which combines nonspecific β- and α-blocker effect (J Nucl Cardiol 2000;7:3)

SSS: Permanent pacer preferably with atrial pacing to reduce emboli, then medications to control tachycardias.

2.5 Congestive Heart Failure

Nejm 2003;348:2007; 1999;341:577; 1999;341:759; Med Hypotheses 2000;54:242

Cause: Subclinical coronary disease; associated with HT in 40% of men and 60% of women, systolic BP > 140; males > females; and inflammation (J Am Coll Cardiol 2000;35:1628); dilated cardiomyopathy; obesity (Nejm 2002;347:305); occasionally valve disease; and more rarely AV malformations. More uncommonly salt water drowning, Paget's disease, hyperthyroidism, beriberi, severe anemia as with pernicious anemia, Fabry disease, multiple myeloma rarely, peripartum (usually secondary to other complications and then idiopathic (Obgyn 1986; 67:157), and NSAID use in the elderly (Arch IM 2000;160:777).

Epidem: In U.S., incidence is 564/100K person yr; 59% 5-yr mortality in males and 45% in females (Nejm 2002;347:1397) and increased mortality from all causes in those with mild diastolic dysfunction and moderate to severe systolic heart failure (Jama 2003;289:194). Elevated plasma homocysteine level correlates to increased risk for CHF (Jama 2003;289:1251); and increased risk of CHF development in blacks with α_{2C} Del 322-325 and β_1Arg389 receptors (Nejm 2002;347:1135).

Pathophys: Most CHF is due to systolic dysfunction with consequent changes consistent with ischemic mitral regurgitation (Nejm 2004;351:1627), but a small percent is due to diastolic dysfunction (Nejm 2004;350:1953; 2004;351:1097), eg, hypertensive pulmonary edema with normal EF (Nejm 2001;344:17), mitral stenosis, constrictive pericarditis, IHSS, etc, conditions that prevent normal diastolic filling. Hypertrophy in response to load creates dysfunctional myocardial cells. Action of ACEIs, β-blockers, and calcium channel blockers may be to relax hypertrophic myocardium as well as decrease afterload. Inadequate production of endogenous atrial natriuretic peptide, an atrial hormone that promotes diuresis (J Cardiovasc Pharmacol 2000;35:129). Cardiac asthma is due to bronchial edema and hyperresponsiveness.

Reversible left ventricular dysfunction may be present in those with emotional stress and is hypothesized to be secondary to a significant sympathetic response (Nejm 2005;352:539).

Sx: Dyspnea on exertion, orthopnea, paroxysmal nocturnal dyspnea, ankle edema, bowel bloating, and sense of fullness pc, nocturia

Si: JVD & S3 gallop each independently associated with worse outcome (Nejm 2001;345:574), pulse > 100, displace point of maximal impulse, dullness in L 5th intercostal space ≥ 10.5 cm from sternum. Central apnea in 45%, especially Cheyne-Stokes respirations.

Crs: 70+% 5-yr mortality if due to HT, 50% 1-yr mortality after starting medications; age > 70, 70% 2-yr mortality after pulmonary edema; increased mortality for those admitted at 30 d and 1 yr if the following clinical bench marks of older age, lower systolic BP, higher respiratory rate, higher BUN, and hyponatremia; or if the following co-morbid conditions of CVA, COPD, hepatic cirrhosis, dementia, or cancer (Jama 2003;290:2581). ADHERE data showed a decision tree of BUN ≥ 43 mg/dL, systolic BP < 115 mm Hg and serum creatinine ≥ 2.75 mg/dL as high risk variables for increased mortality (Jama 2005;293:572).

Cmplc: Sleep apnea (Nejm 1999;341:949).

Diff Dx: Lymphangitic carcinoma; diffuse pneumonia; pulmonary fibrosis; pulmonary arterial HT (Nejm 2004;351:1425)—patients may be on bosentan (Tracleer), epoprostenol (Flolan), treprotinil (Remodulin), or sildenafil (Viagra) for treatment of such.

Lab:
- EKG: look for underlying rhythm, ischemia, acute injury, pericarditis. QRS dispersion (variability in QRS width as predictor of mortality) (Am J Cardiol 2000;85:1212); cardiac resynchronization in those with intraventricular conduction delay and moderate to severe disease is helpful (Nejm 2002;346:1845).
- CXR: redistribution of blood to apices on upright, perihilar haze, Kerley B lines, increased heart size, pleural effusion R > L.
- CBC with diff [assess for anemia and neutrophil percent > 65 post MI associated with risk for CHF (Am Hrt J 2000;139:94)];

CARDIOVASCULAR

metabolic profile; consider ABG and/or continuous O_2 saturations; digoxin level if appropriate; cardiac enzymes if severe, hypotensive or with chest pain; low ESR correlates with acute and severe disease; elevated CRP some correlate with inflammation of CHF; TSH if not previously tested; lactic acid level if chronic CHF and unable to determine current disease severity (Am J Cardiol 1998;82:888). Serum interleukin-6 (> 10 pg/ml) elevation associated with severe disease (J Hrt Lung Transplant 2000;19:419); B-type natriuretic hormone (J Am Coll Cardiol 2001;37:379) with diagnostic accuracy of 83% with cutoff of 100 pg/ml in those with acute dyspnea (Nejm 2002;347:161), although a cutoff of 500 pg/ml may be more appropriate for being highly indicative of CHF and 100-500 pg/ml needing further clinical correlation (Nejm 2004;350:647).

Emergency Management:
- O_2, Airway: Intubate if necessary; consider BiPap (or CPAP) in lieu of intubation with initial settings of 10/4 if patient can tolerate (Cmaj 2000;162:535; Crit Care Med 2004;32:2407); CPAP if coincident obstructive sleep apnea improves left ventricular function (Nejm 2003;348:1233).
- Iv heplock or D_5W if fluid needed; consider bladder catheter to measure urine output.
- Nitroglycerin: sl, iv (Scand J Clin Lab Invest suppl 1984;173: 27), Paste (Circ Res 1976;39:127; Am J Cardiol 1976;38:469). Transdermal routes develop tachyphylaxis (Ann IM 1986;104:295). Effective use of nitrates lowers morbidity when compared to diuretics (Lancet 1998;351:389). Avoid if sildenafil or other drugs for erectile dysfunction, and time of avoidance is specific to the medication—sildenafil needs a 24-hr free window to consider nitroglycerin use, and other drugs in this class require longer waiting periods!

- Dobutamine iv (in combination with iv TNG, nitroprusside, or dopamine if hypotensive) if severe for its positive ionotropic properties, better than dig, or diuretics, no arrhythmias, short half-life; dose at 2.5-15 μg/kg/min (Chest 1980;78:694).
- Nitroprusside iv for afterload reduction, and is effective in those with cardiogenic shock and aortic stenosis (Nejm 2003;348:1756)—beware CN build-up; dose at 1-5 μg/kg/min.
- Nesiritide 2 μg/kg bolus then 0.01 μg/kg/min maintenance infusion if cannot use Nitroprusside and no response to TNG; this is a B-type natriuretic peptide (Med Lett Drugs Ther 2001;43:100; Jama 2002;287:1531). Early ER use helps with morbidity, mortality, and hospital length of stay (Rev Cardiovasc Med 2003;4(7):S13).
- Diuretics: Furosemide, begin dosing at 20-40 mg iv push (Clin Physiol Biochem 1986;4:293), and some data exist that this may help emergently, especially in the very ill (Ann EM 1992;21:669); may consider other loop diuretics such as torsemide 5-20 mg iv (Ann Pharmacother 1995;29:396) or bumetanide 0.5-2 mg iv. Intravenous dosing best for compromised patient because CHF will delay po absorption (Pharmacol 1979;19:121). Furosemide has been studied as continuous iv drip (Chest 1992;102:725) but this elicits a paradoxical pump dysfunction secondary to neurohumoral axis activation (Ann IM 1985;103:1). Elevated serum creatinine, even if a consequence of diuretic therapy, produces poorer patient outcomes (Nejm 2004;351:1285; Clin Nephrol 2004;61:177; J Am Coll Cardiol 2004;44:1301). Spironolactone reduces morbidity/mortality (Nejm 1999;341:709; Am J Cardiol 2000; 85:1207). Replete Thiamine if on long-term furosemide to improve left ventricular function (Am J Med 1995;98:485).
- Amrinone 40 μg/kg/min for 1 hr, then 10 μg/kg/min over 24 hr at least as efficacious as dobutamine (Am J Cardiol

1981;48:170); perhaps augmented with use of inhaled nitric oxide (Eur J EM 1999;6:161).

- Saterinone (PDE III inhibitor) iv at 0.5-4 μg/kg/min combines actions of dobutamine and nitroprusside (J Cardiovasc Pharmacol 1998;32:629).
- β-blockers (eg, metoprolol) if patient can tolerate, especially if rate control is an issue (Jama 2000;283:1295) (Med Lett Drugs Ther 2000;42:54).
- ACEI acutely (captopril 6.25-25 mg sl), as long as no AS and not intubated (Int J Cardiol 1990;27:351). Consider angiotensin II receptor antagonists, as well (Nejm 2001; 345:1667). ACEIs not as efficacious in the black population (Nejm 2001;344:1351).
- Dopamine (with dobutamine) if hypotensive at pressure support doses of 5-20 μg/kg/min, not renal dose. Renal dosing does not help natriuresis (J Am Soc Nephrol 1996;7:1032).
- Carvedilol (Coreg) combines non-specific β- and α-blocker effect (J Nucl Cardiol 2000;7:3) and helpful in all degrees (mild to severe) of CHF (Nejm 2001;341:1651); many drug interactions, eg, with digoxin, cimetidine, SSRIs.
- Dofetilide for CHF and/or Afib conversion, 500 μg dose po for CHF or 250 μg, if in Afib (Nejm 1999;341:857).
- Narcotic of choice prn for pain/anxiolysis.
- Indications for pacing (Cardiol Clin 2000;18:55); consider catheter ablation for those with CHF and Afib to improve left ventricular function, quality of life, and exercise capacity, and this is independent as to whether coincident cardiac disease or adequate rate control is present (Nejm 2004;351:2373).
- Do not use aminophylline, may have early effect that is not sustained (Clin Cardiol 1980;3:268).
- Do not use Isoproterenol as rescue medication, perhaps some use as prognostic challenge (Am Hrt J 1992;123:989).

- Chest tube or thoracentesis if large pleural effusion. CHF (along with cirrhosis and pulmonary embolus) is typically taught as being a condition associated with a transudative effusion, but although rare may present with exudate as well (Am J Med 2001;111:375; Chest 2002;122:1518). Differentiate exudates from transudate (Nejm 2002;346:1971) by using the following data in Table 2.2 and Table 2.3.

CARDIOVASCULAR

Table 2.2   Light's Criteria

Pleural fluid protein level/serum level protein level > 0.5
Pleural fluid LDH/serum level LDH > 0.6
Pleural fluid LDH > ⅔ the upper limit of normal for serum LDH (or > 200 U/L)

(Ann IM 1972;77:507)

Table 2.3   Other Parameters

Pleural fluid cholesterol level > 60 mg/dL
Pleural fluid cholesterol/serum cholesterol level > 0.3
Serum albumin level—pleural fluid albumin ≤ 1.2 g/dL (Chest 1990;546:9)

(Chest 1993;104:399)

Overall, Light's criteria have a sensitivity of 98% for identifying exudates, but its specificity is 83% [77% per Romero (Chest 1993;104:399) and individual criteria range from 82-89% specificity]; this means that some patients with transudates will be thought to have exudates (Chest 1995;107:1604). Thus, the entry of the parameters by Romero et al. By and large, these criteria are more specific (91% specificity) and thus more accurately identify transudates, but their sensitivity is lower (ranging from 54-89%) and thus, a chance exists that an exudate is identified as a transudate. Use both sets of criteria to help determine the most likely cause. Other parameters such as pH, glucose, amylase level, cell count, gram stain, culture, or other specific tests depending on clinical indications may be warranted—our goal here is to deferentiate CHF from everything else.

- Moxonidine (central acting imidazoline) decreases sympathetic output.
- Data for use of an oral non-peptide vasopressin V_2 receptor antagonist (such as Tolvaptan) are very preliminary as far as improvement in vital signs (does not worsen renal function or induce hypokalemia) but more studies needed in regards to morbidity/mortality (Jama 2004;291:1963).
- Adrenomedullin infusion is experimental, with pharmacologic ability for vasodilation, diuresis, and natriuresis (Circ 2000; 101:498).
- Selective adenosine antagonists also experimental, seem to preserve GFR compared to furosemide (J Am Coll Cardiol 2000;35:56).

Chronic Rx (which includes some of the above) (Med Lett Drugs Ther 1999;41:12):

- Digoxin (Eur J Clin Invest 2000;30:285) does not help emergently. Mainstay is for chronic treatment—may begin iv dosing for compromised patient because CHF will delay po absorption (Pharmacol 1979;19:121). Digoxin has been associated with an increase in mortality in females with heart failure and depressed LV function—an absolute difference of 5.8% (Nejm 2002;347:1403) and serum digoxin level in patients with LV dysfunction and EF < 45% is best if it is between 0.5-0.8 ng/ml (Jama 2003:871).
- Fixed dose combination therapy beginning with isosorbide dinitrate 20 mg tid and hydralazine 37.5 mg tid reduces mortality in black patients (Nejm 2004;351:2049).
- Calcium channel blockers for diastolic dysfunction, with even newer agents dangerous if used ubiquitously (Circ 2000; 101:758).

Central apnea:
- Theophylline 250 mg po bid (Nejm 1996;335:562)

2.6 Heart Block and Bradycardia

J Emerg Med 1986;4:25

Cause: Drug toxicity (especially digoxin), ASHD, MI, vasovagal reaction, congenital, granulomatous disease (Eur J Cardiol 1978; 8:349), metastatic calcification.

Electrical rhythm without pulses (Pulseless Electrical Activity—PEA) has a myriad of causes including hypothermia, pulmonary embolus, ineffective perfusion volume, cardiac tamponade, pneumothorax with tension physiology, acidosis, hyperkalemia, and drug overdose.

Epidem: Rarely associated with HLA-B27 and aortic insufficiency; 51% of those with cardiac syncope had some sort of arrhythmia (Nejm 2002;347:878)

Pathophys: See Acute Coronary Syndrome p 7 for ASHD details.

Congenital is associated with maternal autoantibody disease (SLE, Sjogren's, etc.), with anti-SSA (r/o antibodies); parasympathetic and sympathetic function just being elucidated for different etiologies (J Am Coll Cardiol 1988;11:271).

Sx:

1st degree heart block usually causes no symptoms.

2nd degree may cause dizziness or dyspnea.

3rd degree may cause syncope, especially on standing.

Si:

1st degree heart block = PR > 0.22 sec.

2nd degree = some unconducted P waves: Mobitz Type I (Ann IM 1999;130:58) with prolongation of PR interval until dropped beat whereas Mobitz Type II without PR prolongation.

3rd degree = no relationship between P waves and QRS complexes.

Crs: 1st degree heart block usually benign if not associated with organic disease; 60% 5-yr survival if arrhythmia associated with syncope (Nejm 2002;347:878).

Cmplc: R/o Lyme disease if from endemic area (even if no other symptoms) with serology—treat with antibiotics and temporary (not permanent) pacer (Pacing Clin Electrophysiol 1992;15:252).

Low perfusion states can lead to inadequate flow to brain, heart, kidneys, bowel, or any other organ system.

Diff Dx: Vasovagal syncope—pacemaker not indicated even if recurrent and severe vasovagal syncope (Jama 2003;289:2224).

Lab: EKG, metabolic profile, dig level if appropriate, consider cardiac markers; Holter monitor may still miss a majority of intermittent heart blocks.

Emergency Management:

1st degree may not need treatment.

2nd and 3rd degree:

- Atropine 0.5-1 mg iv (temporary solution) (Resuscitation 1999;41:47).
- External pacer until transvenous available, use for 60 min is OK without increased risk for cardiac damage (J Emerg Med 1989;7:1).

External pacer with negative electrode on left anterior chest and positive electrode on left upper back (infrascapular); use lowest current setting until capture and typical range is from 0-200 mAmps—increase slightly post capture; you also set the rate (70-80 beat/min). Transvenous is temporary, although in the setting of inferior MI a permanent pacemaker is usually not needed.

- Isoproterenol iv (Circ 1981;64:427) although controversial—effective yet significant side effects in dig toxicity, acute MI, or those with ASHD

- May consider aminophylline 100 mg/min iv up to 250 mg, although higher doses in chronic therapy (Ann Pharmacother 1998;32:837)
- Consider treatment of excessive β-blockade [reverse with glucagon 1 mg iv (Ann EM 1997;29:181)] or calcium channel blockade [reverse with glucagon 1 mg iv or calcium chloride 10% 10 cc iv (Am J Emerg Med 1985;3:334)], if present.

2.7 Hypertensive Emergencies

Crit Care Clin 1989;5:477; Clin Cornerstone 1999;2:41

Cause: Low calcium, and/or potassium intakes? Genetic by defective angiotensin gene on chromosome #1; red cell membrane Na^+ transport correlates with proximal tubule Na^+ resorption; elevated insulin levels? Drug use such as cocaine or pseudoephedrine (Am J Emerg Med 1986;4:141); increased risk with use of ephedra alkaloids (dietary supplement aka ma huang) (Nejm 2000;343:1833)

Epidem: Increased prevalence in blacks (Clin Cardiol 1989;12:iv13) (perhaps due to G6PD deficiency) and Hispanic males, especially from lower socioeconomic classes (Am J Public Hlth 1988;78:636); in sleep apnea, especially in older men, is this cause or effect?; with > 2 drinks of ethanol qd; with insulin resistance; also increased in those with time urgency/impatience and/or hostility (Jama 2003;290:2138). 90% lifetime risk in middle or older aged adults for acquiring any HT (Jama 2002;287:1003). Increased serum aldosterone levels even within the physiologic range is a risk factor for future development of HT (Nejm 2004;351:33).

Pathophys: Renally secreted prostaglandins protect; renin-aldosterone-angiotensin worsens. Elevated ADH does not increase BP. Calcium and sodium intakes modulate BP via parathyroid hormones and the renin-angiotensin system. "Salt-sensitive" hypertension depends on Na^+ and Cl^- together; BP decreases on Na^+ citrate. Alcohol induces via CRH release. (See Pre-eclampsia and Eclampsia p 303 for pregnancy details.)

Sx: None usually; occasionally causes epistaxis; headache in moderate to severe disease; severe disease may have manifestation of angina, CVA, or other evidence of end-organ dysfunction.

Si: Use correct cuff size.
   a) Mild HT if diastolic 90-105 mm Hg and/or systolic 140-160 mm Hg;
   b) Moderate, diastolic 105-120 mm Hg and/or systolic > 160 mm Hg;
   c) Severe, diastolic > 120 mm Hg and/or systolic > 210 mm Hg. Systolic false increase in elderly due to lead pipe arteries, tell by "Osler's maneuver" (feel artery when occluded above by BP cuff). Controversial significance of "white coat" HT. Assess for bruits to check for systemic vascular disease.

Crs: In elderly, LVH decreases over 6 mon and function improves if treated with verapamil, atenolol, or thiazides, or better with ACEIs as 1st choice, then Ca-channel blockers, then β-blockers, and diuretics. Treatment of isolated systolic HT (> 160 mm Hg) reduces CVAs by ⅓, stroke mortality by 36%, and cardiac mortality by 25%, as does treatment of systolic and diastolic HT up to 85 yr of age. Isolated moderate systolic HT still associated with increased cardiovascular risks of 1.5 times.

Cmplc:
   - Hypertensive crisis: papilledema, obtundation and seizures, renal failure; encephalopathy with stroke; intracranial bleed.
   - Chronic renal failure.
   - LVH.
   - CHF.
   - Diabetes via HT-induced insulin resistance.

Diff Dx: Malignant HT—retinal hemorrhages or papilledema (J Intern Med 1999;246:513); sleep apnea, ethanol and other drug/medicine use, primary renal disease, renovascular causes including coarctation of the aorta (check coincident radial and femoral pulses, rarely need check temporal and radial in proximal type), pheochromocytoma, Cushing's, Conn's toxemia of pregnancy and bcp's, lead-induced renal disease (most "essential" hypertensives with creatinine > 1.5% mg) (Environ Hlth Perspect 1988;78:57), acromegaly.

Lab: CBC with diff, metabolic profile, UA, EKG (3-8% sensitive) or ECHO (100% sensitive, uncertain specificity) for LVH; reversal of LVH on EKG (Jama 2004;292:2343) or ECHO (Jama 2004;292:2350) with antihypertensive treatment associated with improved clinical outcomes.

Emergency Management:

(Drug Saf 1998;19:99)

- HT crisis—severe numbers with evidence of end-organ disease: nitroprusside drip 1-8 μg/kg/min or propranolol 1-3 mg bolus q 5-10 min iv or other β-blocker best; labetalol 20-80 mg over 20 sec, up to 300 mg q 10 min iv; diazoxide 50-150 mg iv q 5 min with propranolol 3 mg/hr and/or diuretic; hydralazine 10-20 mg iv times 1 then, po clonidine or captopril, etc.
- Fenoldopam, a selective dopamine-1-receptor agonist, may be useful and may use this medication for up to 48 hr. Do not use in patients with glaucoma. Dose at 0.1-1.6 μg/kg/min (Nejm 2001;345:1548).
- Nifedipine with substantial complications—not advocated (Circ 1997;95:2368).
- In pregnancy, propranolol OK; so are hydralazine, α-methyldopa, clonidine; avoid teratogenic ACEIs.
- If able to discharge patient to home, arrange early outpatient medical follow-up (Med Care 1984;22:755).

Outpatient treatment (J Hum Hypertens 1999;13:647; 1999;13:803):

CARDIOVASCULAR

Behavior modification—difficult to attain:

- Increase potassium intake (salt substitute)
- Lose weight and regular aerobic exercise (Clin J Sport Med 1999;9:104)
- Increase fruits, vegetables, and polyunsaturated fats (Clin Cardiol 1999;22:iii6)
- Lessen sodium intake—debatable, with and without DASH diet (Nejm 2001;344:3)
- Avoid or stop NSAIDs (Brit J Clin Pharmacol 1990;30:519)
- Perhaps supplemental calcium and magnesium

Drug regimens (Med Lett Drugs Ther 2004;46:53):

- Thiazides, even in diabetics
- β-blockers, all about the same
- ACEIs (Med Lett Drugs Ther 1999;41:105, Nejm 2003;348:583), clearly best in those with NIDDM (preserves renal function in early renal failure). Angiotensin II receptor blockers probably equally good.
- Calcium-channel blockers, long-acting types only; calcium channel blockers (especially short-acting types) associated with higher mortality (Circ 1997;95:2368; Lancet 1997:594; Am J Cardiol 1997;80:1453; Jama 2004;292:2849).
- Direct vasodilators, such as hydralazine or minoxidil, or adrenergic inhibitors like clonidine, α-methyldopa; or α-receptor blockers like prazosin.
- Endothelin receptor antagonist like bosentan—experimental (Nejm 1998;338:784).

2.8 Infectious Endocarditis

Nejm 2001;345:1318; Ann EM 1991;20:405; Emerg Med Clin N Am 1998;16:665

Cause: Streptococcus viridan (47%); Staphylococcus aureus (20%) (usually acute bacterial endocarditis); enterococcus (6%); pneumococcus, nonenterococcal group D streptococcus often misidentified as enterococcus, and rarely anaerobes, fungi, Gramnegatives, lactobacillus, psittacosis organism, and other unusual organisms like *Bartonella* spp. or *Serratia marcescens* (Ann IM 1976;84:29).

Epidem: 4,000-8,000 cases/yr in U.S; 75% in patients with abnormal valves/hearts. Increased in patients with mitral valve prolapse syndrome (yet diagnosis of MVP prior to 1997 with controversial standards), congenital (VSD, PDA, tetralogy of Fallot), CHD especially aortic stenosis both repaired and unrepaired (1.5-20% at 30 yr) and rheumatic heart disease even when given SBE prophylaxis before dental work and surgical procedures.

Pathophys: Less than 5 % are right-sided; higher in iv drug users.

Sx: Fever, hematuria, and weight loss.

Si: Murmur (85% at presentation, 99% eventually; 66% in right-sided type); splenomegaly and/or infarction (25-50%); mucosal petechiae and splinter hemorrhages in nails (29%); clubbing (13%); Roth spots in fundi (2%); Osler's nodes in fingers.

Crs: 100% die without treatment; 80% 10-yr survival with treatment.

Cmplc: CHF (25%) due to chordae rupture and myocarditis; peripheral systemic arterial emboli, mostly with *Streptococcus viridans* type; pulmonary emboli (60% in right-sided type); CNS including TIA, CVA, mycotic aneurysm, abscess, encephalopathy, and bacterial as well as aseptic meningitis (Brain 1989;112:1295); renal failure from diffuse vasculitis, focal "embolic" glomerulonephritis, and renal infarction.

Diff Dx: Acute rheumatic fever, collagen vascular disease, anticardiolipin antibody syndrome (Arch Pathol Lab Med 1989;113:350), acute glomerulonephritis, marantic endocarditis, and rarely atrial myxoma.

Lab: CBC with diff, ESR, UA, CXR, ECHO—TTE OK in those with native valves if negative (Am J Cardiol 1996;78:101), otherwise TEE 95% sensitive (J Am Coll Cardiol 1991;18:391), three 10 cc blood cultures unless antibiotics within 2 wk of presentation—in that case get five 10 cc blood cultures. Consider RA titer. Biopsy and culture of Osler's Nodes (Chest 1987;92:751).

Emergency Management:

- *Therapeutic antibiotics:* Empiric treatment consists of ceftriaxone 2 g iv, vancomycin 1 g iv (Int J Antimicrob Agents 1999;12:191), and gentamicin at 5 mg/kg unless creatinine clearance < 20 ml/min (see p 236), in which case load at 2 mg/kg. Antibiotics to be continued 2-6 wk iv.
- *Surgical interventions:* Rarely needed except for valve ruptures and infections of implanted valves but over time (10 yr) 25% of mitral and 60% of aortic valves need surgery.
- *Prevention:* In those with valvular disease or previous surgery with pre- and post-procedure doses up to 24-48 hr of amoxicillin or alternative antibiotics with equivocal efficacy (Jama 1997;277:1794; Med Lett Drugs Ther 2001;43:98; Lancet 1966;1:686; Circ 1987;76:376).

2.9   Myocarditis/Cardiomyopathy

Emerg Med Clin N Am 1998;16:665; Circ 1999;99:1091; Adv IM 1999;44:293; Nejm 2000;343:1388

Cause:

- Collagen vascular diseases including SLE, polyarteritis nodosa, endocardial fibroelastosis (occasionally seen in children due to a treatable inherited carnitine deficiency), sarcoid, and carcinoid (last two may be restrictive and/or congestive).
- Deficiencies like hypophosphatemia from antacid binding, reversible; thiamine (beriberi), selenium, and carnitine.

- Endocrine: thyrotoxicosis and hypothyroidism; pheochromocytoma; homocystinuria, and hypocalcemia.
- Giant cell (lymphocytic) myocarditis.
- Idiopathic, may be caused by cellular apoptosis (programmed cell death) related to human leukocyte antigen association (J Card Fail 1997;3:97).
- Infectious from any severe bacteremia, eg, meningococcal, shigella, diphtheria, mycoplasma; viral including CMV, influenza, echo, coxsackie B (Scand J Infect Dis 1970;2:25), yellow fever, mumps, polio, rubella, HIV; not Hep C (Cardiol 1998;90:75); parasites including toxoplasma, Chagas' disease.
- Ischemic.
- Neurologic causes including Friedreich's ataxia; dyskalemic myopathies; muscular dystrophies including limb girdle, Emery-Dreifuss, and myotonic; Refsum's disease.
- Peripartum (Obgyn 1986;67:157).
- Toxic agents like ethanol (Am Hrt J 1976;92:561), danorubicin (Daunomycin) and bleomycin, cobalt in beer, arsenic, lead, cocaine, mercury, carbon monoxide, phenothiazines, clozapine (Lancet 1999;354:1841); most reversible except chemotherapy drugs.

Epidem: Idiopathic-type prevalence = 36/100,000: blacks/whites 2.5/1; M/F 25/1.

Pathophys: Dilation of both ventricles; mural thrombi.

Sx: Dyspnea; muscle weakness in alcoholic type, since 83% have skeletal myopathy, as well.

Si: Afib, other supraventricular arrhythmias; S_3 gallop; CHF signs

Crs: Often chronic and indolent, with the degree of microvascular dysfunction on PET scanning correlating with morbidity and mortality—and those with advanced disease may not have significant if any symptoms (Nejm 2003;349:1027). Conversely, may present acutely in infants (Ped Emerg Care 1987;3:110); in alcoholic type, it can rapidly resolve with abstinence; 95% 1-yr, 80% 5-yr survival. Eosinophilic endocardial fibroelastosis, 4% 3-yr mortality. Those with infiltrative types, HIV infection, or doxorubicin related have worse prognosis (Nejm 2000;342:1077). Usually good outcome in children (Heart 1999;82:226).

Cmplc: Systemic emboli from mural thrombi and Afib.

Diff Dx: Hypertrophic (IHSS) and restrictive myocardiopathies: amyloid, hemochromatosis, familial, idiopathic, endomyocardial fibrosis, eosinophilic cardiomyopathy, sarcoid, Gaucher's, Fabry's, and Hurler's disease.

Lab:

- CBC with diff, metabolic profile including phosphate level, CXR, EKG—looking for arrhythmia (20% with Afib), cloven T waves, blocks, Q waves or LVH.
- ECHO most helpful, EF < 45%.
- Endocardial biopsy in peripartum and all types to diagnose infiltrative disease; not helpful in dilated types, IHSS, Wilson's disease, etc; does not correlate well with clinical findings or prognosis once dilated cardiomyopathy has developed (Am Hrt J 1989;117:876).

Emergency Management:

- Anticoagulate acutely and chronically; prednisone treatment even when inflammatory by biopsy is equivocal (Am Hrt J 1989;117:876) or even with immunosuppressive drugs; perhaps human growth hormone 4 IU sc qod or immune globulin 2 g/kg iv (Circ 1997;95:2476); transplantation, 75% 5-yr survival.
- Of CHF using vasodilators (see p 30).
- Indications for pacing (Cardiol Clin 2000;18:55).

2.10 Pericarditis

Emerg Med Clin N Am 1998;16:665; Nejm 2004;351:2195; Am Fam
Phys 2002;66:1695

Cause:

(Arch IM 1979;139:407; Chest 1999;116:1564)
- *Acute:* Post-surgical or traumatic, viral expecially coxsackie,
  mycoplasma, post-MI, bacterial from a subdiaphragmatic
  abscess, post-septicemic, uremia, malignancy invading peri-
  cardium, actinomycosis, candida (Ann Thorac Surg
  1997;63:1200), but probably most commonly idiopathic (Am J
  Cardiol 1995;75:378). Peds includes Kawasaki disease.
- *Chronic:* Tuberculosis, sarcoid, hypothyroidism (Am J EM
  1999;17:176)

Epidem: Coxsackie viral type probably is the most common cause and
occurs in late summer and fall like other enteroviruses.

Pathophys: The stiffening cause restriction of ventricular diastolic
filling; increased heart rate must compensate for decreased stroke
volume; can tolerate 1-3 L, if slowly accumulates; only
300-400 cc, if rapid accumulation.
- Paradoxical pulse if constrictive (exaggeration > 10 mm Hg of
  normal drop of systolic BP with inspiration) due to impaired
  venous return and normal increased pulmonary vascular
  volume with inspiration.

Sx: Dyspnea; chest pain, often pleuritic, and better when sits up.

Si: Ascites, poor heart sounds, no PMI, tachycardia; pleural effusions
on left more often and larger than on right, unlike CHF.
    In constrictive pericarditis: increased CVP with Kussmaul's
sign; paradoxical pulse > 10-20 mm Hg.

Crs: Variable secondary to cause and patient's hemodynamic status;
those with pericarditis within 1 wk of post-MI are likely to have
had an anterior MI, less likely to have atrial arrhythmias, but at

slightly increased risk for ventricular arrhythmias, CHF, and death (Am Hrt J 1974;87:246). Most cases probably resolve within 2 wk, although recurrent pericarditis does occur.

Cmplc: Cardiac tamponade in those progressing to effusive-constrictive pericarditis (Nejm 2004;350:469) (Clin Cardiol 1999; 22:446): Seen in < 1% of thoracic trauma patients who are viable; as complication of pericarditis presents with hypotension as evidence of shock; co-incident pleural effusions may impact noncritical pericardial effusions and make them symptomatic— drain the pleural effusions (Chest 1999;116:1820). Also increased risk in those with a fever > 38°C, subacute (over weeks) onset, immunosuppressed patients, those on anticoagulants, or those with positive cardiac markers (Nejm 2004; 351:2195).

Diff Dx: Acute traumatic cardiac tamponade, those intoxicated may be more difficult to diagnose, but fare no worse (J Trauma 1999; 47:346); severe asthma; Rapid Y descent and rebound, r/o infiltrating myocardiopathy, eg, amyloid.

Lab:

- CBC with diff, ESR, metabolic profile.
- EKG (Chest 1970;57:460; Am J Cardiol 1970;26:471) may show Afib or electrical alternans, ie, alternate QRSs have higher and lower voltages; abnormal P waves; ST elevation, and/or PR depression in limb and precordial leads, which exclude early repolarization, which usually has precordial lead (STs) or limb (PRs) involvement only and isoelectric V_6 (Nejm 1976; 295:523); Ts invert only after STs back to normal. Look for V_6 ST segment elevation/T-wave amplitude of 0.25 or greater to help make the diagnosis (Circ 1982;65:1004). Consider right-sided EKG looking for RV infarct.
- ECHO shows pericardial fluid and may show tamponade hemodynamics.

- CXR shows large heart—may resemble Erlenmeyer flask or "boot-shaped." Normal CXR does not exclude diagnosis (Nephrol Dial Transplant 2000;15:719).

Emergency Management:
- ASA or other NSAID treatment avoiding indomethacin and/or steroids if ASHD and recent MI (Cardiol Rev 2003;11:211)
- Pulsed methylprednisolone (30 mg/kg) iv if Kawasaki disease with impending tamponade (Intensive Care Med 1999;25:1137).
- If constrictive, tap under ECHO or EKG guidance; pulmonary edema can develop if tap too much too fast leading to an overload of a deconditioned heart.
- Uremic pericarditis: Nephrology consult for hemodialysis if patient hemodynamically stable (Am J Kidney Dis 1987;10:2), pericardiocentesis as above if tamponade.
- Cardiac tamponade (Nejm 2003;349:684): pericardiocentesis with 18-gauge spinal needle. If patient responds, emergent pericardial window, reaspirate or place flexible catheter using Seldinger technique, if necessary (may want to use peritoneal catheter). Anticipate ventricular arrhythmias. Apply aspirated blood to 4 × 4 gauze to determine if it is non-clotting.

2.11 Paroxysmal Supraventricular Tachycardia

Cause: Aberrant conduction pathways with different conduction rates within the AV node (AV nodal re-entrant tachycardia—AVNRT), or outside the AV node (AV re-entrant tachycardia or AVRT). Wolff-Parkinson-White syndrome (WPW) is a subset of AVRT. This pathway allows set-up of circus movement continuous stimulation when the aberrant or usual pathway conducts retrograde; or ectopic irritable atrial focus (paroxysmal atrial tachycardia—PAT), often associated with digitalis toxicity, especially if manifest with associated block, eg, 2:1 or 3:1. Different and not as well understood in peds (Brit Hrt J 1990;64:317).

Epidem: AVNRT and AVRT of about equal prevalence and represent about 45% of all PSVTs; PAT constitutes 9%, and rare other syndromes like permanent junctional re-entrant tachycardia (PJRT), the last 1%. Common in infancy (Arch Ped Adolesc Med 1999;153:267). WPW is most common PSVT in China, uncommon in the West (Chin Med J (Engl) 1992;105:284).

Pathophys: Re-entrant tachycardias occur with increased excitability, decreased refractory period, and increased conduction velocity.

Sx: Paroxysmal episodes of palpitations often associated with dizziness, nausea; precipitated by caffeine, alcohol, nicotine, hyperthyroid states, ephedrine in diet supplements, cold/asthma medicines, etc; relieved by Valsalva maneuver by patient often. Neck pounding in AVNRT types, but not accessory pathway (WPW or AVRT) SVT because nearly coincident atrial and ventricular contraction in former cause cannon waves in neck that can be felt.

Si: Rapid tachycardia 150-210 beat/min.

Crs: Recurrent form teenage years on.

Cmplc: Rare permanent junctional re-entrant tachycardia variant associated with myocardiopathy stays in arrhythmia a long time, reversible if treated.
- Post PAT ST depression and T-wave inversions may last days-weeks, correlation with CAD without other symptoms is controversial (Am J Cardiol 1999;83:458,A10).

Diff Dx: Consider Lown-Ganong-Levine (LGL) syndrome if looks like WPW, but no delta waves.

Lab: EKG shows SVT with narrow complexes; AVNRT usually has no apparent P waves, AVRT has Ps closer to the last QRS than the next one, PAT Ps are usually before the next T, and PJRT have Ps closer to the next QRS and beyond the T wave. PSVT is very regular, even when aberrant and wide, unlike Vtach; QRS aberrancy always < 0.14 sec, whereas Vtach often (> 50%) > 0.14 sec, axis is −30° to +120° unlike the LAD with Vtach 60% of the time.

Emergency Management:
- Carotid sinus pressure/massage, if no bruits.
- Adenosine 6-12 mg iv (Brit Hrt J 1986;55:291)—peds 0.1-0.3 mg/kg (Circ 1982;66:504; Ann EM 1999;33:185)—gone in 10 sec, potentiated by dipyridamole and carbamazepine, inhibited by theophyllines—may induce other more malignant arrhythmias in the post-MI period (Pacing Clin Electrophysiol 2000;23:140); or perhaps propranolol 1-5 mg iv or other β-blocker (Brit Hrt J 1977;39:834; Ann Clin Res 1979:34), especially if concerned about ischemia; or verapamil 5-10 mg iv or diltiazem 10-20 mg iv (J Assoc Physicians India 1999;47:969). If QRS is wide, sometimes Ca-channel blockers or β-blockers paradoxically speed up the rate.
- Electrical cardioversion with synchronized mode if meds fail or if unstable—begin with 50 J MPE. (See Afib p 26 for subsequent energy levels.) OK to do even if dig on board as long as levels therapeutic and not toxic, and K+ OK; in resistant cases, implanted atrial burst pacers or catheter ablation of atrial slow pathway works 95% of the time (Circ 1977;56:727) with 77% risk reduction for arrhythmia in those with WPW who have ablation therapy (Nejm 2003;349:1803)

For chronic prevention, avoid stimulants: β-blockers; maybe verapamil or dig, though both can worsen some.

2.12 Shock

Resuscitation 1992;24:55

Cause: Inadequate end-organ perfusion.

Epidem: Has not been quantified; covers multiple disciplines.

Pathophys: Can be multifactorial, but need to consider if due to heart failure (cardiogenic), hypovolemia (hemorrhage, post-surgical) or loss of vascular tone (septic, anaphylactic, spinal cord).

Sx: Dizziness, dyspnea.

Si: Fever in sepsis, hypotension with bradycardia or tachycardia, wheezing is not specific to anaphylaxis, check peripheral limb movement and DTRs to r/o spinal shock and altered consciousness.

Crs: Dependent upon etiology, cardiogenic and spinal cord shock have worse outcomes.

Cmplc: ARDS, ventilator dependent, paralysis.

Lab: CBC with diff, metabolic profile, ABG, consider blood cultures and cardiac markers; consider UA and urine c & s; EKG for acute injury or ischemia; type and crossmatch; and stool guaiac.
- *X-ray:* CXR to check for sepsis source, tension pneumo, pulmonary edema, heart size and morphology, and mediastinum; C-spine evaluation with plain film or CT, if neurogenic shock suspected; abdominal CT, if AAA or other abdominal source suspected.

Emergency Management:
- 2 ivs, consider level 1 warmer for faster infusion.
- Maintain airway.
- Fluid bolus of 20 cc/kg, may repeat ×1 before adding pressors and/or blood products (Jama 1991;266:1242); aggressive resuscitation with PRBCs if hct < 30% (Nejm 2001;345:1368) or hgb < 8 g/dL; type O uncrossmatched blood OK to give emergently (Ann EM 1986;15:1282), try to use Rh negative in females of childbearing age; if more than one volume of blood products given, give FFP to replace factors (Am J Surg;1996: 399). Saline as good as albumin when looking at 28-d outcome (Nejm 2004;350:2247).
- Dopamine (Inotropin) if hypotensive at pressure support doses of 5-20 μg/kg/min. Renal dosing does not help natriuresis, and

is probably not a real entity (J Am Soc Nephrol 1996;7:1032).
Dopamine preferable over norepinephrine if an increase in the
heart rate is desired. May need to combine pressors for hemodynamic support.

- Dobutamine (Dobutrex) iv (in combination with iv TNG,
  nitroprusside or dopamine, if hypotensive and cardiogenic etiology) for its positive ionotropic properties, better than digitalis or diuretics, no arrhythmias, short half-life; dose at 2-20
  μg/kg/min (Chest 1980;78:694).
- Norepinephrine (Levophed), 2-20 μg/min iv (Crit Care Med
  1987;15:687). Norepinephrine preferred over Dopamine if no
  further increase in heart rate desired.
- Phenylephrine (Neo-Synephrine), 0.5-8 μg/kg/min or 50-180
  μg/min iv, may give 50 μg boluses iv (Crit Care Med 1991;
  19:1395)
- Epinephrine, 1-4 μg/min iv, this should be reserved for when
  all other pressors fail (Chest 1990;98:949)
- Perhaps vasopressin, 40 IU iv (J Trauma 1999:699; Ann
  Pharmacother 2000;34:250) or 0.01-0.08 IU per minute drip.
- Isoproterenol (Isuprel), 2-10 μg/min iv (J Oslo City Hosp
  1989;39:23); rarely used.
- If suspect adrenal crisis, hydrocortisone 100 mg iv (Mil Med
  1996;161:624).
- Immediate treatment of underlying cause, with angioplasty or
  CABG to be considered if cardiogenic (Ann IM 1999;131:47).
- Central line for CVP measurement if needed. If Swan-Ganz
  catheter placed [should be used selectively (Chest 1987;92:
  721)], the following indicators can be measured to help define
  the type of shock. CVP, LVEDP, MAP and PCWP are in units
  of mm Hg. CO is in L/min. CI is in $L/min/m^2$. SVR is in
  $dynes/cm^2$. See Table 2.4.

Table 2.4   Central Monitoring Measurements. Cardio, sepsis, and neuro headings refer to types of shock. Remember that those with sepsis may have a fever and those with neurogenic shock will be paralyzed. MAP can be calculated by the following: MAP = (systolic BP + 2 × diastolic BP)/3.

Indicator	Normal	Cardio	Sepsis	Neuro	Hypovolemia
CVP	2 to 8	>8	<8	<8	<4
LVEDP	5 to 10	var*	<5	<5	<5
MAP	70 to 110	var*	<70	<70	<70
CO	4 to 7	<4	>7	>7	<4
CI	2.5 to 4.5	<2.1	>4.5	>4.5	<2.5
SVR	900 to 1200	var*	<900	<900	<900
PCWP	8 to 12	>18	<12	<12	<8

•PCWP is greater than LVEDP if mitral stenosis, left atrial myxoma, pulmonary venous obstruction, or high intra-alveolar pressure as seen with continuous positive pressure ventilation; conversely, PCWP may be lower than LVEDP if stiff left ventricle or high LVEDP such as >25 mm Hg.

*The variability seen in LVEDP, MAP, and SVR with Cardiogenic Shock has to do with the severity of the patient's process. Initially, LVEDP, MAP, and SVR are high and therapy is initiated to return these values to normal. In later stages, LVEDP, MAP, and SVR drop, thus requiring addition of preload, inotropic, and pressor support.

2.13 Thoracic Aortic Aneurysm/Dissection

Circ 1979;60:1619; J R Coll Surg Edinb 1982:195; Am J Emerg Med 2000;18:46

Cause:

Aneurysm: Atherosclerotic; connective tissue defect as seen in Marfan syndrome; now rarely due to syphilis.

Dissection:
(Nejm 1987;317:1060)

Elevated pressures in aorta as seen in HT or cocaine use (Am J Emerg Med 1997;15:507). Defect of connective tissue as seen in Marfan syndrome or Ehler-Danlos syndrome. Traumatic usually at ligamentum arteriosum in chest.

Epidem:

Aneurysm: Usually discovered incidentally during "Other" evaluation unless medical risk factors prompt serial screening. 1.5 times as common as ruptured abdominal aortic aneurysm. 5% surgical mortality for elective repair and 16% mortality for emergency repair; 21% 5-yr survival if no repair (J Thorac Cardiovasc Surg 1985;89:50). More than half of these will be patients > 60 yr of age (Ann Chir Gynaecol Fenn 1967;56:270).

Dissection: Most common acute illness of aorta. If ascending aorta untreated, 50% die within 48 hr and 90% within 12 mon (Am J Cardiol 1972;30:263). Descending aorta with similar medical and surgical outcomes (Circ 1990;82:IV39), and surgery if evidence of end-organ ischemia. Increased incidence with advanced age, HT, pregnancy, cocaine use, Marfan syndrome, Ehler-Danlos syndrome, systemic lupus, Turner syndrome, and Noonan syndrome (J Emerg Med 1997;15:859). Increased risk in those with autosomal dominant polycystic kidney disease (Nephrol Dial Transplant 1997;12:1711).

Pathophys:

Aneurysm: Dilation of vessel, with increased risk of dissection or aortic insufficiency (Circ 1975;52:I202).

Dissection: Medial rupture of vasovasorum causes a dissecting hematoma that ruptures back into lumen, usually, though not always, distally creating a double-barreled lumen.
- Stanford classification: type A = ascending aorta involved; type B = no involvement of ascending aorta, descending only.

Sx (dissection): Severe pain (90%), sudden onset (84%) (Jama 2002;287:2262); thoracic, abdominal, or in back; often migrating.

Si (dissection): Elevated BP (49%); diastolic murmur (28% sensitive) and thus relatively insensitive; BPs in legs and arms unequal or asymmetric pulses (31% sensitivity) and thus relatively insensitive (EMJ 2004;21:589); focal neurologic deficits (17% sensitive) and also insensitive (Jama 2002;287:2262).

Crs: Mortality 1% per hour in type A.

Cmplc: Organ ischemia due to vessel occlusion, including distal neurologic deficits (J Thorac Imaging 1994;9:101).

Diff Dx: Acute coronary syndrome; pulmonary embolus; and pneumothorax.

Lab:

(Ann EM 1996;28:278)

- Plain CXR may show aortic knob widening; normal CXR does not r/o disease
- Spiral CT of chest with iv contrast (94% sensitive, 87% specific) (Radiol Clin N Am 1999;37:575; Clin Radiol 1999;54:38); consider aortogram (Chest 1989;95:124) to define point of origin, aortic insufficiency, and any vessel compromise, but MRI (98% sensitive, 98% specific) + TEE may obviate the need for this.
- Do not do ECHO as 1st test if clinical suspicion is low: transthoracic ECHO (57% sensitive, 83% specific), TEE (97% sensitive, 77% specific), and better specificity if combined with CT (Clin Radiol 1992;45:104) or aortography.

Emergency Management for Symptomatic Dissections:
- 1st nitroprusside 25-50 μg/min with β-blockers, such as lopressor or esmolol 50-200 μg/kg/min (Dicp 1991;25:735), or add α-blocking coverage with labetalol 10-40 mg iv. Goal is systolic BP < 110 mm Hg.

- 2nd trimethaphan (Arfonad) 1-2 mg per min iv
- Surgical for all type A and selected type B

2.14 Ventricular Arrhythmias

Circ 2000;102:I129; Nejm 2001;345:1473

Cause:

Ventricular Fibrillation (Vfib) (Ann Rev Physiol 2000;62:25) is most
likely a terminal rhythm unless noted immediately in hospital
setting, and is the end-stage rhythm in many (if not all) terminal
conditions. Rare chronic Vfib associated with myocarditis (Jpn
Circ J 2000;64:139). Better outcomes now in those post-MI if
definitive intervention available (defibrillation) and treatment of
underlying heart disease (Heart 2000;84:258); out-of-hospital
Vfib associated with acute MI usually implicates left coronary
artery locus (J Am Coll Cardiol 2000;35:144).

Ventricular tachycardia (Vtach): May be due to idiopathic reasons,
scar from myocardiopathy including alcoholic "holiday heart,"
MI with re-entry, CHF, metabolic abnormalities or long Q-T syndrome which may be caused by drugs. Monomorphic is most
common, followed in equal frequency by polymorphic VT and
torsades de pointes (Acad Emerg Med 1999;6:609). Mitral prolapse
syndrome without clear linkage to this arrhythmia.

Torsades de pointes: Is a ventricular tachycardia that has beat to beat
changes along the QRS axis (Nejm 2004;350:1013). Seen in
those with congenital prolonged QT syndrome, heart block, or as
a consequence of drug use. The lengthening of the QT interval
seen as a prognostic risk for development of such an arrhythmia,
with an absolute QT longer than 500 msec implicated as
increasing the risk for development (Nejm 2003;348:1866), and
hypomagnesemia and hypokalemia are also contributing factors
(Am Hrt J 1986;111:1088; J Am Coll Cardiol 1983;2:806; Circ
1996;93:407).

In children and young adults with Vtach, consider IHSS, cardiomyopathies, CHD such as tetralogy of fallot and pulmonic stenosis; long QT syndrome, mitral valve prolapse (conflicting data), cocaine, Marfan's syndrome with aortic dissection, anomalous coronary arteries, Kawasaki's induced coronary aneurysms.

Epidem: Vtach and PVCs increased with nicotine (Am J Physiol Heart Circ Physiol 2000;278:H2124), CO levels > 100 ppm, and subtle ST-T wave electrical alternans. The data for caffeine are equivocal. Decreased 50% with weekly fish consumption. Commotio cordis, and this may even be seen in patients wearing protective padding for the chest (Jama 2002;287:1142). Increased risk of sudden death in those taking erythromycin and strong inhibitors of P-450 3A (CYP3A) isozymes through prolongation of cardiac repolarization so coincident use should be avoided—for example, such inhibitors may be nitroimidazole antifungals, diltiazem, or verapamil (Nejm 2004;351:1089).

Torsades de pointes is commonly associated with female gender (Circ 1998;97:2237; Jama 1993;270:2590), and the following drugs: bepridil, disopyramide, dofetilide (Nejm 1999; 341:857), ibutilide (Circ 1996;94:1613), procainamide, quinidine (Circ 1964;30:17), and sotalol (Circ 1982;65:886). Lower risk associated with the following: amiodarone, arsenic dioxide, some calcium-channel blockers, chlorpromazine, cisapride, clarithromycin, domperidone, droperidol, erythromycin, haloperidol, mesoridazine, methadone, pentamidine, pimozide, sparfloxacin, and thioridazine. Drug-induced *torsades de pointes* with increased risk in those with bradycardia, (Am Hrt J 1986;111:1088; J Am Coll Cardiol 1983;2:806), digitalis therapy (Pacing Clin Electrophysiol 1998;21:1044), CHF (Nejm 1999;341:857), and recent Afib conversion (Am J Med 2002;113:596; J Am Coll Cardiol 1999;34:396).

Pathophys: Vfib is not the asynchronous "Jell-O" as previously thought, but synchronous atrial function is maintained for 8 min after disorganization of ventricular activity (Chest 2000; 117:1118). Most likely a multifactorial phenomenon that is not well elucidated.

For all ventricular arrhythmias, metabolic abnormalities may be myriad, but potassium physiology is the most important. Citing disturbances of calcium and magnesium may be due in part to potassium then having a lower threshold to cause arrhythmias (Clin Cardiol 1992;15:103).

Torsades de pointes occurs because of lengthening of the action potential in some of the ventricular cells (thus, prolonged QT). Different genetic loci have been discovered that can influence the production of different proteins, especially in relation to ion channel proteins (Cell 2001;104:569).

Sx: Syncope that may progress to sudden death; 51% of those with cardiac syncope had some sort of arrhythmia(Nejm 2002; 347:878).

Si: Dizziness, palpitations, unresponsive.

Crs: Of sudden death: 47% 2-yr mortality after first episode; 86% if no MI, 16% if transmural MI; if asymptomatic, prognosis very good even if complex arrhythmias or VT.

Of PVC's in asymptomatic men: 2 ×s the incidence of later MI or other cardiac event.

Of syncope: 60% 5-yr survival if arrhythmia associated with syncope (Nejm 2002;347:878).

Of long-term survival after cardiac arrest: those with rapid defibrillation after community cardiac arrest will have a 72% chance to hospital admission and 40% chance to discharge in good neurologic state (Nejm 2003;348:2626).

Diff Dx: SVT with aberrancy—no clinical data to differentiate this from VT (Ann EM 1987;16:40); dig toxicity; mitral valve prolapse (conflicting data); "slow ventricular tachycardia" is a benign regular accelerated idioventricular rhythm < 100 beat/min and asymptomatic, seen often (30%) in inferior MIs; Brugada syndrome, which is idiopathic Vfib with RBBB and elevated ST segments V1-V3 on baseline EKG (FEBS Let 2000;479:29); Shy-Drager syndrome; and vasovagal syncope.

Lab: EKG:

> *Vfib* has an undulating baseline, no other complexes noted.
> *Vtach* is unlike SVT with aberrancy due to the following:

1) Vtach QRSs are wide (85% > 14 sec—0% false positives, 30% false negatives) with RBBB pattern or > 0.16 with LBBB;
2) Vtach has a left axis deviation;
3) Vtach is not as regular.
4) SVT with aberrancy has initial QRS deflection as per normal QRS complexes—may compare if present earlier on strip or from previous EKGs.

Torsades de pointes is Vtach with a rotating axis.

> *PVCs differ from supraventricular prematures with aberrancy* due to the following:

- PVC QRSs are opposite of the normal beat vector
- T and QRS vectors are in opposite directions
- No atrial depolarization in 70%
- In Afib, if a complex is wide if may be an aberrant conduction rather than a PVC if it follows a previous longer R-R interval.

Bi-directional Vtach—2 ventricular foci alternating in bigeminal pattern—is almost always diagnostic of digitalis toxicity (Acta Cardiol 1976;31:147).

> *Brugada criteria* (98% overall sensitivity) may indicate Brugada Syndrome, which would then suggest Vtach rather than SVT with aberrancy (Heart 2000;84:31):

1) No precordial RS complex (20% sens), or
2) Beginning of R to S nadir > 0.10 sec (52% sens), or
3) AV dissociation present, or

4) RBBB pattern + Left axis deviation, or R/S < 1 in V_6, or positive R forces in V_1 or LBBB pattern + Q in V_6, or in $V_{1\,or\,2}$ > 0.04 sec, or beginning of R to S nadir in V_1 or V_2 > 0.07, or notching of S down stroke in $V_{1\,or\,2}$.

Emergency Management:

- Defibrillation by bystanders using automatic external defibrillators saves lives (Nejm 2000;343:1206; 2000;343:1210; 2002;347:1242); not yet advocated in those < 1 yr of age and pediatric electrodes available for those 1-8 yr of age on some devices; OK to use adult electrodes in those > 1 yr of age, as long as pads do not touch (concern of amount of energy delivered may be offset by risk/benefit of need for this therapy).
- Bystander CPR (response time) is key, but better if in conjunction with AED use (Nejm 2004;351:637). If patient is "down" for greater than some amount of time (3 min, 4 min, 5 min?), then external chest compressions before defibrillation may be useful (Jama 2003;289:1389). Exactly how long a patient needs to be "down" and how long to do chest compressions before defibrillation is not well-delineated. Advocate that CPR be ongoing if defibrillation not immediately available or if responders are "setting up" the machine to defibrillate—in other words, do not withhold CPR (Circ 2003;108:1939; Ann EM 2001;37:602). Do 30 sec of chest compressions between defibrillations to help the AED machines identify Vfib/Vtach (Ann EM 2001;38:256), as well.
- Prehospital intervention of other advanced cardiac life support interventions (endotracheal intubation and medications) did not affect long-term survival (Nejm 2004;351:647).

For Vfib and unstable Vtach:

- Consider precordial thump if defibrillator not available (Am Hrt J 1989;118:248), supposedly delivers approximately 5 J of energy to heart.

- If field defibrillation unsuccessful, ER treatment considered to have low likelihood of success unless other correctable conditions identified.
- Apply O_2 and get iv access.
- Bretylium is equivocally effective (Am J Cardiol 1999;83: 115, A119), not available.

For unstable Vtach:
- Defibrillation sequence of 200 J, then 300 J, then 360 J in adults (AHA recommendations). In peds 2 J/kg, then 4 J/kg × 2. If using biphasic, use manufacturer recommended energy equivalents.
- Drug treatment (post conversion or if stable Vtach):
  1) Lidocaine: 1.0 to 1.5 mg/kg load with repeat dose in 3-5 min if necessary, drip is set at 2-4 mg per min. Peds dose is 1 mg/kg bolus with 20 to 50 µg/kg/min drip. Data are equivocal (Ann EM 1981;10:420).
  2) Amiodarone: 5 mg/kg over 15 min iv drip (Am J Cardiol 1983;51:156) or 150 mg iv bolus, then 0.5-1 mg per min drip.
  3) Procainamide (Clin Cardiol 2000;23:171): Adults 20 to 30 mg/min iv until one of the following:
     a) Arrhythmia suppressed
     b) Hypotension
     c) Widening of QRS > 50%
     d) Max dose of 17 mg/kg given
     In unstable Vtach or Vfib, OK to give 100 mg iv every 5 min
     Drip rate is 1-4 mg/min.
     Peds: Load 2 to 6 mg/min over 5 min, then drip rate of 20 to 80 µg/kg/min; max 2 g per 24 hr.
  4) Consider magnesium sulfate 2 g iv (Chest 1997;111:1454); especially in those who are known to be hypomagnesemic, such as alcoholics, extreme athletes, those on diurectics, or those malnourished.

5) Sotalol: 100 mg iv over 5 min, may be better than lidocaine.
6) Wide complex without pulses is a form of electromechanical dissociation which has a myriad of causes with either narrow or wide complexes (hypovolemia; hypoxia; tension pneumothorax; massive MI; massive pulmonary embolus; acidosis; drug overdose such as TCAs, digoxin, β-blockers, Ca-channel blockers; hypothermia; or cardiac tamponade), but wide complex may be due to hyperkalemia, so consider iv $CaCl_2$ (J Emerg Med 1989;7:109).

For Vfib:
- Defibrillate as above, and one maximum defibrillation after every pharmacologic maneuver. Biphasic waveforms (J Am Coll Cardiol 1989;13:207; Acad Emerg Med 1999;6:880; Circ 2000;101:2968) appear as effective as monophasic with lower energy levels used and 150 J Biphasic with computer adjustment to patient impedance more effective (Resuscitation 2001;49:233)
- Drug Rx:
    1) Epinephrine 1 mg of 1:10,000 iv or et (peds 10 μg/kg, which is 0.1 cc/kg of 1:10,000) every 5 min or vasopressin 40 IU iv single dose (Anesth Analg 2000;90:1067; 2000; 91:627)—both equally effective (Lancet 2001;358:105); high dose epinephrine of no value, even in children (Nejm 2004;350:1722).
    2) Lidocaine, as above.
    3) Amiodarone as above or 300 mg iv bolus, and not proven better than lidocaine re: survival to or neurologic outcome at hospital discharge by Kudenchuk et al (Nejm 1999; 341:871) but increased chance of survival to hospital admission and discharge shown by Dorian et al (Nejm 2002;346:884), but neurologic outcome data are lacking—

this study also confounded by more patients in the miodarone group having a spontaneous pulse prior to use of amiodarone than the patients assigned to the lidocaine group.

4) Procainamide, as above.

5) Magnesium sulfate 2 gm iv—(J Cardiothorac Vasc Anesth 2000:196) vs (Resuscitation 2001;49:245), especially if considering *torsades de pointes* (Herz 1997;22:51)

6) Sotalol, verapamil, and flecainide may all be helpful (Circ 2000;101:1606); verapamil may convert VF to VT (Circ Res 2000;86:684).

- IVF should be wide open (LR or NS).
- Consider pacing if able to induce bradycardia with pulses, not routine for refractory Vfib.
- Perhaps therapeutic hypothermia (32°-34°C) for 12-24 hr to improve neurologic outcome—needs further study in humans (Nejm 2002;346:549; 2002;346:557; Resuscitation 2003;56:9).

For stable Vtach (alert without chest pain, respiratory distress, or hypotension):

- Consider lidocaine, amiodarone, or procainamide—amiodarone and procainamide effective for both supraventricular and ventricular arrhythmias.
- Second, try synchronized cardioversion starting at 100 J, sedate with narcotic and anxiolytic of choice. Fentanyl will more often avoid hypotension seen with other narcotics (minimal histamine release), and midazolam is of quick onset and short acting; etomidate 10-20 mg iv may offer an amnestic response with lower risk of inducing hypotension.
- If pulses lost, see Vfib section above.

For torsades de pointes:

- Magnesium 1-2 gm iv over 10 min (Am J Cardiol 1984;53:528); bolus of 3-12 mg/kg in peds (J Am Coll Nutr 2004;23:497S).

PVC
- No treatment warranted.

Asystole/Pulseless electrical activity (PEA)
- ACLS algorithms available; consider reversible causes of PEA, which include hypovolemia, massive MI, massive PE, hypothermia, drug intoxication, metabolic abnormalities, pericardial tamponade, and tension pneumothorax.
- Airway, breathing, ventilation
- External chest compressions
- Iv NS wide open
- Epinephrine 1 mg of 1:10,000 iv or et (peds 10 μg/kg which is 0.1 cc/kg of 1:10,000) every 5 min or vasopressin 40 IU iv single dose (Anesth Analg 2000;90:1067; 2000;91:627)—both equally effective (Lancet 2001;358:105); vasopressin suggested better for those in asystole but not followed to hospital discharge re: survival or neurologic outcome (Nejm 2004;350: 105); high dose epinephrine of no value, even in children (Nejm 2004;358:1722).
- Atropine 1 mg iv q 5 min to a total of 4 mg in adult—(Ann EM 1981;10:462; 1984;350:815).

N.B. Et tube doses typically double the iv doses and followed with a 10 cc NS flush.

Patient recovery from Vfib, unstable Vtach, PEA, or asystole:
- Some data to recommend hypothermia at 32°-34° C for 12-24 hr to improve post-recovery phase for patients who recover vital signs but are unconscious (Nejm 2002;346:549).

Long-term:
Some are candidates for implantable defibrillators (Nejm 2003:1836)—be sure to document all rhythms and rhythm changes.

Chapter 3
Dental Conditions

3.1 Infection

Compendium 1990;11:492,494,498

Cause: Poor dental hygiene leading to dental and gum disease, or as manifestations of systemic disease as seen in diabetes mellitus, rheumatologic disorders, hematologic diseases, or infectious diseases, such as TB; increase caries with passive smoking (Jama 2003;289:1258)

Epidem: Common as first dental visit for many who come to the ER, especially children < 3.5 yr of age (52%) (Ped Dent 1997; 19:470). Common pathogens include *Streptococcus pyogenes*, *Streptococcus mitis*, *Streptococcus salivarius*, *Staphlococci*, *Streptococcus faecalis*, *Escherichia coli*, and *Klebsiella* (Aust Dent J 1978;23:107).

Pathophys: Breakdown of tooth or gum leading to secondary infectious complication (J Am Dent Assoc 1969;78:1016).
- Periodontal abscess is an abscess between the tooth and gingiva.
- Necrotizing gingivitis are caused by a spirochete very similar to *Treponema pallidum*; it is a *Fusobacteria* spp.

Sx: Halitosis, pain, swelling.

Si: Localized edema, erythema, or tenderness; ulcerations; dental caries; lymphadenopathy.

Cmplc: Tooth loss; secondary abscess in gingivitis.

Lab: None, unless systemic disease sought.

Emergency Management:

(Brit Dent J 1989;166:41)

Periodontal abscess:
- Warm rinses.
- Antibiotics: PCN VK 500 mg po bid to qid, Clindamycin for treatment failures or if PCN allergic—300 mg po qid; perhaps metronidazole for PCN failures (Brit J Oral Surg 1977;14:264).
- I & D, if "pointing," ie, if the abscess has come to a head, perform appropriate block and stab the abscess with a #11 blade.
- Pain medications, with ibuprofen having physiologic advantage over acetaminophen in dental pain (J Endod 1999;25:804).
- Dental referral.

Necrotizing gingivitis:
- Warm rinses.
- Tetracycline 250 mg po qid; or PCN 500 mg tid or qid; or metronidazole 200 mg po tid for 3 d.
- Topical lidocaine (2% viscous) may help, avoid overuse or may precipitate lidocaine toxicity.
- Dental referral.

3.2 Oral Lacerations

Cause: Trauma, usually with tooth or dental hardware as the cutting surface.

Epidem: Common.

Sx: Cut to inside of lip or mouth.

Si: Oral laceration; check for loose tooth or loose dental hardware.

Crs: Usually heals quickly; check carefully for multiple lacerations, especially where mucosa inside of mouth reflects onto the upper or lower jaw.

Cmplc: Infection.

Lab: None, consider x-ray if looking for foreign body.

Emergency Management:
- Update tetanus, if needed.
- Local anesthesia (see p 387).
- Repair with silk, 4-0 or 5-0, after copious irrigation with sterile saline. Place simple sutures loosely and be sure to line up the Vermilion border, if this has been violated.
- May need repair in the operating theater for children.
- Consider 3-5 d of oral antibiotic prophylaxis with penicillin for high risk wounds; may also elect to leave these open if possible.

3.3 Trauma

Compendium 1990;11:526,528,530

Epidem: Incomplete tooth fractures more common in older patient population, complete tooth fractures can occur at any age (J Prosthet Dent 1999;82:226).

Sx/Si:
- Tooth fracture is assigned an Ellis class:
  Class I is a fracture through the enamel.
  Class II involves the dentin, as evidenced by air and cold sensitivity.
  Class III involves the pulp, evidenced by central blood spot when tooth is gently sponged with a gauze.
- A subluxed tooth is a loose tooth, with a spectrum of subluxation possible.
- An avulsed tooth is a tooth that is missing.
- All but Ellis Class I fractures will involve pain.

Cmplc: Loss of tooth or secondary infection for all but Ellis Class I.

Lab: X-ray if avulsed tooth cannot be located (r/o gingival location) or if tooth fragments suspected in soft tissues; tooth may be in stomach.

Emergency Management:

(Otolaryngol Clin N Am 1972;5:273)

- Ellis Class I:

File edges if necessary, elective dental referral.

- Ellis Class II:

Cover the dentin with CaOH and bandage (foil or dry gauze) and
avoid hot or cold foods—if minimal dentin showing in adolescents or older patients, may just need dietary changes for a few
wk. Next day dental referral.

- Ellis Class III:

Cover tooth with foil and give immediate dental referral—same
day, next day at the most. Oral analgesics, nothing on the
pulp!

- Subluxed tooth:

If minimal, reassurance—if an anterior tooth, explicit instructions to seek dental attention if pain worsening or tooth loos-
ening. Anterior teeth with somewhat tenuous anchoring re:
neurovascular bundle. Soft diet for 2-3 wk.

If grossly unstable, immediate dental referral for stabilization.

- Avulsed tooth (Endod Dent Traumatol 1986;2:1; Otolaryngol
  Clin N Am 1991;24:165; Am J EM 1990;8:351):

Re-implant permanent teeth. Gentle rinsing with tap water,
avoid touching roots. If unable to re-implant, place in moistened gauze, glass of milk with ice if available, or Hank's solution ideally. Re-implant at ER, and immediate dental referral.

N.B. Periodontal dressings are widely available for temporary stabilization in the ER.

Chapter 4
Endocrinology

4.1 Acute Adrenal Insufficiency

Ann Clin Biochem 1999;36:151; Nejm 2003;348:727

Cause: Primary adrenal insufficiency (Addison's disease) can be atrophic in nature as seen in idiopathic or autoimmune with suppressor T-cell defect; or it can be characterized as destructive as seen in primary or metastatic cancer (Ann Hematol 1999;78:151); antiphospholipid syndrome (Chest 1998; 113:1136); infection, especially in TB or in peds with sepsis (Arch Dis Child 1999;80:51); and meningococcemia with Friderichsen-Waterhouse syndrome; in amyloidosis; or in severe hemorrhage with hypotension (Arch Surg 1999;134:394). Secondary adrenal insufficiency occurs in those who may be panhypopit, those who are on chronic steroids—including the possibility of inhaled beclomethasone (J Allergy Clin Immunol 1999;103:956), or those who have just come off of corticosteroids and are now under stress; or autoimmune disorders in general (Clin Endocrinol (Oxf) 1998;49:779). Also seen in HIV in AIDS patients.

Epidem: In Addison's Disease, peak incidence age 20-40 yr. Associated with HLA-B8 and DR 3/4, and thereby with pernicious anemia, myasthenia gravis, islet cell antibody IDDM, myxedema, vitiligo, alopecia, and primary gonadal failure.

Pathophys: 80% of gland must be destroyed to get symptoms. ACTH and MSH similar, hence increased pigmentation; both mineralocorticoid and glucocorticoid deficiencies create si/sx.

Sx: Loss of sense of well-being; nausea, vomiting, and diarrhea; salt craving and weight loss; galactorrhea, rarely; increased pigmentation if chronic.

Si: Hypotension; cachexia; hyperpigmentation, vitiligo, longitudinal nail pigment streaks if chronic; diminished axillary and pubic hair; remember not to rely on abdominal exam for acute abdomen if patient is on exogenous steroids.

Crs: 40% of those with Addison's disease will develop other glandular failure (especially thyroid and gonadal).

Diff Dx:
- Hyporeninemic hypoaldosteronism: hyperkalemia and metabolic acidosis due to depressed prostaglandin synthesis.
- Adrenoleukodystrophy: in boys, a sex-linked abnormality of fatty acid metabolism.

Lab: Chemistry profile with low Na^+, low HCO_3, elevated K^+, order a cortisol level—if < 15 μgm%, then diagnosis most likely; check TSH (J Clin Endocrinol Metab 2000;85:1388), CBC with diff looking for eosinophilia (Lancet 1999;353:1675), consider steroid-21-hydroxylase antibody and very long chain fatty acids serum levels looking for elevation for diagnosis of idiopathic (J Clin Endocrinol Metab 1998;83:3163), consider pan culture and other ID evaluation for hypotension; EKG; Graded ACTH stimulation test diagnostic (J Endocrinol Invest 2000;23:163).

Emergency Management:
- IVF with 20 cc/kg bolus.
- Hydrocortisone 100 mg iv (and may repeat in 6 hr) (Mil Med 1996;161:624).
- Methylprednisolone 1-2 mg/kg iv if additional glucocorticoid boost needed (respiratory distress, hypotension).

4.2 Diabetic Ketoacidosis

Acta Paediatr suppl 1999;88:14; Emerg Med Clin N Am 1989;7:859

Cause: IDDM with noncompliance and/or secondary infection most likely.

Epidem: Approximately 5% mortality (Med J Aust 1989;151: 439,441,442)

Pathophys: Coma from CSF acidosis, hence rarer in metabolic than respiratory acidosis because CO_2 crosses blood-brain barrier easily; HCO_3 treatment may paradoxically induce/worsen coma. Atrial natriuretic peptide suppressed in children to maintain fluid and sodium (J Peds 1987;111:329).

Sx: Malaise, confusion, nausea, vomiting, abdominal pain.

Si: Kussmaul's respirations; stupor; coma; hypotension; dehydration.

Crs: Onset over 2-3 d.

Cmplc: Cerebral edema leading to coma with 90% mortality 6-10 hr after starting treatment—especially in children (Nejm 1967; 276:665) with low $PaCO_2$ and high serum BUN (Nejm 2001; 344:264). Secondary infection with *Pseudomonas pseudomallei* (Melioidosis), ubiquitous in Asia (Arch IM 1972;130:268).

Diff Dx: Hypoglycemia; infection; drug intoxication; appendicitis; acute renal failure; Non-ketotic, nonacidotic hyperosmolar coma—seen in the elderly with NIDDM.

Lab: Chemistry profile and blood gas, specifically looking for bicarb < 10 and pH < 7.2 (Ped Emerg Care 1996;12:347). Look for anion gap (AG) > 15 calculating the following: Na − (Cl + CO_2) = AG (Nejm 1977;297:814). ABG vs venous blood gas— venous just as useful (Ann EM 1998;31:459). CBC with diff, and > 10% bandemia warrants search for secondary infection (Am J EM 1987;5:1). UA as quick test for ketones and hydration status and if secondary UTI. Consider pan culture and other ID evaluation if source or febrile. Consider serum ketones or acetone level (Diabetes 1986;35:668). Consider measured and/or calculated osmoles—calculated osmoles = glucose/18 + 2 × Na + BUN/2.8.

Emergency Management:

- Adults with iv NS with 1 L bolus then 1 L per hr.
- Peds with 20 cc/kg IVF bolus and may repeat × 1 before maintenance rate if needed; studies that call into question the use of IVF because of cerebral edema are just selecting those that are the sickest who required the most fluid resuscitation and these patients have increased water diffusion in the brain (J Peds 2004;145:164).
- Regular insulin 0.33-0.44 U/kg iv push, then 7 U/hr iv continuous until glucose < 250 mg%; then 2-6 U/hr iv until glucose < 150 mg%; then routine maintenance (Arch IM 1977;137:1377); check K^+ before infusing insulin unless EKG changes such as wide QRS.
- Insulin for peds: 0.1-0.2 U/kg iv push, then 0.1-0.2 U/hr.
- Fluids: After first liter, NS or change to ½ NS if osmoles elevated with 40 mEq KCl/L at 1 L/hr until serum glucose < 250 mg%, then change to D_5W or D_5NS depending on the serum sodium (high sodium, go more hypotonic, and vice versa).
- TNG if vomiting (treatment for gastroparesis).
- HCO_3 iv only if HCO_3 < 5 mEq/L or pH < 6.9 (Crit Care Med 1999;27:2690); gives paradoxical CNS acidosis, and right shift of hemoglobin dissociation curve; avoid more so if possible in peds (Nejm 2001;344:264)
- PO_4 treatment rarely needed; maybe as K_2PO_4 if low (PO_4 < 0.1-0.5 mg%) to prevent insulin resistance.
- Medical consult for admission

4.3 Hyperosmolar States

Nejm 1974;290:1184; West J Med 1980;132:16

Cause:

Diabetes Insipidus (DI) (Endocrinol Metab Clin N Am 1993;22:411):

- Central DI from idiopathic, sarcoid, eosinophilic granuloma, CNS insult—tumor, trauma, surgery; ethanol ingestion is transient but aggravates all other causes.
- Nephrogenic DI, including drug induced by lithium, demeclocycline (Declomycin), transient in pregnancy due to increased vaopressinase, renal tubular damage from hypercalcemia, hypokalemia, chronic pyelonephritis, chronic partial obstruction, sickle cell anemia, lead poisoning, and renal tubular acidosis.

Dehydration from one of the following:

Loop Diuretics

Inability to drink

Betadine treatment of burns

Peritoneal or hemodialysis

Diminished urine concentration and diminished thirst in elderly, especially with AODM as a comorbid diagnosis which leads to nonketotic hyperosmolar coma (Drugs 1989;38:462; Curr Ther Endocrinol Metab 1997;6:438). Perhaps precipitated by glucocorticoids, β-blockers, or diazoxide.

Epidem: DI is 3:100,000 (Ped Rev 2000:122)

Pathophys: Both types of DI associated with ADH deficiency or resistance [nephrogenic (J Mol Med 1998;76:326)]—normally ADH dilates splanchnic arterioles, increases renin, and stimulates factor VIII clotting factors while causing water resorption in kidney. Dehydration as per etiology.

Sx: Confusion.

Si: Confusion, stupor, coma, hypotension, dehydration.

Crs: Worse prognosis in those who have normal or elevated corrected serum sodium (Ann IM 1989;110:855); and 1.6 mmol/L to the serum sodium for every 100 mg/dL of serum glucose over 100 mg/dL.

Cmplc: Mortality > 40% in elderly patients.

Lab: CBC with diff, chemistry profile, measured or calculated osmoles (formula above). Consider UA and pan culture to search for ID reasons for hypotension; EKG
- *X-ray:* Neuroimaging such as CT/MRI (J Clin Endocrinol Metab 1999;84:1954) to evaluate pituitary in Central DI, may not be necessary in isolated idiopathic DI or those with growth hormone deficiency only (Lancet 1999;353:2212).

Emergency Management:
- O_2; IVF
- Replace H_2O, but at less than 12 mEq Na change per 24 hr (cerebral edema) or change serum osmolality at < 2 mOsm/l/hr. Water deficit = 0.6 × (ideal body weight) $[1 - 140/(\text{measured serum sodium})]$.
- Central DI treated with Desmopressin (vasopressin analog) 5-20 µg nasal, subcutaneous, or iv q 4-20 hr for complete types. Desmopressin is resistant to vasopressinase. Perhaps indapamide 2.5 mg qd (Arch IM 1999;159:2085). For incomplete type, treat the same way or treat like nephrogenic.
- Nephrogenic treated with thiazides, carbamazepine, or chlorpropamide; amiloride 5-10 mg bid (0.3 mg/kg/d tid in peds) (Arch Dis Child 1999;80:548).
- NSAIDs (indomethacin) for lithium-induced DI (Ren Fail 1997;19:183).
- Non-Ketotic Hyperosmolar Coma with 0.15 U/kg iv bolus of regular insulin, followed by regular insulin infusion in ½ NS at

5-7 U per hr. NS for iv fluid resuscitation, avoid hypokalemia (Diabetes Care 1982;1:78).

4.4 Hypoglycemia

Cause:

Exogenous:
- Insulin: low plasma C peptide levels; prolonged hypoglycemia with use of β-blockers (Diabetes Care 1984;7:243)
- Sulfonyureas
- Endotoxic Shock (Circ Shock 1982;9:269).
- Drug List from Ann IM 1993;118:536, including fluoro-quinolones (Med Lett Drugs Ther 2003;45:64).

Fasting:
- Pancreatic functioning tumor (Diabetes 1981;30:377)
- Nonpancreatic functioning tumor (Arch IM 1972;129:447)
- Liver disease
  Acquired, especially from CHF
  Congenital glycogen storage disease or galactosemia (J Clin Invest 1998;102:507)
  Hepatoma
- Ethanol (Endocrinol Metab Clin N Am 1989;18:75) and/or poor nutrition, from decreased gluconeogenesis; eg, in diarrheal disease in children.
- Endocrine deficiencies, eg, Addison's, hypopituitarism, decreased pancreatic α-cell function.
- Normal physiologic responses in women and children.

Reactive (postprandial) (Diabetes 1981;30:465): oral GTT no help, get blood glucose prn symptoms; ≤ 60 mg% is significant:
- Rapid gastric emptying
- Fast absorption
- Prediabetes

- Dumping syndrome (Peds 1987;80:937)
- Leucine sensitivity
- Hereditary fructose intolerance

Sx: Confusion, epinephrine release symptoms—sweaty, pale, nausea.

Si: Tachycardia, pallor, diaphoresis, intoxication, coma.

Cmplc: CNS insult, coma.

Lab: Glucoscan, chemistry profile.

Emergency Management:

- O_2; iv access.
- 25 g of glucose (50 cc of 50% solution—D50 1 amp) (Prehospital Disaster Med 1998;13:44)—give with 100 mg of thiamine iv if ethanol abuse related or suspected. Repeat as needed. Peds: 2 cc of a 50% soln or 4 cc of a 25% soln (1 g)/kg iv.
- Or may try Glucagon 1 mg iv (Diabetes Care 1987;10:712), im OK if no access.
- May give juice or glucose paste if patient alert and able to swallow (Diabetes Care 1982;5:512); rectal glucose not effective (Acta Paediatr Scand 1984;73:560).
- Feed when alert.
- Outpatient follow-up if short-lived reason for hypoglycemia and patient recovers, otherwise medical admission.

4.5 Myxedema Coma

Jama 1974;230:884; Med Clin N Am 1995;79:185; Am Fam Phys 2000;62:2485

Cause: Untreated hypothyroid state, with the hypothyroidism due to any factor, such as I_2 deficiency or excess, autoimmune (Ann IM 1985;103:26), surgical excision, radiation, or iodide after treatment of diffuse toxic goiter (Nejm 1969;28:816). Less likely from lithium therapy or secondary (pituitary or hypothalamic failure) hypothyroidism.

Epidem: Rare, with 50% mortality in elderly even if recognized and treated (J Am Board Fam Pract 1995;8:376); more common in cold climates.

Pathophys: Lack of T3 and T4 has global influence on the body. Autoimmune Hashimoto's has associations with pernicious anemia and insulin-dependent diabetes; phenytoin and carbamazepine may precipitate hypothyroidism (Acta Neurol Scand 1980;61:330).

Sx: Hair loss and coarseness; skin coarseness; fatigue; swollen tongue; constipation; and/or muscle cramps.

Si: Hypothermia; goiter; surgical scar on neck; hung-up reflexes (J Psych Res 1967;5:289) or areflexia; diminished PMI from pericardial effusion; psychosis; respiratory depression; seizures; or coma.

Crs: Imminent death if not recognized early and treated.

Cmplc: Environmental cold, trauma, secondary infection, and drugs as listed above may all be complicating factors. Cardiac arrhythmias may occur with rewarming. Cardiac tamponade (Clin Cardiol 1982;5:459).

Lab: Chemistry profile, CBC with diff, TSH (Nejm 1971;285:529), Free T4, EKG, ABG if significant neuro or respiratory compromise, UA and/or pan culture if considering other reasons for mental status change, CXR—may show Erlenmeyer flask sign, as seen in pericardial effusion, consider head CT to r/o intracranial process, if change in mental status.

Emergency Management:
- Coma protocol of O_2, and iv narcan, dextrose, thiamine, if appropriate. Consider iv pyridoxine, if Hazmat event and/or hydrazine exposure.
- Secure airway if necessary, intubate for hypoxemia.

- 500 µg iv of T4 or 40µg iv of T3, if possible—give ASAP, but be cautious of cardiac effects.
- Rewarm gradually and medical consult for admission.

4.6 Thyroid Storm

Jama 1974;230:592

Cause: Untreated hyperthyroid state, which may have a heightened physiologic response due to cessation of antithyroid meds (Metabolism 1968;17:893), radiation thyroiditis, infection, trauma, surgery, acidosis, or toxemia of pregnancy.

Epidem: Those with previous surgical treatment for hyperthyroidism may relapse (16%) (Brit J Surg;1983;70:408)

Pathophys: Unopposed hyperthyroid state, with T3 and T4 influencing the physiology of the whole body. Autoimmune thyroiditis (Graves disease) is a classification of many different subtypes (Clin Endocrinol (Oxf) 1992;36:75); rarely Hashimoto thyroiditis (Metab Ped Ophthalmol 1981;5:213).

Thyroid cancer present in approximately 6% (World J Surg 1998;22:473,477), more often found in those with solitary adenoma.

Sx: Hot and sweaty; smooth skin; diarrhea from steatorrhea, polyphagia of fat, and decreased gi transit time.

Si: Fever; muscle wasting; resting tachycardia; tremors; hyperactivity; weakness; confusion; psychosis; coma; and/or hepatomegaly.

Crs: Death is imminent unless recognized and treated.

Cmplc: Treatment induced hypothyroidism (Clin Endocrinol (Oxf) 1997;46:1) or hypocalcemia.

Diff Dx: Physical signs of chorea may also be seen in medication reaction, neurologic lesion, or psychiatric disorder (Am J Psych 1979;136:1208).

Lab: Metabolic profile, CBC with diff, TSH, Free T4, Free or Total T3 (J Am Ger Soc 1988;36:242), consider ID evaluation with UA and pan culture for fever and mental status changes, EKG, ABG if neuro changes and/or respiratory compromise.

Emergency Management:

- IVF, have D$_5$NS ready for bolus with treatment, as below,
- β-blockade: Propranolol 2-10 mg iv—go slow, or Esmolol (Brevibloc) 50-200 μg/kg/min; not in heart failure (BMJ 1977;1:1505).
- Hydrocortisone 100 mg iv (q 6 hr) and consider dexamethasone to prevent T4 to T3 peripheral conversion.
- PTU 1 gm po or via NG tube.
- Iodine as Lugol's solution, 10 gtts po tid or organic iodide 1 gm qd—not ideal for long-term use.
- Consider lithium 300 mg po tid instead of SSKI.
- Cooling blanket for hyperthermia; cool mist with fan works quicker to cool patient.
- Digitalis, if necessary (afib).

Chapter 5

Environmental

Some basic environmental facts:
- When we speak of elevation (high altitude), we generally mean > 8,000 ft above sea level, although high altitude is anything > 5,000 ft.
- A person gets colder faster in water.
- Hypothermia is also a summertime problem.
- Hyperthermia has a myriad of causes besides environmental.
- When unable to explain neurologic problems or constitutional symptoms, think CO.

5.1 Altitude (AMS, HAPE, HACE)

Am J Emerg Med 1985;3:217; Emerg Med Clin N Am 1984;2:503; Nejm 2001;345:107

Cause: Being above altitude (8,000-10,000 ft above sea level) with or without appropriate acclimatization. To prevent: "Climb high, sleep low." (Aviat Space Environ Med 1976;47:512; N Z Med J 1998;111:168)

Epidem: Getting to altitude is easier today than in the past, even extreme altitude (18,000 ft above sea level) is attainable at a cost.

Pathophys:
- Hypoxia is the problem, with the partial pressure of O_2 decreasing as we attain higher elevations. Initial hyperventilation—due to decreased Pa_{O_2}—is blunted by an ensuing respiratory alkalosis. Peripheral vasoconstriction leads to central

venous pooling, which causes a diuresis and increasing osmo-lality. Pulmonary hypertensive tendencies (Adv Exp Med Biol 1999;474:93) will be exacerbated by altitude due to the global pulmonary hypoxia, and perhaps pulmonary vasoconstrictors such as endothelin-1 (Circ 1999;99:2665). Cerebral blood flow will increase in an attempt to increase oxygen flow to the brain, yet this increase in cerebral blood volume may lead to an increase in intracranial pressure. Perhaps this is due to edema and ischemia (J Appl Physiol 1995;79:375). Cerebral blood flow is important in high altitude cerebral edema, but probably not the significant physiologic problem in Acute Mountain Sickness (J Appl Physiol 1999;86:1578).

- Acclimatization may offset some of the problems with attaining altitude, but this is not always certain. Climb high, sleep low—with no more than 2,000 to 2,500 ft increase being allowed in altitude on a single day.
- The three major problems with altitude are acute mountain sickness (AMS), high altitude pulmonary edema (HAPE) (Wilderness Environ Med 1999;10:88), and high altitude cerebral edema (HACE) (Wilderness Environ Med 1999;10:97).

Sx:

AMS: Headache, fatigue, nausea, vomiting, anorexia.
HAPE: Same as AMS with cough and dyspnea on exertion.
HACE: Same as AMS and HAPE with change in mental status.

Si:

AMS: Nonspecific.
HAPE: Rales; irregular, nocturnal breathing patterns (Aviat Space Environ Med 1989;60:786).
HACE: As with HAPE as well as stupor, coma, focal cranial nerve deficit.

Crs: Rapid physiologic decline in all categories unless rapid diagnosis and treatment.

Table 5.1 AMS Self Assessment

Headache	0	None at all
	1	A mild headache
	2	Moderate headache
	3	Severe headache, incapacitating
Gastrointestinal symptoms	0	Good appetite
	1	Poor appetite or nausea
	2	Moderate nausea or vomiting
	3	Severe, incapacitating nausea and vomiting
Fatigue and/or weakness	0	Not tired or weak
	1	Mild fatigue/weakness
	2	Moderate fatigue/weakness
	3	Severe fatigue/weakness, incapacitating
Dizziness/lightheadedness	0	None
	1	Mild
	2	Moderate
	3	Severe, incapacitating
Difficulty sleeping	0	Slept as well as usual
	1	Did not sleep as well as usual
	2	Woke many times, poor night's sleep
	3	Could not sleep at all
Total		(Score of 3 or more consistent with AMS)

Cmplc: AMS may progress to HAPE or HACE or both, and symptoms may worsen with use of ethanol, respiratory depressants, inadequate fluid intake, and overexertion.

Diff Dx: Hypothermia, dehydration, drug side-effect or OD (specifically CO poisoning), infection, PE, CVA, diabetic reaction, or simply fatigue or bronchitis.

Scoring System: Lake Louise AMS Scoring System (Hypoxia and Molecular Med 1993;66:272; Aviat Space Environ Med 1995:963). See Table 5.1.

Lab: None for mild episodes.

More severe episodes, begin treatment and gather the following: metabolic profile, glucoscan, ABG, CO level, CBC with diff, CXR, EKG, UA with pan culture if ID evaluation considered, head CT without contrast if CNS insult considered, ethanol level or urine toxic screen, if drugs of abuse considered.

N.B. Low resting SaO_2 is a risk factor for developing AMS and HAPE (Aviat Space Environ Med 1998;69:1182).

Emergency Management:
- Descent, then rest (J Appl Physiol 2000;88:581) and warm patient.
- O_2; Gamow Bag if necessary and available (Am J Emerg Med 1996;14:412; Biomed Sci Instrum 1989;25:79); perhaps hyperbaric bag in ERs that treat many with altitude illnesses and that are at altitude.

Mild AMS will resolve with some descent (1,000 ft), further evaluation per patient symptoms. All other cases should do the following:
- As above.
- Good oral hydration; iv access if needed (Aviat Space Environ Med 1999;70:867).
- Maintain/secure airway; possible use of PEEP valve for prevention (Eur J Appl Physiol 1998;77:32).
- Acetazolamide (Diamox) 5 mg/kg/d divided tid (Nejm 1968;279:839; Nejm 1969;280:49; Lancet 1981;1:180; Ann IM 1992;116:461).
- Dexamethasone 4 mg q 6 hr any route (po/im/iv) (West J Med 1991;154:289).
- Acetazolamide + Dexamethasone better than Acetazolamide alone which is better than Dexamethasone alone (Aviat Space Environ Med 1998;69:883).
- Data on theophylline are equivocal (Eur Respir J 2000;15:123).
- Potential role of magnesium (orally) (Aviat Space Environ Med 1999;70:625).

HAPE:
- Loop diuretics such as furosemide 60-80 mg iv, paucity of data.

- Nifedipine 10 mg po, data equivocal (Med Sci Sports Exerc 1999;31:S23).
- Hydralazine10 mg iv or phentolamine, data equivocal (Int J Sports Med 1992;13:S68)
- Consider CPAP (Chest 2003;123:49).
- Whether narcotics facilitate splanchnic pooling is equivocal, and if using for anxiolysis and wish to avoid inducing hypotension, narcotic of choice would be fentanyl 25 μg iv in an adult every 10 min—obviously use with caution in those with respiratory distress.

HACE:
- Consider mannitol and loop diuretics—data equivocal.

Prevention:
- Acetazolamide, Dexamethasone, good hiking habits, Salemterol Inhaler 125 μg q 12 hr (Nejm 2002;364:1631)

5.2 Electrical Injury

Emerg Med Clin N Am 1992;10:211; Ann EM 1993;22:378; J Emerg Med 1999;17:977; 2000;18:181; 2000;18:27

Cause: Children playing around electrical sockets or broken electrical cord; non-grounded tools; lack of appropriate barrier secondary to material breakdown, sweat, or water.

Epidem: 3-5% of burn center admissions, 1000 deaths/yr (Ann EM 1993;22:378)

Pathophys: More than 1000 volts is significant to humans, with as little as 20 mAmps causing significant morbidity if alternating current. Ohm's law: amperage = voltage/resistance. The electrical injury can cause conduction problems in nerve or cardiac cells, as well as thermal destruction.

Sx: Tingling in body part in contact, inability to relax grip, shortness of breath, localized pain.

Si: Tissue destruction, respiratory distress, arrhythmias, mental status changes, paralysis, or sudden death.

Crs: Variable

Cmplc: Sudden death from delivery of current on ventricular repolarization phase—analogous to R on T phenomenon. Children who bite electrical cords may have delayed labial artery hemorrhage resulting from sloughing mucosa as underlying tissues heal—delay may be as much as 2 wk.

Lab:
- If localized hand tingling with no other symptoms and no evidence of entrance and exit wounds on opposites sides of the body, nothing specific.
- All other cases: EKG; CMP, PT/PTT, CPK, UA, and urine for myoglobin if suspect significant muscle destruction; check LFTs and amylase if intra-abdominal path; head CT if mental status changes.

Emergency Management:
- Iv access.
- Airway management if facial or neck burns with declining respiratory function, or if burns noted in mouth or oropharynx.
- Treat cardiac arrhythmias if lethal pattern. Continuous cardiac monitoring is not needed if normal EKG and no acute problems (J Emerg Med 2000;18:181), including loss of consciousness (Burns 1997;23:576). Perhaps 24-hr observation if exit and entrance wounds through thorax (Brit Hrt J 1987;57:279).
- Iv fluid for burn resuscitation if significant burns noted during physical or laboratory evaluation (South Med J 1996;89:869).
- Update tetanus, if necessary.
- NG tube if intra-abdominal process with ileus.
- Fracture management as appropriate.

5.3   Envenomations

Nejm 2002;347:347; Ann EM 2001;37:189; 2001;37:196; 2001;37:181; Am Fam Phys 2002;65:1367

Cause: Bites from spiders and reptiles or scorpion stings

Epidem: Annual number of significant spider envenomations in the U.S. is not well known but about 50 species in the U.S. are considered dangerous. Approximately 8000 envenomous snakebites occur per year in the U.S., with about 19 species being responsible. Scorpion stings are also difficult to track, but only *Centruroides exilicauda* produces a significant systemic envenomation response. C. *exilicauda* is also known as the black scorpion.

Pathophys: Anywhere from local to systemic reactions may occur. The venom may carry a variety of proteins that may cause local tissue destruction due to proteases, phosphatases, lipase, and complement system inhibitors, such as seen in the *Loxosceles reclusa,* or Brown Recluse spider (Nejm 2005;352:700). Neurotoxic proteins may also play a factor, such as in the Black Widow spider venom. Other venoms may carry a combination of local tissue destructors and neuroproteins, such as seen in rattlesnake venom. The Black scorpion venom carries proteins that activate sodium channels— the resultant neurologic sequelae is that of firing of sympathetic, parasympathetic, and somatic efferent nerves. Others such as scorpions may carry proteins that disrupt K^+ channels (Methods Enzymol 1999;294:624).

Sx: Pain, edema, and erythema. Possibly systemic reaction, including blurry vision, difficulty breathing, difficulty swallowing, dizziness, muscle fatigue, or stiffness.

Si: Puncture wound, ulceration, local tissue necrosis, muscular rigidity, ptosis, respiratory distress, drooling, nausea, vomiting, hypotension, tachycardia.

ENVIRONMENTAL

Crs: Variable course depending on type of envenomation, dose and depth of wound.
- Spider and snakebites generally respond to general supportive measures, with severe respiratory and neurologic problems waning after 2-3 d, and hematologic complications taking longer to resolve. Antivenin will be covered below.
- Scorpion stings initiate neurologic compromise that should respond to airway management and antivenin—scorpion sting antivenin (Toxicon 1999;37:1627) vs (J Toxicol Clin Toxicol 1999;37:51).

Cmplc: Shock, airway edema, coagulopathy (coagulopathy not seen in scorpion stings).

Lab:
- CBC with diff, metabolic profile, PT/PTT, ABG, CPK, UA.
- ELISA for Loxosceles species (brown reclucse) which works best (less cross reactivity) at a 40 nanograms quantity (Ann EM 2002;39:469).
- R/o other causes of airway compromise and shock: ethanol level, urine toxic screen, EKG, consider lateral neck x-ray, consider head CT (consideration of CNS insult with neurogenic pulmonary edema); if coagulopathy suspected: d-dimer, fibrin split products, fibrinogen.

Emergency Management:
- Airway and shock management, with specific antivenin therapy if indicated.
- Absolute rest, and consider splinting and lymphatic constriction bands (Ann EM 2001;37:168)
- Consider pretreatment with iv methylprednisolone 1 mg/kg and/or diphenhydramine 25 mg for antivenin pre-treatment, or iv midazolam for muscle fasciculations (Ann EM 1999;34:620).
- Contact state poison control for specific guidelines; American Association of Poison Control Centers 1-800-222-1222;

Wyeth Labs at 1-800-934-5556, if questions regarding use and availability of antivenin, such as CroFab for crotaline envenomation.

- Local measures for wound cleaning; perhaps constriction band between bite and torso although not proven effective; specific antivenom measures such as suction (Ann EM 2004;43:181), incision, ice, or electric therapy have not been shown to be effective, nor nitroglycerin for brown recluse spider bites (Ann EM 2001;37:161). Specifically, fasciotomy in a porcine model worsens the myonecrosis seen with crotaline (pit viper) envenomation (Ann EM 2004;44:99).

5.4 Frostbite

J Trauma 2000;48:171

Cause: Tissue destruction from cold exposure.

Epidem: Seen frequently in those with ethanol abuse or psychiatric issues.

Pathophys: Peripheral vasoconstriction to maintain core temperature, leaving extremities at risk for cold exposure without rewarming. Local tissue destruction from cell lysis and ice crystal formation. Distal destruction is irreversible with venous and arterial thrombosis, proximal injury is noted by erythema, with an unknown extent of destruction between these two extremes.

Sx/Si:

First Degree: Erythema, edema, border erythema
Second Degree: Partial thickness with blisters and black eschar
Third Degree: Full thickness with subcutaneous involvement, hemorrhagic blisters with skin necrosis
Fourth Degree: Full thickness with subcutaneous involvement, as well as tendon, muscle, and/or bone involvement.

Cmplc: Refreezing and inadequate treatment leading to extension of tissue destruction is a possible problem. Peripheral vascular disease, diabetes mellitus, dehydration, trauma, and infection all worsen outcome.

Lab: As dictated by patients' co-morbid diagnoses; consider CBC with diff, ESR, and appropriate x-ray to diagnose osteomyelitis.

Emergency Management:
- Rapid rewarming in warm (not hot) water 40°C (104°F) for 10-30 min
- Avoid refreezing
- Do not open intact blisters, opening them is controversial
- Ibuprofen (Ann EM 1987;16:1056)
- Topical aloe vera (Postgrad Med 1990;88:67,73)
- Narcotics iv for pain management
- Update tetanus, if necessary
- Intra-arterial thrombolysis experimental
- Prophylactic antibiotics controversial
- Dextran and heparin controversial
- Hyperbaric O_2 controversial
- Pentoxifylline is experimental (Arch Otolaryngol Head Neck Surg 1995;121:678)

5.5 Heat-Related Illnesses

Trans R Soc Trop Med Hyg 1977;170:402; 1977;70:412; 1977;70:419; Lancet 1998;352:1329; Crit Care Clin 1999;15:251

Cause: Inability to handle endogenous heat production with exogenous heat augmentation. Anticipatory intervention (Pub Hlth Rev 1985;13:115; Jama 1996;276:593) and monitoring weather extremes key in prevention (Jama 1998;279:1514). Children at risk when left in cars (Peds 1976;58:101).

Epidem: Heat-related problems increase markedly if environmental T > 91°F. Potentially exacerbated by being very young or very old, using drugs of abuse, or being on anticholinergic or neuroleptic medications (see Neuroleptic Malignant Syndrome on p 282).

Perhaps risk of malignant hyperthermia if episode of heat stroke; or heterozygote status for cystic fibrosis, if significant episode of heat exhaustion (J R Army Med Corps 1995;141:40).

Pathophys: Although dehydration a component of pathophys, exact mechanisms for these problems not fully elucidated (Int J Sports Med 1998;19:S146), perhaps neuro (J Sports Sci 1997;15:277) or immune dysfunction (Crit Rev Immunol 1999;19:285).

- Usual cooling methods of conduction, convection, and evaporation are overwhelmed. Evaporation is major cooling mechanism, followed by convection, and finally conduction.
- Heat exhaustion is an overheating problem but sweating is still intact, and is considered a diagnosis of exclusion. May be accompanied by a myriad of minor heat-related problems, eg, heat cramps, heat syncope, prickly heat, etc.
- Heat stroke is the clinical triad of hyperpyrexia (T > 40°C), mental status changes, and anhidrosis (anhidrosis is not a hard and fast finding) (Nejm 2002;346:1978).

Sx: Dizzy, weak, tired, nausea, vomiting, headache.

Si: Hypotension (commonly asymptomatic in extreme athletes [Med Sci Sports Exerc 1995;27:1595]), core temp elevated (may be normal in heat exhaustion), diaphoresis, anhidrosis in heat stroke (+/−), and mental status changes is the *sine qua non* of heat stroke.

Crs: Difficult to discern heat exhaustion from early heat stroke.

Cmplc: Worse with the very young and very old; associated cardiovascular disease; dehydration; secondary drug use such as sympathomimetics, β-blockers, Ca-channel blockers, MAOIs or TCAs, etc; high body mass index; inappropriate clothing; and altered skin physiology.

ENVIRONMENTAL

Diff Dx: Neuroleptic malignant syndrome (NMS); infection or sepsis; CVA; DKA; thyroid storm; malignant hyperthermia; seizures; drug (ethanol or benzodiazepine) withdrawal; drug abuse, such as ethanol, cocaine, amphetamines, LSD, or phencyclidine (PCP).

Lab: Core Temp, CBC with diff, metabolic profile—specifically hyponatremia (Am J Emerg Med 1999;17:532), Mg, PT/PTT, ABG, TSH, ethanol level, salicylate level, UA, urine toxic screen, urine for myoglobin, pan culture, CXR, head CT with and without iv contrast (iv contrast to r/o abscess)—MRI better for intracranial abscess or other nontraumatic diagnoses, LP.

Emergency Management:
- Remove heavy clothing
- Cool thermal windows (neck, axilla, groin); consider sponge bath/cool mist that is water at 30°-40°C, *not cold*.
- Iv access, consider fluid bolus
- O_2
- Cooling methods:
  - Thermal windows with cool packs
  - Cool mist with fan blow by
  - NG tube with cool saline
  - Peritoneal lavage
  - Immersion cooling
  - Treat shivering with benzodiazepines or phenothiazines, if not contraindicated.
- Discontinue aggressive cooling measures when core temperature is < 40°C, goal is core temperature < 39.4°C.

5.6 Hypothermia

Aviat Space Environ Med 1983;54:425; Ann EM 1993;22:370; Jama 2000;283:878

Cause: Core temperature < 35°C (95°F) due to environmental, physiologic, or functional problem.

Epidem: Seen all year round, with about 780 deaths per year in U.S. Infants fare better than all others unless co-incident septicemia (Intensive Care Med 2000;26:88). Core temp < 26°C associated with 50% mortality (Ann EM 1982;11:417). Associated in those with dementia or psychiatric problems if it impairs judgment or protective instincts.

Pathophys: Mild hypothermia is 32°-35°C (90°-95°F). Shivering stops below 32°C. Metabolism slows after an initial and short-lived increase in an attempt to stay warm.

Sx: Shivering early, then just cold.

Si: Early tachycardia followed by bradycardia, bronchospasm, hypotension, mental status changes, decreased core temperature (use appropriate thermometer).

Crs: Trauma and submersion may be coincident problems that have worse prognosis and longer hospital stays independent of age (Eur J Emerg Med 1995;2:38). Co-incident shock has a multiplicative effect on hemodynamic and coagulation problems (Am Surg 2000;66:348).

Cmplc: The very young and very old (Clin Ger Med 1994;10:213) are at risk of more sequalae from this problem, perhaps secondary to elevated bacterial lipopolysaccharide concentrations from ischemic gut (Undersea Hyperb Med 2000;27:1). Data are equivocal for noncardiogenic pulmonary edema (Chest 1993;103:971).

Diff Dx: Hypothyroidism; hypopituitarism, hypothalamic, or other CNS insult; hypoglycemia; drug abuse such as ethanol, barbiturates, phenothiazines; sepsis; altered skin physiology such as burn victims; chronic disease including metabolic and functional movement problems.

Lab: Core temp, CBC with diff, glucoscan, metabolic profile, PT/PTT, amylase, ethanol level, UA, urine for myoglobin, urine toxic screen, consider pan culture for ID evaluation, CXR, head CT,

ENVIRONMENTAL

EKG—interval prolongation and Osborn waves (which are positive deflections just after the QRS following the R waves usually seen in the precordial leads) (Circ 1996;93:372; Acad Emerg Med 1999;6:1121) may be present as well as many other potential abnormalities. ABG of equivocal help, with tendency toward acidosis, but perhaps induced alkalosis (Arch IM 1988;148:1643), and even if corrected for temperature will give little prognostic information (Arctic Med Res 1995;54:76).

Emergency Management:

(Aviat Space Environ Med 1983;54:487; Arctic Med Res 1986;41:16; 1991;50:28; Ann EM 1987;16:1042)

- Rewarm, attain iv access
  - Remove wet clothing and place in dry clothes or sleeping bag as insulator.
  - Inhalation rewarming and peripheral rewarming of no benefit in the field (Ann EM 1991;20:896).
  - The field treatment of mild hypothermia (T > 33°C) with shivering, external heat and exercise are all about equivalent (J Appl Physiol 1987;63:2375).
  - Heating blanket, such as a forced air torso blanket (eg, Bair Hugger) more effective than simple insulating procedures (Aviat Space Environ Med 1994;65:803; Resuscitation 1999;41:105; Ann EM 2000;35:337).
  - Thermal window warm packs (neck, axilla, groin)
  - Warm inhaled gases (O_2)
  - Warmed iv fluids (eg, Level 1 warmer)
  - NG tube with warm saline lavage
  - Bladder lavage with Foley catheter
  - Two chest tubes on one side (left) with lavage
  - Peritoneal lavage/dialysis (Jama 1978;240:2289)
  - Thoracotomy with mediastinal lavage
  - Warm water immersion

- Extracorporeal warming via extracorporeal circuit (Intensive Care Med 1999;25:520), dialysis, or cardiopulmonary bypass
- Check pulses for 1 full min before considering CPR
- Cardiopulmonary bypass for the atraumatic cardiac-arrested patient, if immediately available (Lancet 1995;345:493).
- Beware of cardiac arrhythmias, Afib is a stable rhythm in hypothermia.
- Treat co-morbid problems as they are determined.
- May declare death if active rewarming and ½ hr with ALS; or active rewarming and 1 hr with BLS. This is a reasonable pre-hospital guideline.
- Vfib refractory to countershock when T < 30°C, limit total number to 3 until T > 30°C.

5.7 Lightning

Emerg Med Clin N Am 1992;10:211; Ann EM 1993;22:378; J Emerg Med 2000;18:181

Cause: Random strikes, but may be augmented by holding onto metal items and not wearing rubber-soled shoes.

Epidem: 150-300 fatalities per yr.

Pathophys: Higher energy delivery over a shorter period of time when compared to manmade electrical energy.

Sx/Si: Depending on the pathway, any organ system may be affected, with consequent acute injury symptoms for that system; extent of burns, and coincident superior and inferior wounds (one being entrance, and the other exit) should be noted. **N.B.** More than one system may be involved, and the hematologic system may be involved as well, and may manifest DIC.

Crs: Common to see neurologic and otologic problems after a lightning strike.
- Although paralysis may be a factor, a subset of patients have keraunoparalysis, which is a lower extremity flaccid paralysis

that may resolve over days to hours—acute injury to the spinal cord should still be entertained, though.

- Tympanic membrane rupture is very common as well ($> 50\%$)—always check for this if patient unconscious and history unclear. TM rupture also very common in closed space blast injuries.

Cmplc: Mainly from cardiac or neurologic sequalae, may have sudden death or permanent paralysis (Ann EM 1992;21:575). A single strike may involve multiple victims (J Trauma 1999;46:937).

Lab: EKG, CBC with diff, consider metabolic profile if fluid resuscitation or cardiac arrhythmia are problems, CPK, UA, urine for myoglobin, ABG if respiratory compromise or coma, PT/PTT if acute neuro or cardiac event suspected, neuroimaging of head or spinal column, as appropriate.

Emergency Management:
- Supportive measures including airway support. Warm, if hypothermic.
- Coma protocol, if presentation unclear (O_2, naoloxone, thiamine, glucoscan)
- Treat underlying arrhythmias.
- Suspect cardiac involvement if wounds on superior and inferior aspect of body (Crit Care Med 1990;18:293)
- Fluid resuscitation rarely needed secondary to tissue destruction, consider blunt trauma, extrinsic blood loss or spinal cord shock.
- 24-hr cardiac monitoring for all patients is not advocated (J Trauma 1986;26:166).

5.8   Near-Drowning

Ped Clin N Am 1993;40:321; Ann EM 1993;22:366

Cause: Immersion in water with some degree of suffocation.
Associated with ethanol use and high rates of speed in watercraft.

Epidem: Exact numbers unknown, hypothesized that > 4000 deaths per year. Fresh water > salt water—swimming pools. Less ethanol use associated with some decrease in incidence of drowning (Jama 1999;281:2198).

Pathophys: Hypoxia secondary to aspiration of water or from laryngospasm, leading to neurologic and other end-organ ischemia.

Sx: Coughing, shivering, confusion, not responsive.

Si: Hypothermia, cold skin, piloerection, tachypnea or apnea, rales, tachycardia or bradycardia, confusion, obtundation, coma.

Course: Poor neuro function in ER after warm water drowning is controversial as to whether extended resuscitation has a better prognosis in children—(Can Anaesth Soc J 1980;27:201; Am J Dis Child 1986;140:571) vs (Peds 1977;59:364; Am J Dis Child 1981;135:1006; Ped Emerg Care 1997;13:98)—vs adults (J Trauma 1982;22:544); case reports of extended submersion with "good" outcomes in children is in cold water (< 20°C) or core temp < 32°C (Jama 1980;244:1233).

Cmplc: Some patients have delayed respiratory insufficiency after appearing stable—aka Secondary drowning which usually manifests in 4-6 hr (Ann EM 1986;15:1084); Pulmonary edema in salt water drowning (Am Rev Respir Dis 1992;146:794), fresh water is hypothesized to absorb into the bloodstream since it is isotonic (Med J Aust 1966;2:1282).

Lab: CBC with diff; ABG; metabolic profile; PT/PTT; ethanol level; UA; UTS; EKG.
  • X-ray—C-spine single view lateral, CXR; CT—C-spine CT and Head CT if neuro insult.

Emergency Management:
  • Safe removal of patient from water, maintain open airway.
  • Rescue breathing or CPR if needed.

ENVIRONMENTAL

- Airway, O_2; perhaps warm butyl alcohol vapor 7.5% for aspirated sea water near-drownings (Am J Emerg Med 1993;11:20); Heimlich maneuver probably not helpful (J Emerg Med 1995;13:397).
- Treat underlying arrhythmias. Role of calcium channel blockers post resuscitation not well elucidated (Am J Emerg Med 1984;2:148).
- Remove wet clothing, warm patient, if necessary.
- Warm, if hypothermic; perhaps use of cardiopulmonary bypass (Arch Surg 1992;127:525).
- Fluid resuscitation, if necessary.
- Pressors, if fluid ineffective.
- Consider NG tube and Foley catheter.
- May discharge children to home if GCS $\geq$ 13 and SaO_2 > 95% after 4-6 hr of observation (Am J Emerg Med 2000;18:9).

Chapter 6

Gastroenterology

6.1 Diverticulitis

Gastroenterol Clin N Am 1988;17:357; Dis Colon Rectum 2000:289

Cause: Diverticulosis with secondary infection.

Epidem: Diverticulosis present in almost all patients age > 40 yr in U.S. if on a low-bulk diet. Increased risk in alcoholics (Brit J Surg 1999;86:1067).

Pathophys: Low-residue diet leads to increased intracolonic pressures causing outpocketings.

Sx: Left lower quadrant pain, usually, although may be anywhere.

Si: Localized abdominal tenderness (LLQ in 67% < 40 yr of age); fever; tachycardia (Am J Emerg Med 2000;18:140).

Crs: Variable, with obesity as risk for accurate diagnosis and surgical treatment, if needed.

Cmplc: Perforation; peritonitis; partial obstruction; abscess; fistulas; and/or bleeding from diverticulosis alone.

Diff Dx: Intestinal gas; gastroenteritis; abdominal wall muscle strain; colitis; hernia; right-sided angiodysplasia of the colon, often seen in elderly and associated with aortic stenosis.

Lab: CBC with diff showing leukocytosis in 91%, consider UA in atypical cases.
* *X-ray:* Plain films if looking for free air (Dis Colon Rectum 1970;13:444); CT delineates site/process.

Emergency Management:

- Iv with parenteral narcotics, if needed for pain control, this does not obscure the diagnosis (J Am Coll Surg 2003;196:18).

- Antibiotics for acute disease (TMP/SMX DS 1 pill bid + metronidazole 500 mg tid; ciprofloxacin 500 mg bid + metronidazole; or amoxicillin/clavulanate 875 mg bid) for 2 wk of oral therapy. May use intravenous equivalents for those needing admission, such as ciprofloxacin 400 mg, metronidazole 500 mg, or ampicillin/sulbactam 3 gm iv.

- Surgical staged colonic resection with temporary colostomy for recurrent disease, perforation, or abscess. Perhaps primary surgical therapy in those < 40 yr of age (Am J Surg 1997;174:733). Prevent with high fiber diet.

6.2   Esophageal Foreign Bodies

Gastroenterol Clin N Am 1991;1:691

Cause: Inadvertent ingestion of foreign body or large food bolus.

Epidem: 80% peds.

Pathophys: Pediatric esophagus with 5 natural narrowings, adults may have rings, webs, dysmotility, or mass lesions.

Sx: Foreign body sensation anywhere from oropharynx to epigastrium, inability to swallow saliva.

Si: Drooling is almost pathognomonic.

Crs: If no foreign body on exam or plain film, no hypersalivation, and no obstruction or foreign body on barium swallow, then expectant management OK (Jacep 1979;8:101), except as noted under "Cmplc."

Cmplc:

- Button batteries (Ann Otol Rhinol Laryngol 1984;93:364) and sharp objects may need removal even if they have passed through the esophagus—erosion and laceration are still potential complications. Button batteries are given 48 hr to pass through the pylorus (Jama 1983;249:2495). Sharp objects past the esophagus may be managed expectantly as long as they are small (relative to patient size) and not causing secondary problems (perforation). All sewing needle ingestions should be referred to a surgeon or gastroenterologist.

- Cocaine packet ingestion (these patients referred to as "mules") may warrant surgery, Golytely or expectant passage.
- Aspiration
- Tracheal compression in peds (Am J Roentgenol Radium Ther Nucl Med 1974;122:80)

Lab: CXR to r/o aspiration, and to identify location if radio-opaque. Consider lateral neck film or abdominal film if unable to locate object in chest. Barium swallow if still uncertain.

Emergency Management: For esophageal foreign bodies without an acute abdomen:

- INT (heplock)
- TNG 0.4 mg sl (Nejm 1973;289:23).
- If unsuccessful, glucagon 1 mg iv (Radiology 1986;159:567; Jacep 1979;8:228), or consider pulse doses every 30 min of 20-100 μg iv (GE 1975;69:160).
- Perhaps effervescent drink to push bolus forward or facilitate regurgitation (Radiology 1983;146:299; Ann EM 1988;17:693).
- If unsuccessful, gi consult for EGD; surgery consult if acute abdomen.
- Potential use of radiologists with balloon catheter extraction in selected patients with proximal foreign bodies (Am J Roentgenol 1979;132:441; Arch Otolaryngol 1983;109:323), but not first choice (Gastrointest Endosc 1993;39:626).

6.3 Esophageal Rupture

Chest Surg Clin N Am 1994;4:819

Cause: Full thickness esophageal tear, known as Boerhaave's syndrome (named after the Danish physician who first diagnosed this after the Danish grand admiral had vomited portions of a duck). May occur secondary to a weakened esophagus or after violent emesis, but the hx is nonspecific most of the time. Ingested sharp or corrosive foreign bodies, or direct penetrating trauma are also risk factors.

Epidem: Uncommon, many diagnoses made postmortem. If diagnosis made promptly, outcome as good as with esophageal perforation secondary to endoscopy (Chest 1987;92:995).

Pathophys: Cause as above, leakage of enteric contents causes the secondary mediastinitis. One hypothesis is lack of muscularis mucosa at site of rupture (Am J Surg 1989;158:420).

Sx: Hx of vomiting; chest pain, abdominal pain, fever, otherwise nonspecific.

Si: Rales; subcutaneous emphysema.

Crs: Worse with delayed diagnosis; classic triad of vomiting, chest pain, and subcutaneous emphysema is not common (Am Surg 1999;65:449).

Cmplc: Mediastinitis—mortality > 70% with delayed diagnosis.

Diff Dx: Stomach rupture (Jama 1982;247:811); tension pneumothorax; bronchial tear; pulmonary embolus.

Lab: Low SaO_2; pleural fluid for food particles if radiographic studies equivocal (Chest 1992;102:976).
- *X-ray:* CXR—pneumothorax, pleural effusion, pneumomediastinum, or subcutaneous emphysema (Am J Gastroenterol 1978;69:212); Gastrografin swallow (Brit J Surg 1985;72:204) or CT (Arch IM 1988;148:223) confirmatory.

Emergency Management:

- Treat/anticipate shock—iv access with fluid resuscitation.
- Immediate surgical consult.
- Anecdotally, conservative treatment has worked in some patients (Am J Surg 1981;141:531).

6.4   Esophageal Varices

Gastrointest Endosc Clin N Am 1999;9:175; Drug Ther Bull 2000;38:37; Nejm 2001;345:669)

Cause: End-stage hepatic failure has many etiologies, one of the four major complications is hemorrhage, and esophageal bleeding is the most life threatening. Other complications are ascites, renal failure, and encephalopathy.

Pathophys: Portal hypertension leading to varices; bleeding from depressed prothrombin and fibrinogen; depressed platelets from bleeding and hypersplenism; perhaps diminished platelet function from increased BUN; increased plasminogen activators due to diminished hepatic filtration.

Sx/Si: Hematemesis, melena.

Crs: Cause of death in 20% of patients with cirrhosis.

Complc: Coagulopathy; encephalopathy.

Diff Dx: See Upper GI Bleed p 127.

Lab: Hemoccult emesis and stool, CBC with diff, PT/PTT, type and cross for PRBCs.

Emergency Management:

(Gastrointest Endosc Clin N Am 1999;9:287)

- Iv, with fluid resuscitation if necessary to keep sys BP > 100 mm Hg
- FFP, if coagulopathy
- Somatostatin 250 μg iv bolus, then 250 μg/hr continuous drip (GE 1990;99:1388); or, octreotide 25 μg/h iv drip (Can J

Gastroenterol 1997;11:339) or 50 μg iv over 20 min then 50 μg/h drip.

- Consider TNG via transdermal (Hepatology 1990;11:678) or sublingual (Hepatology 1986;6:406) routes.
- Vasopressin no longer advocated, somatostatin or its analog (such as terlipressin) with less transfusion requirements (Hepatology 1993;18:61). Terlipressin and nitroglycerin better than balloon tamponade (Hepatology 1990;11:678).
- Sengstaaken-Blakemore tube (Surg Gynecol Obstet 1976;142:529) with accessory NG tube until endoscopy available if pt hemorrhaging—applying external traction not necessary (GE 1978;75:566); not a substitute nor should it delay endoscopy (Surg Gynecol Obstet 1988;167:331).
- Endoscopic ligation as good as surgery (50% survival), better than medical treatment using Nadolol and isosorbide mononitrate after a bleed—(Hepatology 1997;25:1101) vs (Nejm 2001;345:647) yet best to use both for bleeding control (Nejm 2001;344:23); do not use ligation prophylactically if patient has never bled, and is better than sclerosis (Surg Gynecol Obstet 1985;161:438; Endoscopy 1997:241). Sclerotherapy better than medical therapy (Hepatology 1989;9:274), and better hemorrhage control when combined with octreotide (Nejm 1995;333:555).
- Perhaps eventual portocaval or splenorenal (Ann Surg 1982;195:393) surgical shunting.

6.5   Gallbladder Disease

Emerg Med Clin N Am 1996;14:719

Cause: Cholelithiasis may cause lodging of stones in the cystic duct, the common duct, or they may pass to the duodenum. Colic (misnomer) is an obstructed gallbladder, usually due to stones but may be due to a mass lesion. Cholecystitis is inflammation/

infection of the gallbladder; acalculous cholecystitis is inflammation without stones. Cholangitis is infection of the biliary system, and may be due to a gallstone lodged in the common duct.

Epidem: Cholecystitis is F/M 2:1, with stones present in 10% of adult women in U.S., 70% of Southwestern Native American women. Higher incidence of stone with the following:

- Increasing age
- Multiple pregnancies
- During pregnancy, but later reverting to normal
- +/− Chronic thiazide treatment
- Hemolytic disease
- Birth control and other estrogen use
- Ethanol abuse
- Cirrhosis
- Vagotomy
- TPN—100% have sludge at 6 wk
- Prolonged starvation/fasting
- Obesity, especially during weight loss
- Ileal disease
- Elevated triglycerides

Pathophys: Stones are usually mucin protein + cholesterol, less often with bilirubin and calcium.

Sx: Steady epigastric or right upper quadrant pain (colic is a misnomer in this case), radiates to right scapula, nausea, vomiting—temporary relief after vomiting.

Si: Fever, pressure at the right subcostal area inhibits patient from taking deep breath when prompted secondary to pain [Murphy's sign—97% sensitivity (Ann EM 1996;28:267)].

Crs: Those with stones will have a 10-20% chance of having symptoms over 20-30 yr; after first symptoms, 50% will recur over 20 yr, with 25-50% getting complications—these are the low numbers, it may be higher.

Cmplc: Pancreatitis; cholangitis; hydrops, emphysema, or empyema of gallbladder; perforation and peritonitis; gallstone ileus is rare—a small bowel obstruction from a gallstone that has lodged at the ileocecal valve after eroding through the gallbladder into the duodenum; perhaps gallbladder cancer—cause and effect in these cases is uncertain.

Diff Dx: Chronic acalculous cholecystitis [seen mainly in white females (Jsls 1999;3:221)]; hepatitis; PUD; pyelonephritis; Saint's triad—hiatal hernia, colonic diverticulosis, and cholelithiasis.

Lab: CBC with diff, LFTs, amylase, lipase—the elderly may have moderate to severe disease with little supportive serum laboratory data, age ≥ 65 yr (Acad Emerg Med 1997;4:51); Perhaps CRP (Eur J Surg 1992;158:365); gallbladder US (Gastrointest Radiol 1986;11:334); consider HIDA scan (Radiology 1982;144:369), if US equivocal—No dye in gallbladder is consistent with cholecystitis, no dye into duodenum is consistent with common duct stone. Abdominal x-ray usually not helpful, even for emphysematous cholecystitis (Brit J Radiol 1997;70:986)—US better. If UA obtained, may show WBCs, but should lack bacteria.

Emergency Management:

- Iv access for nausea, vomiting, and pain control—some consider MSO_4 to cause spasm at the sphincter of Oddi, but is not supported by good evidence. Perhaps NSAIDs of use, such as diclofenac 75 mg im (Dig Dis Sci 1989;34:809). Doubt the efficacy of glycopyrrolate for pain control (Ann EM 2005;45:172).
- Parenteral antibiotics such as ampicillin/sulbactam, cefotetan, cefoperazone, or ceftriaxone (Chemotherapy 1988;34:30) for acute cholecystitis with fever and/or elevated white count, and surgical consult.
- Parenteral antibiotics as above for cholangitis, and gi consult to consider ERCP. Would also get gi consult if concerned about common duct stone for any other reason.

- If simple biliary colic, and/or mild cholecystitis (fever < 101°F and no abnormal white count), consider outpatient follow-up with explicit instructions for surgical follow-up (1 wk), and si/sx to monitor which would necessitate immediate ER follow-up.

6.6   Hepatitis, Acute Viral

Am J Clin Pathol 2000;113:12; hep A (Vaccine 1992;10:S15); hep B (Nejm 2004;350:1118; Vaccine 1998;16:S11; Microbiol Mol Biol Rev 2000;64:51); hep C (Cmaj 2000;102:827; J Clin Gastroenterol 2000;30:125)

Cause: Hepatitis in general is inflammation of the liver from infectious, autoimmune, toxin, or metabolic disorder. Common causes are mononucleosis, hepatitis A, hepatitis B, hepatitis C, ethanol, and autoimmune hepatitis (Biomed Pharmacother 1999;53:255).

Epidem:
Hepatitis A is usually a fecal-oral passage. Higher in parents of day care children and common in developing countries.

Hepatitis B and *hepatitis C* is parenteral or via sexual contact.

Hepatitis C is the leading cause of chronic liver disease (J Hepatol 2000;32:98).

Other hepatitides are of a more chronic basis and most will be outpt work-up.

Pathophys:
Hepatitis A is an RNA enterovirus, with peak incidence in late summer and early winter.

Hepatitis B is a DNA virus that may incorporate into liver genome, associated with liver carcinoma—perhaps due to secondary carcinogenic exposures (Cancer Surv 1986;5: 765). Hepatitis D (delta particle) (Antivir Ther 1998;3:37) can only infect in conjunction with hepatitis B.

Hepatitis C is an RNA virus that appears to merit no protective antibody response

Sx:

Hepatitis A with 15-40 d incubation period. Only 5-15% of children get symptoms, with malaise, anorexia, abdominal pain, nausea, vomiting, diarrhea, light colored stools, and dark-colored urine being found in symptomatic children and adults.

Hepatitis B has a 60-160 d incubation period, with arthralgias, arthritis, urticaria, and other rashes being common.

Hepatitis C has a 2 to 20-wk incubation period (6-7 wk being average).

Chronic hepatitis associated with autoantibodies (Prog Liver Dis 1994;12:137).

Si:

Hepatitis A with jaundice, although anicteric form also common and more benign.

Hepatitis B with many cases anicteric.

Hepatitis C with 80% anicteric.

Crs:

Hepatitis A is usually benign, with 15% morbidity and 0.3% mortality, symptoms peak 2 wk after onset and take about 4 wk to clear; 6% of patients will relapse in 1-3 mon.

Hepatitis B has many possibilities with acute hepatitis, typical or cholangitic, leading to the following:

- Benign course, recover or relapsing, or chronic persistent (portal) or mild hepatitis; or
- Acute liver necrosis, where all pts die; or
- Submassive hepatic necrosis (bridging) pts 60% die or go on to postnecrotic cirrhosis, the balance of patients recover completely; or

- Chronic active hepatitis, usually with a progressive down-hill course over 5-10 yr; or
- Asymptomatic carrier state in about 90% newborns, 20% school age children, < 1% young healthy adults (WWII vaccine epidemic)

Hepatitis C also has a variable course. 60-70% of patients still have elevated LFTs 12 mon later, but overall mortality over decades is not increased. Acute hepatitis, typical or cholangitic, leads to the following:

- Chronic active hepatitis in most; or
- Benign course, recover or have relapsing, or chronic persistent (mild or "portal") hepatitis; or
- Acute liver necrosis, where all pts die; or
- Submassive hepatic necrosis (bridging) pts 60% die or go on to postnecrotic cirrhosis; the balance of patients recovering completely.

Cmplc:

Hepatitis A with fulminant hepatitis or relapsing hepatitis.

Hepatitis B with hepatoma; 10% go on to chronic active hepatitis (Ann IM 2000;132:723); facilitates secondary infection with delta agent (hepatitis D) which is an RNA virus and this leads also to acute hepatitis or a severe chronic active hepatitis; fasting hypoglycemia; serum sickness; polyarteritis (J Clin Invest 1975;55:930); and nephritis, especially membranous GN.

Hepatitis C with 80% going onto chronic active hepatitis over 10 yr, and 20-35% of these people go onto cirrhosis over 20 yr; hepatocellular carcinoma over 30 yr independent of hep B; and may develop mixed cryoglobulinemia.

Diff Dx:

With fever: Mononucleosis, Q fever (GE 1982;83:474), toxoplasmosis, CMV, Fitzhugh-Curtis syndrome, psittacosis, hepatitis E, and other viral hepatitides

Without fever: Drugs (Nejm 2003;349:474; Baillieres Clin
Gastroenterol 1988;2:385)—ethanol, acetaminophen,
NSAIDs, other toxins; chronic autoimmune hepatitis;
hemochromatosis; Wilson's disease; α-antitrypsin deficiency;
α-methyldopa (Aldomet)-induced hepatitis; oxyphenisatin
laxative induction; primary biliary cirrhosis; diabetes;
myxedema; hepatitis G and other viral hepatitides;
myopathy.

Lab: CBC with diff, LFTs, amylase, lipase, monospot; PT/PTT, if suspect fulminant hepatitis (Vaccine 1992;10:S21); Get CPK, especially if LDH > AST (SGOT) > ALT (SGPT) to r/o
myopathy—may also check aldolase.

Serologic Markers (see Table 6.1):
- Hepatitis A shows IgM first, this later goes negative as IgG
  appears and stays positive (J Virol Methods 1980;2:31).
- Hepatitis B with HBsAg first, and then anti-HBs—If both negative but high suspicion, then retest. A small window exists
  when both may be negative. Those vaccinated usually mount
  an anti-HBs response.
- Hepatitis C antibody elevated 4-50 weeks after LFTs abnormal,
  may check sera for hep C viral RNA via PCR.
- Hepatitis E serology accurate (Clin Infect Dis 1995;21:621).

X-ray: Get US of abdomen for imaging study, if concerned about
anatomic or obstructive problem with liver, especially suspect if
patient elderly. Abdominal CT may further delineate anatomy.

Emergency Management:
- *Hepatitis A* exposures should prophylax with 0.02 cc/kg of IgG,
  max dose 2 cc IM. A vaccine does exist [Havrix, or Vaqta; or
  Twinrix which is a combination with Hep B Vaccine (Nejm
  2004;350:476; Med Lett Drugs Ther 2001;43:1110)] for travel
  or high risk prophylaxis—booster needs unknown. Vaccine does
  prevent secondary cases (Lancet 1999;353:1136).

Table 6.1 Viral Hepatitis

Type	Clinical Features	Transaminases	Serologic Findings: Acute Disease	Serologic Findings: Immunity
A (RNA)	Acute self-limiting; fecal-oral transmission; no carrier state	Markedly elevated 3+ to 4+	IgM anti-HAV	IgG anti-HAV
B (DNA)	Acute or chronic; often asymptomatic 5% infected blood and body fluids	1+ to 3+ (acute); variable; chronic	IgM anti-HBc; HBsAg; HBeAg; HBV DNA	IgG anti-HBs; anti-HBe
C (RNA)	Usually chronic	Mild to moderate elevation even in acute cases	Total anti-HCV; HCV RNA	Unknown
D (RNA)	Requires HBV coinfection; acute or chronic; rate in United States	Often markedly elevated	IgM anti-HDV; total anti-HDV; may require multiple assays	Unknown
E (RNA)	Epidemic similar to HAV; acute self-limiting; water borne and enteric; transmission in India and Southeast Asia	Variable	Testing not widely available; reference laboratory; CDC	Unknown
G (RNA)	Close homology to HCV; high prevalence (2% of US donors); usually mild disease; if at all; disease spectrum uncertain	Variable	HGV-RNA and EIA (reference laboratory only)	Unknown
Non-A-E, Exclude EBV and CMV	Possibly acute or chronic	Variable	None	Unknown

Adapted from Sacher RA, Peters SM, Bryan JA. Testing for viral hepatitis. A practice parameter. Am J Clin Pathol 2000;113:12-17. Reprinted with permission.

- *Hepatitis B* exposures should receive hep B immune globulin (HBIG) if not vaccinated—dose is 0.05 cc/kg times two doses 30 d apart within 24-72 hr of exposure. The vaccination series is recommended for everyone not already vaccinated and is 3 injections on d 0, d 30, and d 180. If acute exposure, the vaccine should be given as well. Active disease should be referred to GI for consideration of peginterferon α-2a or -2b, or possibly lamivudine (3TC) (Nejm 1998;339:61), but no steroids.
- *Hepatitis C* as with Hep B except immune globulin is ineffective, and perhaps use of other nucleoside analogues (Nejm 1998;339:1493; Lancet 1998;352:1426) such as peginterferon α-2a (Nejm 2000;343:1666) or peginterferon α-2b (Nejm 2001;345:1452); also, consider adding ribavirin in those with coincident HIV infection (Nejm 2004;351:438; 2004;351:451; Jama 2004;292:2839). Perhaps vaccine (Proc Natl Acad Sci USA 2000;97:297).
- OK to give hep A and hep B vaccines together (Vaccine 2000:1074).

N.B. Universal precautions advocated for everyone, wear gloves, wash hands, and get screened, if you have a body fluid exposure. If patient has active disease, high risk behaviors discouraged—iv drugs, sexual promiscuity, blood donation.

6.7 Infectious Diarrhea

Nejm 2004;350:38; 2004;351:2417; Medicine (Baltimore) 1979:95; Arch Dis Child 1984:848

Cause: Inadequately prepared or maintained food, fecal-oral contamination or water supply [*Campylobacter* (Lancet 1983;1:287)]; resistant *Salmonella,* due to antibiotics in animal stock (Nejm 2001;345:1147). Possibly air-borne, as well (Am J Epidemiol 1988;127:1261).

Epidem: Most common in United States is *Staphylococcus* spp.,
Salmonella spp., *Clostridium perfringens* (Mmwr 1994;43:137,143),
Shigella, Campylobacter jejuni (common), *C. upsaliensis* (rare) (Ped
Infect Dis J 1999;18:988), *E. coli*—both invasive (Mmwr
1991;40:265) and toxigenic, and *Listeria monocytogenes*
[uncommon (Nejm 2000;342:1236)]. Potential current omeprazole use as risk factor for *Camylobacter* infection (Br Med J
1996;312:414). *Cryptosporidiosis* may occur most commonly
during the summer and yersiniosis most commonly during the
winter months, although both are relatively uncommon (Ann
EM 2000;35:92).

 Many outbreaks are episodic, or possibly referable to water
supply, daycare setting, hospital ward (J Infect Dis 1982;146:727),
or other common variable. United Kingdom evaluating small
round structed viruses as predominant factors in outbreaks (J Med
Virol 2000;61:132).

Pathophys: In U.S., acute diarrhea is usually due to a viral agent (gastroenteritis or enteritis) with some specific exceptions, as noted
below. The most common viruses are Rotavirus, Norwalk virus,
enteric adenovirus, Calcivirus, and Astrovirus.

- *Staphylococcus* spp. forms a heat stable toxin, does not stick to
  bowel wall.
- *Salmonella* spp. invades bowel wall.
- *Clostridium perfringens* produces a toxin.
- *Shigella* spp. demonstrates wall invasion (Infect Dis Clin N Am
  2000;14:41).
- *Campylobacter* spp. invades bowel wall and produces a heat-
  labile toxin.
- Invasive *E. coli* (O157:H7, eg) invades colon wall and pro-
  duces toxin (Infect Dis Clin N Am 2000;14:41).
- Toxigenic *E. coli* may produce both heat-labile and -stable
  toxins.

- *Clostridium difficile*—seen after antibiotic use, specific risks of advanced age and/or clindamycin use. Asymptomatic carrier state in peds < 1 yr of age, even after antibiotic use (Ped Infect Dis 1984;3:433) and increased likelihood with bottle-fed infants (J Clin Microbiol 1983;17:830).
- *Giardia lamblia (intestinalis)*—seen after exposure to untreated fresh water supply, such as mountain lakes or streams.
- *Yersinia* spp. colitis—household pets, as well as food or water borne exposures, as proposed transmission.

Sx: Abdominal discomfort, vomiting, diarrhea. Bloating, gaseous, and profuse and foul-smelling diarrhea in *Giardia*.

Si: Fever in those with rotavirus, *Salmonella*, *Shigella* spp., *C. diff* and *Yersinia* spp.; less likely or low grade fever in *Campylobacter* spp. and invasive *E. coli*; no fever in *Staphylococcus* spp., *Clostridium* spp. or toxigenic *E. coli*.

Crs: Viral causes usually self-limited. Some with persistent problems consistent with irritable bowel syndrome (Br Med J 1997;314:779).

Cmplc:
- Dehydration; for gastroenteritis, oral rehydration is effective in both children (Arch Ped Adolesc Med 2004;158:483) and adults—should be considered first line treatement.
- *Shigella* spp. (Clin Diagn Lab Immunol 1996;3:701) and invasive *E. coli* (Peds 1992:616) may be complicated by the Hemolytic-Uremic syndrome (HUS);
- *Shigella* spp. may also be complicated by Reiter syndrome, reactive arthritis, myocarditis (J Peds 1993;122:82), or erythema nodosum (Scott Med J 1984:197).
- *Salmonella* with some multiresistant clones (J Lab Clin Med 2002;140:135), and this may become more prevalent with continued use of antibiotics in the food supply.

Diff Dx: *Cryptosporidiosis* spp., *Listeria monocytogenes*, Vibrio, Scombroid (Nejm 1991;324:716; Jama 2000;283:2927) and ciguatera (J Toxicol Clin Toxicol 1993;31:1; Med J Aust 2000;172:176) poisoning if fish eaten; perhaps sorbitol or olestra (large doses) consumption (Regul Toxicol Pharmacol 2000;31:59).

Risk factors predispose to other etiologies as listed below:
- Male homosexual: Herpes II, gonorrhea, and Chlamydia colitis.
- Immunocompromised individuals: *Cryptosporidium* spp., *Cyclospora cayetanensis*, *Enterocytozoon bienensis*, *Isospora belli*, *Plesiomonas* spp., and *Aeromonas* spp.
- World travel: *Entamoeba histolytica*, *Bacillus cereus*, *Vibrio cholera*, *Vibrio parahaemolyticus*.
- Handlers of seawater: *Vibrio mimicus*.
- Radiation enteritis.
- Chemotherapeutic-induced, specifically fluoropyrimidines and irinotecan (J Pain Symptom Manage 2000;19:118)

Lab: Consider stool culture if bloody diarrhea or if symptoms > 72 hr; stool for leukocytes is not sensitive and nonspecific (Diagn Microbiol Infect Dis 1993;16:313); other laboratory tests rarely alter treatment or disease course (Ann EM 1989;18:258; Dig Dis Sci 1996;41:1749; Acta Paediatr 1999;88:592).

C. *difficile*—stool toxin; perhaps useful in patient with antibiotics within last month, significant diarrhea, abdominal discomfort or recent hospitalization (and > 1 yr of age) (Diagn Microbiol Infect Dis 2000;36:169).

Campylobacter spp. perhaps PCR (Epidemiol Infect 1998; 121:547).

Giardia spp. stool antigen, 3 O&P samples if antigen test not available.

Yersinia spp. stool culture, antibody titers with 30% false negative.

Rotavirus—latex agglutination (fast) and stool ELISA test available—sensitivity > 90% and specificity approximately 99%, if used in first week of the illness (J Clin Microbiol 1985;22: 846; 1982;16:562).

Emergency Management:

- Iv hydration, if oral rehydration solution (ORS) not possible po. Oral rehydration with WHO ORS (8:1 sugar to salt solution such as 2 tsp sugar, $\frac{1}{4}$ tsp salt, and a squeeze of citrus per 8 oz of boiled water) or with one of the many ORS available that contain sodium, potassium, chloride, base, and glucose with osmolality 311 mMol/L or less (Nutr Rev 2000;58:80). OK to iv hydrate children at 20-30 cc/kg over 1-2 hr and then send home if able to take po (Ann EM 1996;28:318).
- Antiemetics, decreased use of iv fluid (and makes ORT possible) (Ann EM 2002;39:397); caution with all antiemetics in children < 3 yr of age.
- Anti-diarrheals—does not worsen clinical picture and prevents ongoing fluid losses, such as bismuth subsalicylate [Bismuth subsalicylate (Pepto-Bismol) 60 cc in adults or 1.14 cc/kg (100 mg/kg) in children qid] or loperamide (Jama 1986;255:757).
- Zinc gluconate 20 mg po qd within first 3 d in peds in developing countries.
- TMP/SMX DS bid is better than ampicillin 500 mg po qid for 5 d for *Shigella* in areas of ampicillin-resistance (Antimicrob Agents Chemother 1980;17:961).
- Cipro 500 mg po bid for 3-5 d covers all pathogens (Eur J Clin Microbiol 1986;5:241), including traveler's diarrhea, where *E. coli* is prevalent (Ann IM 1991;114:731), both *Staphylococcus* spp. and *Clostridium perfringens* are self-limited in this setting. This does limit duration and severity of illness (Clin Infect Dis 1996;22:1019).

- Consider rifaximin (Xifaxan) 200 mg tid for 3 d, which is a non-absorbed form of rifampin—OK in those > 12 yr of age and non-pregnant women with noninvasive *E. coli* (Traveler's diarrhea); fewer systemic effects than absorbed antibiotics (Med Lett Drugs Ther 2004;46:73).
- *C. difficile:* Metronidazole orally, oral Vancomycin if no response or if severe illness; perhaps the probiotic *Lactobacillus* GG (Am J Gastroenterol 2000;95:S11).
- *Giardia:* Metronidazole (Flagyl) 250 mg tid for 5 d; nitazoxanie (Alinia) 500 mg bid for 3 d and liquid is available for children (Med Lett Drugs Ther 2003;45:29); tinidazole (Tindamax) 2 gm single dose therapy (Med Lett Drugs Ther 2004;46:70).
- *Yersinia* spp: consider tetracycline.
- Children with mild to moderate diarrhea may fare better with homeopathy (J Altern Complement Med 2000;6:131), although this group of patients would do OK with WHO ORS and all the children received individual (different) homeo-pathic medication.

Oral Rotavirus tetravalent vaccine at 2, 3, and 4 mon of age available (Mmwr 1999:1).

6.8   Lower GI Bleed

Am J Roentgenol 1993;161:703

Cause: Consider upper gi bleed, but lower gi bleed causes included hemorrhoids, diverticulosis, ischemic colitis, AV malformations, polyps, cancer, stercoral ulcer (hard stool with constipation) and Meckel's diverticulum. Rarely TB (Am J Gastroenterol 1999;94:270).

Epidem: Less common than upper gi bleeds; more common in older age and if male (Am J Gastroenterol 1997;92:419).

GASTROENTEROLOGY

Pathophys: Erosion through mucosa may herald bleeding in ischemic colitis and AV malformations, and the arterial bleeding of diverticulosis is secondary to the diverticula outpouching occurring at the site of weakness from the perforating mucosal vessels. Meckel's diverticulum may have gastric tissue and consequent ulcer formation.

Sx: Painless hematochezia usually, may have pain with external hemorrhoids.

Si: Bright red blood on rectal exam, obvious hemorrhoids.

Crs: Worse prognosis if ongoing bleeding, systolic BP < 100 mm Hg, elevated PT (INR > 1.2), change in mental status, or other unstable disease process (Crit Care Med 1997;25:1125).

Cmplc: If significant anemia, secondary cardiac (Chest 1998;114:1137) or neurologic compromise.

Diff Dx: Carcinoma, Inflammatory bowel disease, polyps, and infectious (including TB) enteritis may cause lower gi bleeding, but not usually hemorrhage unless some sort of trauma—inadvertent shearing of a polyp, for example—or coagulopathy, such as seen with liver dysfunction or ASA use.

Lab: Guaiac stool, CBC with diff, PT/PTT, type and cross, metabolic profile to look for BUN/Cr ratio (see p 127), EKG to r/o silent ischemia if this is an issue.

Consider anoscopy at bedside as diagnostic test.

- *X-ray:* barium enema not superior to colonoscopy.

Emergency Management:

- O_2
- 2 large bore ivs, at least one with NS to be compatible with blood
- Blood, if no response to fluid resuscitation. **N.B.** Tachycardia with no fever or pain in an elderly patient necessitates resuscitation even with no hypotension or orthostasis.

- Nuclear tagged red cell scan (Radiology 1981;139:465; Ann Surg 1996;224:29) if pt is stable, consider Meckel scan if previous evaluation has been complete and without source. Only those patients with immediate blush on technitium scan most likely to have useful angiography (Dis Colon Rectum 1997;40:471).
- Surgical and gi consult for the unstable patient, perhaps urgent angiography (Ann Surg 1989;209:175; Am J Roentgenol 1992;159:521) or colonoscopy (Gastrointest Endosc 1995;41:93).

6.9 Pancreatitis

Gastroenterol Clin N Am 1999;28:571

Cause:
- Gallstones in 45-75%, biliary sludge is an ultrasound diagnosis that is underappreciated (Nejm 1992;326:589).
- Ethanol use is responsible for 10-35% of cases via 10-35% sphincter of Oddi spasm and increased pancreatic secretion via secretin.
- Hereditary types I and V, hyperlipidemia.
- Idiopathic in 10-30%, perhaps association with cystic fibrosis gene (Nejm 1998;339:653).
- Posterior duodenal ulcer.
- Accidental trauma or inadvertent during surgery.
- Hyperparathyroidism with calcium stone formation.
- Infectious such as mumps, coxsackie, many viruses including HIV, ascariasis (Brit J Surg 1992;79:1335), clonorchiasis.
- Cancer of duodenum, pancreas, or ampulla; diabetes seen with pancreatic cancer most likely of recent onset, diabetes not a risk factor for pancreatic cancer (Nejm 1994;331:81).
- Anatomic variants such as choledochal cysts, duodenal diverticula, or pancreatic divisum.
- Pregnancy

- Protein starvation.
- Vasculitis, specifically with anticardiolipin antibodies (Am J Emerg Med 1993;11:230).
- Drugs such as thiazides, steroids, sulfasalazine (Azulfidine) and other sulfas, furosemide, azathioprine.
- Post pump after bypass surgery, probably from iv $CaCl_2$ given.

Epidem: M/F: 2:1; incidence approximately 400/million/yr, but in AIDS, 5-20 per 100 per year.

Pathophys: Autodigestion perhaps due to trypsin and lipase, hypocalcemia from calcium soap formation, or perhaps glucagon-induced.

Sx: Epigastric abdominal pain relieved by leaning forward, radiates to back/flank; abdominal distention, nausea, and vomiting.

Si: Ileus; guarding; fever, or hypothermia at times; erythema nodosum-like lesions due to focal fat necrosis; Grey-Turner sign is flank ecchymoses with retroperitoneal bleeding and Cullen's sign is periumbilical ecchymoses from extension of pancreatic enzymes along falciform or round ligament (Gastrointest Radiol 1989;14:31).

Crs: 50-80% never recur. Worse prognosis with age > 55 years, male gender and idiopathic or alcoholic pancreatitis (Hepatogastroenterology 1998;45:1859).

Ranson (Am J Gastroenterol 1974;61:443) and modified Ranson criteria (see Table 6.2): mortality < 1% if ≤ 2 risk factors, 16% if 3-4 risk factors, and 100% if ≥ 7 risk factors; APACHE III and modified Glasgow Coma score also predictive (Crit Care Med 1999:901).

Cmplc: ARDS; ATN; tetany with hypocalcemia; shock; pancreatic abscess (4%); pancreatic pseudocyst formation (Am J Surg 1996;172:228), which can result in infection or rupture into peritoneal cavity, spleen or dissection along body planes; gi bleeding and splenomegaly from splenic vein thrombosis rare.

Table 6.2   Early Objective Prognostic Signs Used to Estimate the Risk of Death or Major Complications from Acute Pancreatitis—Ranson Criteria

At admission or diagnosis
    Age > 55 yr
    Serum WBC count > 16K/mm3
    Serum glucose > 200 mg/dL
    Serum LDH > 350 IU
    SGOT > 250 sigma Frankel Units %
During initial 48 hr
    Hct fall > 10 percentage points
    BUN rise > 5 mg/dL
    Serum Calcium < 8 mg/dL
    Arterial pO2 < 60 mm Hg
    Base deficit > 4 mEq/L
    Estimated fluid sequestration > 6 L

Adapted from the AJG American Journal of Gastroenterology, v100.i1, Etiological & Prognostic Factors in Human Acute Pancreatitis; 1982:63 tb.5 Reprinted with permission from Blackwell Publishing.

Diff Dx: Amylase elevation from 5 sources: pancreas, parotid/salivary glands, small bowel, fallopian tubes, and macroamylasemia—the molecule is too big to filter through kidney.

Lab: CBC with diff; metabolic profile, including calcium, magnesium, phosphorous; amylase and lipase (J Emerg Med 1999;17:1027); urine for trypsinogen-2 dipstick positive is 92% sensitive/specific (Nejm 1997;336:1788); perhaps phospholipase A_2, pancreatitis-associated protein (Ann Med 1998;30:169), or interleukin-6 (Clin Chem 1999;45:1762) and interleukin-8 (Am J Gastroenterol 2002;97:1309).

- Amylase serum levels up for 3 d, > 225 IU is 95% sensitive and 98% specific; Lipase peaks at 4-7 d, and correlates with hypertriglyceridemia that follows acute attacks and is more sensitive (95% vs 79%) in direct comparison study (Am J Emerg Med 1994;12:21).

GASTROENTEROLOGY

- Glucose may be elevated form transient glucagon release.
- ALT $\geq$ 3 times normal indicates gallstone etiology with 95% certainty.
- Isoamylase equally as good as lipase as a confirmation test.
- X-ray: Gallbladder US to evaluate common duct, cystic duct, and to look for stones. Intravenous cholangiography may be better (Jama 1979;242:342). CT is best for delineating intra-abdominal processes in those with complicated courses (J Gastroenterol Hepatol 1990;5:103).

Emergency Management:
- Iv fluid, patient will most likely be volume contracted secondary to plasma loss from third spacing.
- Antiemetics and parenteral narcotics for pain management.
- NG tube if significant ileus or obstruction.
- Iv H_2 blocker, controversial as far as helping pancreatitis resolve, but helpful for gastritis associated with pancreatitis.
- Consider iv antibiotics, such as ampicillin sulbactam or imipenem, if patient appears septic (this is debatable).
- Gi consult—consideration of ERCP (this is where the US helps).

6.10 Peptic Ulcer Disease (PUD)/Gastritis

Dig Dis Sci 1988;33:129; Am Surg 1990;56:737; Gut 1993;34:580

Cause: Due to *Helicobacter pylori* infection; or endogenous or NSAID-induced (GE 1989;96:640) increased acid/pepsin secretion, compounded problem with use of corticosteroids (Nejm 1983;309:21; BMJ (Clin Res Ed) 1987;295:1227; Ann IM 1991;114:735); and/or decreased pancreatic or duodenal HCO_3 secretion; or a decrease in other gi defenses.

Epidem:
- *Duodenal ulcer:* 90% associated with chronic *H. pylori* infection that often begins early in life, but 28% with NSAIDs if > age

60, occurs in 10% of people, M/F = 4:1 < 60 yr; positive family history in 50% < 30 yr, 20% in those > 30 yr at age of onset.

- *Gastric ulcers* have an 80% association with chronic *H. pylori* infection (Nejm 1989;321:1562) found in 3% of people, F > M.
- *Meckel's diverticulum* in <1% of people, usually ulcerates in childhood.

N.B. Only 15-20% of those chronically infected get duodenal or gastric ulcers.

Pathophys:

Increased acid production in the following:

- Zollinger-Ellison syndrome
- Neurogenically increased secretion, eg, burn or CVA patients
- Nicotine users
- Coffee users, but it's not the caffeine
- TPN patients from the iv amino acids
- Hypersecretors, who can be divided into hypersecretors and hypergastrin responders
- ASA, NSAID, and ethanol users

Diminished pancreatic secretions in the following:

- 10% of those with cystic fibrosis, maybe first symptom in heterozygote
- Perhaps with nicotine
- Perhaps with steroids

Impaired gi defenses include the following:

- *H. pylori* infection which tolerates high acid environment
- ASA and NSAIDs in elderly, especially if concomitant steroid use.
- Ethanol use increases permeability of mucosa to H^+ and produces direct mucosal damage.
- Smoking inhibits duodenal HCO_3 secretion.

Sx: Epigastric pain especially 1-2 hr pc and 2 am; gi bleeding, occult, melena, or hematemesis

Si: Epigastric tenderness; stool guaiac-positive.

Crs:

- *Duodenal ulcer* recurs in 10% except in smokers where 72% recur in 1 yr; r/o Zollinger-Ellison syndrome if does recur and not a smoker; eradication of H. *pylori* reduces rate of rebleeding (Gastrointest Endosc 1995;41:1).
- *Gastric ulcer* recurs in 50%; takes approximately 8 wk to heal with treatment.
- H. *pylori* may be chronic, recurrent, and resistant to multiple treatment attempts, but 96% do not recur after cleared with antibiotic course.

Cmplc: Persistent bleeding, perforation, obstruction, pain; possibly adenocarcinoma and non-Hodgkin's gastric lymphoma in patients with H. *pylori.*

Diff Dx: Gastroesophageal reflux esophagitis (GERD); gastric carcinoma—document healing; celiac artery compression/obstruction give pc pain—aka, abdominal angina.

Lab: CBC with diff, LFTs, PT/PTT if bleeding, consider amylase and lipase, consider UA if considering genitourinary etiology; H. *pylori* antibody titer if considering empiric treatment with proton pump inhibitor, although poor test for screening for ulcer (Aliment Pharmacol Ther 2000;14:615).

- *X-ray:* 3-view abdominal series if suspect perforation to r/o free air.

Emergency Management:

If active bleeding, consider immediate endoscopy and possibly iv octreotide (see p. 128).

If no active bleeding, consider the following options:

- Gi cocktail:

Silver Slider: 10 cc viscous lidocaine with 20 cc Mylanta.

Green Goddess: 10 cc each of viscous lidocaine, Mylanta and Donnatal.

- H_2 blocker of choice: cimetidine 300-400 mg po bid or 800 mg po QHS, ranitidine 150 mg po bid or 300 mg po QHS, famotidine 20 mg po bid or 40 mg po QHS, or nizatidine 150 mg po bid or 300 mg po QHS.

- Proton-pump inhibitor of choice if patient already failed H_2 blocker: lansoprazole 30 mg po qd (Nejm 2002;346:2033); omeprazole 20 mg po qd or bid (Digestion 1990;47:64; Aliment Pharmacol Ther 1989;3:83); rabeprazole 20 mg po qd (Med Lett Drugs Ther 1999;41:110); or pantoprazole 40 mg po qd for GERD (Med Lett Drugs Ther 2000;42:65) or pantoprazole 40 mg iv for upper gi bleed.

- Antacids work the quickest, such as Maalox or Mylanta (Nejm 1966;274:921)—avoid those with $CaCO_3$ because of acid rebound seen 1 hr after ingestion.

- Black licorice helpful (Scand J Gastroenterol suppl 1979;55:117); propantheline (Pro-Banthine) 15 mg ac appear equivocal (Am J Gastroenterol 1967;47:124)

- Sucralfate (Carafate) 1 gm po qid 1 hr ac (Pharmacotherapy 1982;2:67) as benign and as good as cimetidine.

- Behavioral treatment: stop tobacco, ethanol, NSAIDs, coffee (Nejm 1974;290:469).

- Outpt referral for consideration of *H. pylori* treatment, radiographic upper gi imaging or endoscopy.

6.11 Proctitis

Gastroenterol Clin N Am 1987;16:157; Clin Infect Dis 1999;28:S84

Cause: Seen in inflammatory bowel disease (Ulcerative Colitis) and as a sexually transmitted disease (STD). Less common from trauma (Sex Transm Dis 1979;6:75), iatrogenic from gold

(J Rheumatol 1987;14:142) or radiation therapy (Am J Gastroenterol 1996;91:1309).

Epidem: Unsure.

Pathophys: Seen in ulcerative colitis as an autoimmune phenomenon, which is usually refractory to therapy.

As an STD, occurs from direct anal intercourse or as contiguous spread sometimes in *Chlamydia trachomatis* (Lymphogranuloma venereum) or *Neisseria gonorrheae*. The same organisms implicated in common STDs are seen here—*Herpes* type II, HIV, papilloma virus, and *Treponema pallidum*.

Sx: Pain, itching [pruritus ani (Dis Colon Rectum 1994;37:670)] and discharge.

Si: Erythematous mucosa, possible discharge.

Cmplc: Ulcerative proctitis may go onto carcinoma, stricture, or be associated with other autoimmune phenomenon. STDs as covered on p 153.

Diff Dx: Perirectal abscess, hemorrhoids, fissure, neoplasm, fistula, pruritus ani (commonly from pinworm—scotch tape test at night and treat with Mebendazole).

Lab: If not consistent with STD, CBC with diff.

If STD considered, anoscopy with gram stain, culture; serum test for syphilis—eg, VDRL or RPR; HIV counseling and/or testing.

Emergency Management:

If ulcerative proctitis, GI consult—timing depends on how symptomatic pt feels.

If STD, refer to p 153 for females and p 491 for males. All partners should be evaluated.

6.12 Upper GI Hemorrhage

Digestion 1999;60:47

Cause: Most commonly seen in esophageal varices (p 103), Mallory-Weiss Tear, Peptic Ulcer Disease (p 122), Erosive esophagitis and gastritis, and less commonly in arteriovenous malformation, carcinoma, or pure arterial bleed (Dieulafoy's lesion). Those with previous aortic repair are at risk for aortoenteric fistula. Rarely TB (Am J Gastroenterol 1999;94:270).

Epidem: Greater than 60 yr of age usually with less ethanol use, and greater likelihood of PUD; < 60 yr of age with more Mallory-Weiss tears and variceal problems (Am J Gastroenterol 1997;92:42).

Pathophys: Mallory-Weiss tear is a partial thickness tear at the GE junction usually following vomiting. Erosive esophagitis is a mucosal problem with usually self-limited hemorrhage seen in those who use tobacco, ethanol, and NSAIDs, and may or may not have a coincident hiatal hernia—seems as if a variant of PUD/gastritis.

Sx: Hematemesis, melena, abdominal pain.

Si: Epigastric tenderness.

Crs: Worse prognosis if older, co-morbid disease processes, tachycardia or hypotension, or if ongoing bleeding (Scand J Gastroenterol 1995;30:327).

Cmplc: Secondary to hemorrhage, ischemic/infarcting cardiac (Chest 1998;114:1137; Mayo Clin Proc 1999;74:235) and/or neurologic events.

Diff Dx: Upper pharyngeal hemorrhage.

Lab: Guaiac positive stools, hemoccult positive emesis, CBC with diff, PT/PTT, metabolic profile—look for BUN/Cr > 23/1 (Am J Gastroenterol 1997;92:1796) although not solely discriminatory, type and screen, consider EKG.

GASTROENTEROLOGY

Emergency Management:

- Iv, with fluid resuscitation if necessary to keep system B/P >100 mm Hg.
- Blood products if fluid bolus ineffective, consider pressors.
- FFP, if coagulopathy.
- Consider somatostatin 250 μg iv bolus, then 250 μg/hr continuous drip (Digestion 1989;43:190; 1999;60:1); or, octreotide 50 μg iv over 20 min, then 50 μg/hr iv drip.
- H_2 blockers of no help emergently (Scand J Gastroenterol 1984;19:885).
- Sengstaaken-Blakemore tube with accessory NG tube until endoscopy (Gastrointest Endosc 1999;49:145) available, if patient hemorrhaging.
- If due to peptic ulcer disease, proton pump inhibitor to prevent recurrence may be helpful but not clear if iv or po dosing is the best despite these study conclusions (Epidemiology 1999;10:228; Crit Care Med 2004;32:1277; Aliment Pharmacol Ther 2004;20:195).
- Non-variceal bleeding that is not persistent and without significant anemia, no orthostasis or baseline vital sign abnormalities, no liver disease or coagulopathy, and in a non-disabled young patient (< 60 yr of age) may be considered for outpatient follow-up and treatment (Acad Emerg Med 1999;6: 196).

Chapter 7
General Surgery

7.1   Abdominal Aortic Aneurysm

Cause: Arteriosclerotic disease or genetic cause (Ann IM 1999; 130:637) most likely, such as Marfan syndrome; less likely due to trauma or infection [syphilis, TB (Ped Radiol 1999;29:536)].

Epidem: Male:Female 10:1.

Pathophys: Proposed that degenerative changes in the media of the arterial wall responsible for the aneurysm formation with rupture causing a surgical emergency.

Sx: Abdominal pain, radiating to or originating in the back, flank, or genital area.

Si: Presence of pulsatile mass not as significant as the width—with > 5 to 5.5 cm being significant (Can Fam Physician 1999; 45:2069; J Vasc Surg 1999;29:191), loss of femoral pulses. Check for systemic vascular disease by checking for bruits.

Crs: Spontaneous rupture of this aneurysm increases with size, with aneurysms between 4 to 7 cm in diameter having a 25% chance of rupture (Circ 1977;56:II161). Elective repair of aneurysms < 5.5 cm in diameter not associated with increased long-term survival (Nejm 2002;346:1437; 2002;346:1445), but elective repair of those > 5cm in diameter may have decreased 30-d mortality (Nejm 2004;351:1607).

Cmplc: Vascular collapse resulting in death; this is higher in AAA repairs done emergently after symptoms start (Ann Vasc Surg 1999;13:613).

Diff Dx: Myocardial infarction, aortitis (J Vasc Surg 1999;30:189), pneumonia, pancreatitis, nephrolithiasis, bowel obstruction, diverticulitis, sickle cell crisis, mesenteric thrombosis, porphyria, diabetes, cholecystitis, perforated viscus, splenic infarct, incarcerated hernia.

Lab: CBC with diff with abnormal platelets (Eur J Vasc Endovasc Surg 1999;17:434), PT/PTT, type and cross 10 units PRBCs for repair, UA may show hematuria (hypothesized with dissection into renal arteries but this may occur in infrarenal aneurysms as well).

- X-ray studies: May be seen on plain abdominal lateral shoot-through, or look for more horizontal positioning of psoas muscle shadow on AP film as indication of retroperitoneal hemorrhage which could be due to AAA or iliac artery aneurysm; ultrasound for screening (Eur J Vasc Endovasc Surg 1999;17:472); abdominal CT gives the most information (Am J Roentgenol 2000;174:181) and may be better than aortography (J Endovasc Surg 1998;5:222); MRI may have role (Magn Reson Imaging 1990;8:199).

Emergency Management:
- 2 large bore ivs.
- Fluid resuscitation if necessary, consider pressors and blood products.
- Judicious use of pain medications (because of hypotension)— may want to preferentially use fentanyl [minimal histamine release thus low incidence of hypotension caused by fentanyl (Ann EM 1989;18:635)].
- To operating theater in a timely fashion even with ongoing resuscitation.

7.2 Appendicitis

Emerg Med Clin N Am 1996;14:653; Am Fam Phys 1999; 60:2027

Cause: Obstructed appendix from fecolith, lymphoid hyperplasia from viral illness or infiltrative disease.

Epidem: Seven percent lifetime risk; male to female 1.5:1; incidence is 23 per 10,000 population/yr if between second and third decade of life. Suggestion of ulcerative colitis protection if done before 20 yr of age (Nejm 2001;344:808).

Pathophys: As above.

Sx: Nausea, anorexia; periumbilical pain at first that moves to the RLQ; > 36 hr (Am Surg 1999;65:453) but < 72 hours of duration; sense of constipation and urge to defecate.

Si: Fever 37.5°-38.5°C; < 101°F (Am Surg 1999;65:453). RLQ guarding, rebound, and cough tenderness; right-sided rectal tenderness not helpful (World J Surg 1999;23:133; Ann R Coll Surg Engl 2004;86:292). Iliopsoas, obturator internus, and heel pounding signs may also be positive.

Crs: 12-24 hr.

Cmplc: Perforation with peritonitis (20-33%—pre CT) (Peds 1979;63:36); perforation increases prevalence of infertility × 5.

Diff Dx: UTI; urolithiasis; incarcerated inguinal or femoral hernia; intussusception in children < 4 yr of age; cecal mass (World J Surg 1999;23:713) including neoplasm; tuberculosis; schistosomiasis; mesenteric adenitis including *Yersinia* spp. pseudoappendicular syndrome; diverticulitis; epiploic appendagitis; typhilitis, a cecal colitis seen with aggressive chemotherapy for leukemia; Streptococcus throat infection in children.

Gynecologic: Ruptured ovarian cyst, ectopic pregnancy, ovarian torsion, tubo-ovarian abscess, PID.

Obstetrical: Difficult diagnosis during pregnancy, with clinical and serum markers of little help in diagnosis (Acta Obstet Gynecol Scand 1999;78:758).

Lab: CBC with diff [WBC usually 10K-13K, but not sensitive nor specific—perhaps low normal WBC helpful in excluding diagnosis, ie, < 8K (World J Surg 1999;23:133)]; +/− CRP with elevation (large grey zone between 10-50) indicative of acute complicated disease, eg, abscess or perforation (Brit J Surg 1999;86:501); UA, hematuria does not necessary implicate nephrolithiasis with appropriate history for appendicitis, or AAA—and WBCs may be seen in UA with appendicitis, but should be lacking bacteria; pregnancy test, if of childbearing age.

- *X-ray:* KUB not helpful, but presence of appendicolith will necessitate surgery; helical CT with rectal contrast helpful with up to 98% sensitivity and 98% specificity (Nejm 1998;338:141; Am J Roentgenol 1997;169:1275) or unenhanced (Am J Roentgenol 1993;160:763), or with iv and oral gastrograffin contrast (BMJ 2002;325:1387). CT also helps with gyn diagnoses (Obgyn 1999;93:417), +/− gastrografin enema. US not helpful (World J Surg 1999;23:141). Possible use of a technetium labeled antibody fragment, sulesomab [91% sensitive, 92% specific (Surgery 1999;125:288)].

Emergency Management:
- Place iv, give pain medicines and anti-emetics; surgery is curative. Pain medicines do not obscure diagnosis (J Am Coll Surg 2003;196:18; Ann R Coll Surg Engl 1986:209; Am J Emerg Med 2004;22:280).

7.3 Bowel Obstruction

Cause: Inability of intraluminal intestinal contents to be moved forward via peristalsis.

Epidem: Complications and death have decreased since 1961 with more timely diagnosis, now being less than 10% if younger than 80 yr of age (Ann Surg 2000;231:529).

Pathophys: May be due to previous surgery with either defect in the mesentery or the development of adhesions causing problems; herniation through the femoral canal, inguinal area or anterior abdominal wall; inflammatory bowel disease or radiation enteritis with luminal stenosis; volvulus due to medications or loss of ganglion cells (J Surg Res 1996;60:385); neoplasm; or less likely a foreign body or gallstone ileus or ascaris.

Sx: Abdominal pain, nausea, vomiting, bloating, constipation.

Si: Diffuse abdominal pain with peritoneal signs, increased or lack of bowel sounds, distended or tympanic abdomen.

Crs: May pass spontaneously, others will require surgery.

Cmplc: Perforation.

Diff Dx: Ileus, Ogilvie's syndrome (Arch Surg 1977;112:512), Partial small bowel obstruction.

- Peds: Intussusception, Hirschsprung disease, atresia or stenosis.

Lab: CBC with diff, metabolic profile to exclude reasons for an ileus, type and cross if surgery considered.

X-ray:

- Consider radiographs if at least two of the following (Eur J Surg 1998;164:777):
  (1) Distended abdomen,
  (2) Increased bowel sounds,
  (3) History of constipation,
  (4) Previous abdominal surgery,
  (5) > 50 yr of age, or
  (6) Vomiting.
- Abdominal series may disclose no air in the rectum (helpful if x-rays previous to rectal exam), dilated bowel with paucity of

bowel gas in distal colon, air/fluid levels on upright film; CT is better (Am J Surg 1999;177:375), some obstructions have no obvious dilation nor air/fluid levels on plain film secondary to the intraluminal regions having no air; small bowel follow-through (SBFT) if CT is not diagnostic—SBFT does not provide treatment (Eur J Surg 2000;166:39).

Emergency Management:
(J Pain Symptom Manage 2000;19:23)

- Iv access with hydration and consider NG tube.
- Parenteral antiemetics and narcotics, if necessary.
- Consider dexamethasone 6-16 mg im for malignant bowel obstruction due to gi or gyn cancer (Cochrane Database Syst Rev 2000;2).
- Surgical consult.

7.4 Incarcerated Hernia (Abdominal)

Am J Surg 1967;114:888; Emerg Med Clin N Am 1996;14:739

Cause: Outpouching of intra-abdominal contents through wall defect produces a hernia. If complete defect with no covering of contents—including parietal peritoneum—then this is evisceration. Usually due to genetic defect, post-surgical site or augmented by peritoneal dialysis (Surg Gynecol Obstet 1983;157:541).

- *Inguinal:* Consider femoral hernia in this area, as well. A direct inguinal hernia goes through Hesselbach's triangle, which is defined as the area lateral to the lateral border of the rectus abdominus, superior to the inguinal ligament, and medial/inferior to the inferior epigastric artery. An indirect inguinal hernia lies lateral to the inferior epigastric artery and above the inguinal ligament. A femoral hernia lies below the inguinal ligament in the empty space below the inguinal canal, and this type of hernia is more common in females. An inguinal hernia in pediatrics calls for either laparoscopic or direct inspection of the contralateral side according to some authors.

- *Umbilical:* Location as name implies, could be congenital or post surgical. More common in females, and in those who are obese, have ascites, or women who are pregnant. Although troublesome in adults, watchful waiting is OK in children. In neonates, consider patent urachus and/or omphalocele.
- *Ventral:* May have gastric involvement (Gastrointest Radiol 1984;9:311). Consider Spigelian hernia—this is a potential defect where the inferior border of the posterior rectus sheath (linea semicircularis) and the lateral border of the rectus abdominus muscles intersect. Seen commonly in post-operative sites. In children, consider a diastasis recti—a condition where the linea alba does not form a tough sheath—which is amenable to watchful waiting.

Pathophys: Inability to reduce contents back to correct cavity is incarceration, and this may be acute or chronic. Cutting off the blood supply is strangulation. If the hernia sac includes one wall of a hollow viscus so that intraluminal contents can still pass unimpeded, then this is called a Richter (sliding) hernia.

Sx: Mass felt at site of herniation, pain; nausea and vomiting if incarcerated, even with or without obstruction.

Si: Palpable mass, may be erythematous if acute incarceration or strangulation, bowel sounds may be present. Increase in intra-abdominal pressure with cough, lifting head from pillow or valsalva may make lesion more noticeable and may be diagnostic.

Crs: If bowel involved, this may go onto obstruction (Gastrointest Radiol 1984;9:311).

Cmplc: Perforation possible if bowel involved and if obstructed. Abscess or peritonitis may also ensue. Strangulation induces ischemia, which may cause bowel necrosis.

Diff Dx: Testicular problems in males such as torsion, tumor, hydrocele, or epididymitis; lymphadenopathy in the inguinal area.

Lab: Clinical diagnosis—CBC with diff may help delineate degree of inflammation, as well as give you the hgb/hct for pre-op.

- X-ray: Abdominal series may show obstruction. CT can help delineate anatomy if diagnosis is in question (Br J Surg 1999;86:1243). Perhaps US with tangential plain films (Clin Radiol 1991;44:185) or herniography if site uncertain (Radiographics 1995;15:315), although CT has largely supplanted this.

Emergency Management:

- If patient has a chronic incarceration and is not ill or obstructed, may elect outpatient surgical follow-up. To avoid activities which increase intra-abdominal pressure.

Otherwise:

- IVF, NG tube, and parenteral antiemetics and narcotic analgesia, if necessary.
- May try gentle reduction if peritonitis not present, advocate the use of iv midazolam if reduction attempted. Gently direct hernia toward defect and feed contents back into abdominal cavity starting with the contents at the site of the defect.
- Iv antibiotics if peritonitis or sepsis present, consider ampicillin/sulbactam 1.5-3 gm iv or cefoxitin 2 gm iv or imipenem.
- Surgical referral.

7.5 Ischemic Bowel

Dis Colon Rectum 1970;13:275; 1970;13:283; Radiol Clin N Am 1993;31:1197

Cause: Atherosclerotic or other arterial or venous disease with low flow states, also consider embolic disease. Rarely post-traumatic (ischemic stenosis) (Arch Surg 1980;115:1039) or drug-related such as ergotamine (GE 1977;72:1336), oral contraceptives (Gastrointest Radiol 1977;2:221), or pitressin (Am J Roentgenol 1976;126:829).

Epidem: Should increase as population ages.

Pathophys: Watershed areas most susceptible, if global arteriosclerotic disease of bowel—ileocecal area, splenic flexure of colon, for example. May be seen with occlusion of celiac, superior mesenteric, or inferior mesenteric artery.

Mesenteric ischemia is a different disease than colonic ischemia, with mesenteric ischemia having a younger average age (~61 yrs) and presenting with pain. Those with colonic ischemia are on average a little older (~77 yrs) and present with a lower gi bleed. Mesenteric ischemia will most likely eventually lead to a lower gi bleed (J Emerg Med 2004;27:1).

In neonates, systemic hypoxia or incomplete bowel generation may be the nidus for ischemic problems (Perspect Ped Pathol 1976;3:273).

Sx: Crampy abdominal pain, blood in stools

Si: Abdominal exam usually underwhelming (Can J Surg 1974;17:435); have a high index of suspicion in the elderly.

Crs: After initial episode, will develop scarring with consequent lumen narrowing as part of the healing process.

Cmplc: Strictures; those with SMA lesions fare poorly.

Diff Dx: Lower gi bleed, see p 117.

Lab: Guaiac positive stool, CBC with diff, PT/PTT, metabolic profile, type and cross; EKG if considering global ischemic disease.
- *X-ray:* Consider nuclear red cell tagged scan if unsure of lower gi bleed etiology; Abd CT will give most info if considering primary working diagnosis of ischemic bowel (Radiology 1988;166:149), especially in those with SLE (Radiology 1999;211:203); Barium enema will show "thumbprints."

Emergency Management:
- Iv access, fluid resuscitation if necessary; parenteral antiemetics and narcotic analgesia, as needed.
- Gi consult if stable, possibly considering endoscopy or arteriography/angioplasty (J Vasc Interv Radiol 1995;6:785).
- Surgery consult as well, if patient hemorrhaging or unstable.

7.6 Perforated Viscus

Surg Clin N Am 1972;52:231

Cause: May be seen in peptic ulcer disease, especially at the duodenum; trauma, also in regards to the duodenum and proximal jejunum; inflammatory bowel disease, being more common in ulcerative colitis compared to Crohn's disease; diverticulitis; appendicitis; bowel obstruction from any cause with subsequent perforation—most common at cecum when diameter greater than 10 cm; bowel ischemia; and neoplasm.

Epidem: Non-traumatic small bowel perforation with mortality of approximately 29%, irrespective of timeliness of diagnosis (Am J Surg 1987;153:355).

Pathophys: Erosion/defect through bowel wall resulting in leakage of intraluminal contents into peritoneal cavity.

Sx: Diffuse abdominal pain, nausea, vomiting.

Si: Acute abdomen signs with decreased bowel sounds, rebound tenderness, cough tenderness, percussion tenderness

  N.B. Acute abdomen symptoms and signs may be lacking in those with diabetes and/or being treated with corticosteroids (Ann Surg 1980;192:581).

Crs: Suspect perforated viscus in those with gunshot wounds to the spine (Spine 1989;14:808).

Cmplc: Peritonitis, sepsis, abscess formation, multi-organ failure that is not associated with etiology of perforation (Arch Surg 1996;131:37).

Diff Dx: Gangrenous cholecystitis, abdominal aortic aneurysm, bowel obstruction, ischemic bowel, pancreatitis, nephrolithiasis; more uncommonly—Ogilvie's syndrome—nonobstructive massive cecal dilatation (Arch Surg 1977;112:512), sickle cell crisis, porphyria

Lab: CBC with diff, metabolic profile with LFTs, amylase, lipase, UA.
- *X-ray:* Abd series with free air under the diaphragm on upright or along the liver edge on left lateral decubitus—less sensitive in those with atraumatic small bowel perforation (approximately 17%); in those without obvious free air or bowel dilatation, an ileus may be a positive sign if patient with the clinical exam of an acute abdomen (Am J Roentgenol Radium Ther Nucl Med 1973;117:275); Abd CT in stable patient will also disclose free air, even if not seen on plain films, and may help define etiology (Gastrointest Radiol 1984;9:133)—use gastrografin if giving oral contrast.

Emergency Management:
- Iv fluid, parenteral antiemetics, parenteral narcotics as needed, and consider NG tube.
- Parenteral antiemetics or narcotics if needed, consider iv antibiotics, such as ampicillin/sulbactam 1.5-3 gm iv or cefoxitin 2 gm iv pre-op.
- Surgical consult.

7.7 Perirectal Abscess

Am J Surg 1973;126:765; Ann EM 1995;25:597

Cause: Infection of anal glands with subsequent loculation forming an abscess.

Epidem: Associated with previous abscess, inflammatory bowel disease (Dis Colon Rectum 1990;33:933), and diabetes mellitus. Association with hemorrhoids may be linked to prior misdiagnosis.

Pathophys: Inoculation with cutaneous and enteric organisms, such as *Staphylococcus* spp., *Streptococcus* spp., *Escherichia coli*, *Bacteroides* spp., *Peptostreptococcus* spp., *Clostridium* spp., and the like (Peds 1980;66:282).

Sx: Rectal/perirectal pain, purulent drainage.

Si: Possible palpable mass, tenderness, erythema, warmth; exquisite pain on rectal exam—clinical exam can diagnose this abscess approximately 95% of the time. Anoscopy.

Crs: I & D is curative, if uncomplicated presentation in a healthy pt.

Cmplc: May progress to a secondary cellulitis, fasciitis, or even septicemia. Some may develop fistula-in-ano.

Diff Dx: Perianal is most common and easiest to diagnose and treat—if no apparent mass on exam, consider ischiorectal abscess or an abscess between the internal and external sphincter muscles or an abscess above the levator ani muscle(s) as the cause.

Consider fissure, inflamed hemorrhoids, inflammatory bowel disease, perianal hematoma (Lancet 1982;2:467), infectious proctitis, uterine pathology, endometriosis, rectal foreign body [po (Dis Colon Rectum 1975;18:407) or pr source], referred pain from sacral plexus, or neoplasm (Arch Surg 1985;120:632).

Lab: None for uncomplicated perianal abscess, otherwise do the following:

CBC with diff (not sensitive or specific), and specimen culture for fasciitis and/or septicemia to direct antibiotic therapy.

- *X-ray:* CT of pelvis to delineate anatomy if perirectal abscess suspected, but cannot define on physical exam; better than US.

Emergency Management:

For perianal abscess:

- Pretreat with antibiotics if pt with congenital heart or valvular disease who would receive pretreatment for dental and/or other invasive procedures.

- Iv access if narcotics and/or midazolam necessary for procedural sedation or if iv antibiotics necessary.
- Prep the area with betadine, then drape.
- Anesthetize with 1% or 2% lidocaine buffered with bicarb.
- Cross hatch incision over the abscess, trim all edges to keep wound patent—you should end with a hole in the skin tracking directly to the abscess. Either pack or place a drain: 1-2 d follow-up with surgery.
- Consider outpatient oral antibiotics for patients who required pretreatment, those with secondary cellulitis, or those with compromised immune function—eg, diabetes mellitus.
- If patient is systemically ill, has an ischiorectal fossa abscess, or cannot tolerate procedure in ER, surgical consult.

7.8 Pilonidal Cyst Abscess

Brit J Surg 1990;77:123; J Wound Care 1998;7:481

Cause: Ingrown hair that becomes secondarily infected.

Epidem: Most come to medical attention in second to fourth decade of life.

Pathophys: Anaerobic bacteria in all cases with mixed aerobic (*Escherichia coli,* group D strep, α-hemolytic strep, *Proteus*) co-infection in ~32% of cases, with *Bacteroides* species, Gram-positive anaerobic cocci, and *Fusobacterium* predominating (Am J Dis Child 1980;134:679)—peds study.

Sx: Pain in coccyx area, worse with sitting, even worse with driving.

Si: Mass at coccyx area that is tender, erythematous, warm, and may have a sinus tract with drainage. Early on, may only be tender.

Crs: Repeated infection if not removed, surgical referral for removal once acute episode has waned.

Cmplc: Rare cases of CSF involvement with leakage and meningitis (Clin Neurol Neurosurg 1985;87:131).

Diff Dx: Coccydynia; coccygeal sinus or cyst with secondary infection.

Lab: None.

Emergency Management:

(J Emerg Med 1985;3:295)

- Iv access if procedural sedation necessary to I & D, consider narcotics and/or midazolam.
- Prep area with Betadine, drape, and local anesthesia as per p 387.
- Cross hatch over abscess, trim edges to prevent closure.
- Place drain if deep—may use either Penrose or simply pack with plain Nu-Gauze.
- Antibiotics not necessary unless significant secondary cellulitis.
- Have wound rechecked in 2 d to ensure healing and remove/change drain/packing.
- Surgical referral electively once healed.

7.9 Thrombosed Hemorrhoids

Practitioner 1974;2:221

Cause: External rectal hemorrhoids are equivocally associated with constipation (Am J Gastroenterol 1994;89:1981), straining at stool, and dehydration, but probably have more to do with increased sphincter tone (Dis Colon Rectum 1998;41:1534).

Internal hemorrhoids usually present with bleeding, and are only covered here as advocating surgical referral for persistent bleeding, internal hemorrhoid prolapse through rectum, or incarceration of internal hemorrhoids.

Epidem: Common.

Pathophys: Some external hemorrhoids thrombose secondary to the stasis that develops in the protruded tissue.

Sx: Pain with defecation and sitting, blood in stools, palpable mass.

Si: Palpable mass with solid-feeling clot in hemorrhoidal tissue.

Crs: Behavioral modification usually curative.

Cmplc: Recurrent bleeding, incarceration of tissue.

Diff Dx: Fissure, cryptitis, rectal foreign body, infectious proctitis, fistula-in-ano, abscess, inflammatory bowel disease, neoplasm.

Lab: None if diagnosis obvious on exam, H/H if anemia is a concern. No reason to look for systemic hypercoaguable state (Dis Colon Rectum 1971;14:331).

Emergency Management:

If not thrombosed, then do the following:
- Stool softener, such as colace.
- Suppository with steroid (Med Lett Drugs Ther 1968;10:105), such as Anusol HC—equivocal data.
- Increase bulk in diet.
- Drink liberal amount of fluid, ie, 6-8 8 oz cups of H_2O per day.
- Sitz baths.

If thrombosed, do the following:
- Iv access if patient requires procedural sedation with parenteral narcotics and/or midazolam for incision procedure.
- Tape Buttocks if necessary for better exposure.
- Left lateral decubitus position, prep, drape, and local anesthesia per p 387.
- Incise directly on top of thrombosed hemorrhoid the entire length of the protruded tissue, and express clot with Mosquito forceps. Explore the entire length of the hemorrhoid, and if clot not expressed, may have to unroof the mucosa and the hemorrhoid still needs to be lanced (Dis Colon Rectum 1990;33:249).
- Place pads in area for the expected bleeding.
- Follow instructions as above for when thrombosis not present, and pain meds for home, as well.

Chapter 8

Gynecology

8.1 Bartholin Cyst Abscess

Brit J Clin Pract 1978;32:101

Epidem: 80% of acute episodes associated with *Neisseria gonorrheae*, and may also be associated with *Chlamydia trachomatis*, *Escherichia coli*, or mixed flora. Seen predominantly in Hispanic or black women 20-29 yr of age, with multi-gravid and multi-parity as protective (South Med J 1994;87:26).

Pathophys: Obstruction of Bartholin duct with abscess formation.

Sx: Labial pain and swelling.

Si: Usually unilateral lower labial swelling with erythema, warmth, and tenderness.

Crs: Recurrence may be treated/prevented with marsupialization of cyst.

Cmplc: Work-up and treat as with other STDs—see p 153.

Lab: Gram stain of abscess contents, gc/chlamydia from cervix (urine for chlamydia could be considered), test for syphilis (RPR, VDRL, etc), consider HIV and partner testing.

Emergency Management:
- Iv access if procedural sedation with parenteral narcotics and/or midazolam necessary for procedure.
- Lithotomy position, prep with Betadine, then drape.
- Anesthetize with 1-2% lidocaine buffered with bicarb.

- Incise on mucosal surface, and place gauze packing or Word catheter (South Med J 1968;61:514); the Word catheter works by placing needle on syringe filled with 3-5 cc of saline through the rubber on the flat end of the catheter so that the needle tip now sits inside the closed "balloon," and once incision is cross-hatched, place the curved end of the balloon into the wound and inject approximately 3 cc of saline into balloon so that it does not come out and keeps the wound open—remove 1 cc q wk until this heals from inside out.
- To marsupialize, cross hatch on mucosal surface and carry cross hatch down to the cyst. The four corners of the incised cyst will be sewn to the superficial mucosal surface, so that the cyst cannot reocclude, and will heal by secondary intention.
- Consider silver nitrate for sclerosis (Eur J Obstet Gynecol Reprod Biol 1995;63:61).
- Sitz baths.
- Refer to STD section for specific STD treatments.

8.2 Ovarian Cyst Rupture

Cause: Rupture of cyst, which may be physiologic, benign or malignant. Some examples are follicular cysts, mucinous or serous cystadenomas, endometriomas, or cystic teratomas—usually benign.

Epidem: 2-5% in prepubertal females (Obgyn 1993;81:434)

Pathophys: The size of the unruptured cyst does not correlate with physical symptoms, and a ruptured cyst of any size may cause significant pelvic pain.

Sx: Pelvic pain of sudden onset, nausea.

Si: Abdominal exam may be non-specific, pelvic exam may disclose localized tenderness with or without a mass, cervical motion tenderness (Chandelier sign) should be lacking, but not 100%.

Crs: Most will be self-limited and respond to pain treatment and others will be recurrent. Cysts > 5 cm or complex need further evaluation, or if other concerning aspects are noted during a patients evaluation—eg, ectopic tooth.

Cmplc: Hemoperitoneum (hemorrhage) (Abdom Imaging 1999;24:304), peritonitis.

Diff Dx: Ectopic pregnancy [pseudo-ectopic pregnancy (W V Med J 1989;85:488)], appendicitis, tubo-ovarian abscess, ovarian torsion, PID, nephrolithiasis, UTI, endometriosis, or Mittelschmerz.

Endometriosis is difficult to qualify as to whether it is an individual's cause for pelvic pain. It may be found gross or microscopically in either women with chronic pelvic pain or found incidentally during other procedures without correlation to pain hx (Hum Reprod 1996;11:387).

Lab: Urine pregnancy test—serum quantitative if positive; UA, CBC with diff if considering infectious etiology, gc/chlamydia for all women of childbearing age and/or if cervix inflamed or chandelier sign.

- *X-ray:* This discussion is for a non-pregnant patient. If unsure of diagnosis or if palpable mass, US may show a cyst coincident with pain locale, or free fluid with no other lesions which may be consistent with a ruptured cyst. US may also define simple vs complex cysts. Hemorrhagic ovarian cyst may be better elucidated with transvaginal ultrasound (Gynecol Endocrinol 1991;5:123). Right-sided pain may not be easily explained with free fluid but no other lesions noted—this may be consistent with appendicitis, as well.

Emergency Management: If patient is pregnant, go to Ectopic Pregnancy, p 292. If not, then:

- If patient afebrile, and left-sided pain, may elect to treat with NSAIDs and narcotics for breakthrough pain—US as outpt with referral to primary care physician or gynecologist.

- If pain is right-sided, must consider appendicitis. Using Bayseian reasoning, consider the H&P and CBC with diff (UA and urine pregnancy test should both be unremarkable, although ureteral irritation sometimes occurs) to decide whether diagnosis needs to be made immediately, or have the patient return in 6-8 hr for a recheck. Abdominal CT for cases with high index of suspicion for appendicitis—do not rely on US to r/o appendicitis although it may rule it in (not as good as CT). Iv medications for pain control (narcotics) and nausea/vomiting are OK.
- Cysts > 5 cm refer for gyn follow-up, for either aspiration (Brit J Obstet Gynaecol 1989;96:1035), laparoscopy or laparotomy.

8.3 Ovarian Torsion

Ann EM 2001;38:156

Cause: Enlarged ovary (cyst) that twists on itself usually in a woman of childbearing age; perhaps Tamoxifen a risk (Gynecol Obstet Invest 1999;48:200); rarely due to leiomyomatosis peritonealis disseminata (Abdom Imaging 1998;23:640).

Epidem: Incidence approximately 7%; more common on the right side and in pregnancy (Int J Gynaecol Obstet 1989;28:21) and with h/o ovarian cyst or pelvic surgery.

Pathophys: The enlarged ovary will asymmetrically grow in relation to its position in the meso-ovarium. This will allow it to twist on its axis, and this will threaten its blood supply, which may cause necrosis to the ovary.

Sx: Pelvic pain, nausea, vomiting.

Si: Pain upon palpation, palpable mass (80%).

Crs: Necrosis with non-viable ovary if not repositioned, with 50% gangrenous in operating theater.

Cmplc: Loss of ovary.

Lab: Check urine pregnancy test, and consider CBC with diff and UA.
- *X-ray:* US with large and eccentric ovary > 5 cm, perhaps with Doppler to determine viability (Ultrasound Obstet Gynecol 1995;5:129); may also be seen with CT (J Reprod Med 1998;43:827).

Emergency Management:
- Iv access for parenteral anti-emetics and narcotics, if necessary.
- Gynecologic consult.

8.4 Pelvic Inflammatory Disease

Mmwr 1998;47:1

Cause: Chlamydia causes over half of mild cases (Ann IM 1981;95:685); Neisseria gonococcus in 13-20% of cases (Am J Obgyn 1980;138:909); anaerobes (Clin Infect Dis 1999;28:S29); cytomegalovirus; mycoplasma. All via sexual intercourse, especially with multiple partners. IUD use previously thought to increase risk, but this is equivocal—presenting with febrile PID is probably higher in those with IUDs (Jama 1976;235:1851).

Epidem: Approximately 1 million cases/yr in U.S.; associated in those with induced abortion and harboring chlamydia or bacterial vaginosis (Am J Obgyn 1980;138:868), specific prophylaxis is helpful (Am J Obgyn 1992;166:100; Infection 1994;22:242).

Pathophys: Lower genital tract infections ascend cervical canal, usually just before or during menses, with infection spreading to tubes and ovaries.

Sx: Pain in lower abdomen; nausea; vomiting; anorexia; dyspareunia; dysuria; tenesmus; dysmenorrhea.

Si: Adnexal mass (20%) and tenderness; cervical motion tenderness—Chandelier sign; fever; cervical discharge; mild cases have no specific clinical criteria to aid in diagnosis (Sex Transm Dis 1986;13:119).

Crs: Bilateral tubal ligation is not protective (Ann EM 1991;20:344), but perhaps milder course (Am J Emerg Med 1997;15:271). Pregnancy is not protective in adolescents (J Ped Adolesc Gynecol 1996;9:129).

Cmplc: Infertility—15+% with each episode; ectopic pregnancy; pelvic abscess; septic thrombophlebitis; surgical excision of reproductive organs. No difference in outcomes for reproductive abilities in those with mild-moderate disease when comparing inpatient and outpt treatment (Am J Obgyn 2002;186:929).

Diff Dx: Ectopic pregnancy; appendicitis—presentation to the ER in the latter 2 wk of the menstrual cycle (Am J Emerg Med 1993;11:569), within 2 d of symptom onset, and with both nausea and vomiting may favor appendicitis (Am J Surg 1985;150:90); septic abortion; endometriosis; adenomyosis.

Lab: CBC with diff, UA, urine pregnancy test, gc and chlamydia screens, test for syphilis (Jacep 1978;7:93), consider HIV testing; consider ESR or CRP to follow for resolution (Arch Gynecol Obstet 1987;241:177) if there is a concern.

- *X-ray:* Pelvic ultrasound or CT scan for abscess if clinically suspected.

Emergency Management: Initiate treatment based on pain and tenderness.

Outpatients

- First: Cefoxitin 2 gm im + probenecid 1 gm po, or ceftriaxone 250 mg im; then tetracycline 500 mg po qid or doxycycline 100 mg po bid for 14 d.

- Second: Ofloxacin 400 mg po bid + clindamycin 450 mg po qid or metronidazole 500 mg po bid for 2 wk.

Inpatients

Hospitalize if:
- Dx uncertain, gyn consult for laparoscopy (J Reprod Med 1993:53).
- Mass is present.
- Unable to keep po meds down.
- Peritoneal signs present.
- Output treatment failure.
- If compliance is poor.
- First: Doxycycline 100 mg iv + cefoxitin 2 gm iv q 6 hr, or cefotetan 2 gm iv q 12 hr, or metronidazole 1 gm iv bid.
- 2nd: Gentamicin + clindamycin iv until better, then f/u with po clindamycin for 14 d.

N.B. Treat partners.

8.5   Sexual Assault

Rev Infect Dis 1990;12:S682; Ann EM 1995;12:728; Emerg Med Clin N Am 1999;17:685

Best if entire exam is done with dedicated nurse or forensic examiner (Ann EM 2000:353) present at all times since chain of evidence will need to be preserved. Sexual assault kits are available to help preserve the chain of evidence and guide you through key exam points. Epidemiology F:M is approximately 96%:4%.

W/u:
- Medical history
- Exact detail of events, including times, names, recollection of physical area, and whether drugs, weapons, or threats were used.

- Specifically ask if assailant ejaculated on victim's body, throat, vagina, or rectum, and ask whether a condom was used.
- Evaluate and treat physical injuries—coincident trauma is common (Ann EM 2000;35:358); better medicolegal outcomes with injury documentation (Ann EM 2002;39:639).

For exam, some specifics are as follows—place all collected items in separate envelopes:
- Use Woods lamp to look for semen on body. Use sterile gauze moistened with saline to collect any samples.
- All of victim's clothes should be collected and placed in separate paper bags and taped closed.
- Take 12 hairs from head and genital area.
- Scrape under fingernails into envelope, and then clip nails into each envelope.
- Gc culture of throat.
- DNA swab of oral mucosa.
- Have patient spit on gauze and place in its own envelope.
- Only saline for speculum exam, and collect DNA swab from vagina and rectum separately, as indicated, as well as gc and chlamydia cultures.
- Take photos of any specific injuries.

Lab: (Mmwr 1998;47:1) Consider testing for syphilis, HIV, Hepatitis B_SAg and Hep B_SAb, pregnancy, blood type. *STD testing for gc and chlamydia is not in the best interest of the patient because if positive, can lead to a stigma and we are treating for this anyway.* (B. Covey, 2001).

High incidence of coincident drug use in cases (J Anal Toxicol 1999;23:141). Ethanol is most prevalent but including cannabinoids, cocaine, amphetamines, and gamma hydroxy butyrate (GHB = liquid ecstacy) (Am Fam Phys 2000;62:2478). GHB, along with ketamine and rohypnol, have been implicated as "date rape" drugs. Consider testing for these substances. GHB similar to 1,4-butanediol, an industrial solvent (Nejm 2001; 344:87).

Emergency Management (Mmwr 1998;47:1): As above, but also include the following:

- "Morning After Pill"—use one of the following: 2 each of 50 μg estradiol bcp, or 35 μg estradiol bcp po q 12 hr × 2; or levonorgestrel 0.75 mg (Plan B) po q 12 hr × 2 (Lancet 1998;352:428; Med Lett Drugs Ther 2000;42:10; Am Fam Phys 2000;62:2287)
- Prophylactic antibiotics if indicated or requested (Obstet Gynecol Surv 2000:51)—Ceftriaxone 125-250 mg im or spectinomycin 2 gm im; plus doxycycline 100 mg po bid for 7 d; or single dose therapy with azithromycin 1 gm po + metronidazole 2 gm po.
- Immunize with hep B vaccine and HBIG, unless contraindicated.
- Antiemetic of choice for ensuing nausea from treatment.
- HIV counseling re: AZT use prophylactically; useful for high-risk cases (Cmaj 2000;162:641)
- Rape support counseling, police report, and f/u with primary physician in 2-4 wk.

8.6 Sexually Transmitted Diseases

Mmwr 1998;47:1

As pertaining to females.

Cause:

- *Chlamydia trachomatis.*
- *Neisseria gonorrhoeae.*
- Human papilloma virus—HPV or venereal warts, as common name.
- Herpes simplex Types I and II (Jama 2000;283:791; Nejm 2004;15:1970).
- Chancroid (J Am Acad Dermatol 1986:939)—*Haemophilus ducreyi.*

- Treponema pallidum (syphilis)—covered on p 214.
- Human immunodeficiency virus—covered on p 186.
- Trichomonas—covered on p 159.

Epidem:
- All may be spread even when no active lesions.
- Gc and chlamydia coincident 15% of the time; gc may be present in girls < 12 yr of age who are Tanner Stage I without history of abuse, but have vaginal discharge (Peds 1999;104:e72).
- Chancroid associated with syphilis in 15% of cases.
- HSV Types I and II may both be venerally spread; active lesions associated with increased HIV transmission (Arch Dermatol 1999;135:1393); epidemics of Type I among wrestlers is termed *Herpes gladiatorum* (Jama 1965;194:993).
- HPV with higher prevalence in HIV + women and cause of laryngeal papillomas from aspiration at delivery of infant

Pathophys:
- Gc infects membranes of genitourinary tract, with possible septicemia and rash secondary to systemic spread, and arthralgias secondary to immune complex disease—negative taps.
- Chlamydia and gc commonly asymptomatic and difficult to diagnose clinically (Acad Emerg Med 1997:962).
- HPV present in normal as well as wart skin, highly infective.
- HSV Type I tends to be orolabial with complications of encephalitis, whereas Type II tends to be genital and neonatal with complications of meningitis, but clinically full overlap exists.

Sx:
- Gc or chlamydia may present with sore throat with fellatio, labial tenderness, vaginal discharge, dysuria, abnormal vaginal bleeding associated with endometritis, and/or pelvic pain, or chlamydia may cause no symptoms.
- HPV with 1-6 mon incubation with pain at site.

- HSV with sicker primary course, with fever, sore throat, and/or genital lesions.
- Chancroid with painful ulcer after 2-15 d incubation.

Si:
- Gc or chlamydia may disclose pharyngitis, abdominal pain, cervical motion tenderness—Chandelier sign, or pus on cervix.
- HPV with warts on genitalia that are seen better with acetic acid swabbing.
- HSV with adenopathy, gingivostomatitis, pharyngitis, cervicitis, external genital lesions that are painful; recurrent type with classic genital sores.
- Chancroid with tender adenopathy—bubos; also with tender, necrotic ulcers.

Crs:
- Gc with 2-7 d or more latent period.
- HSV with primary infection lasting 10 d, recurs 1-2 times per yr lasting 4 d.
- Chancroid with self-limited course.

Cmplc:
- Gc and chlamydia may go onto PID, endometritis, or sterility—higher chance of sterility with chlamydia.
- GC (BMJ 1970;3:420) with bacteremia with purpuric or vesicular pustule on broad erythematous base or hemorrhagic bullae; those with endocarditis will have 80% chance of arthritis as well; Glisson's capsule inflammation—Fitzhugh-Curtis syndrome; polyarthritis; tenosynovitis; and newborns may acquire vertical transmission conjunctivitis.
- Chlamydia may have perihepatitis analogous to Fitzhugh-Curtis syndrome.
- HPV associated with cervical intraepithelial neoplasia often within 2 yr of contagion; also associated with vaginal, endometrial, vulvar, anal, laryngeal, and conjunctival cancers.

- HSV ocular keratitis by self-inoculation; colitis; aseptic meningitis—or recurrently as Mollaret's meningitis; urinary hesitancy and sacral paresthesias; disseminated forms with encephalitis.

Diff Dx: (Other than gc, chlamydia, syphilis, HSV, HPV, or HIV)
gc and chlamydia: trichomonas, Candida, Reiter's syndrome, appendicitis.

HPV: *Molluscum contagiosum*.

HSV: erythema multiforme, hand-foot-mouth disease (where the base is not erythematous); monkey herpes in monkey handlers.

Lab: Screen for associated STDs, if STD suspected [syphilis (Ann EM 1991;20:627)], but specific tests listed below. Some results may not be available at end of visit and mechanism should be in place to ensure treatment for positive test results (Sex Transm Dis 1999;26:496).

- Gc (Cutis 1981;27:249): Gram stain of D & C of cervix to look for > 3 polys/hpf with intracellular Gram-neg diplococci, has a 67% sensitivity, 98% specificity. Culture or antigen screen (Am J Clin Pathol 1985;83:613), or DNA probe (J Clin Microbiol 1989;27:632), if negative.
- Chlamydia: Single swab culture is 100% specific, 66% sensitive (Genitourin Med 1994;70:300). Gram stain shows 10+ polys/hpf (at 1,000 X) with 17% false positive, 10% false negative (Am J Epidemiol 1988;128:298). Monoclonal antibody immunofluorescence is 93% sensitive and 96% specific (Nejm 1984;310:1146). Pap smear detection is unreliable (Obgyn 1986;68:691). ELISA on secretions or urine is 80% sensitive and 98% specific (APMIS suppl 1988;3:35); urine testing in sexually active adolescent girls is helpful in screening (all visits) (Jama 2002;288:2846). PCR is accurate, availability may be an issue.
- HSV (J Med Virol 1998;55:177): Culture is 77% sensitive in primary herpes. Skin biopsy shows inclusion and giant cells; scraped

Tzanck prep of skin lesion is sensitive and specific. Rapid slide prep kits < 1 hr results, but culture if negative. PCR most sensitive.

- Chancroid culture is difficult and best with specialized media and sampling with sterile plastic loop (J Med Microbiol 1998;47:1023). PCR the best (J Clin Microbiol 1995;33:787).

Emergency Management:

Med Lett Drugs Ther 1999;41:85

All partners should be tested, barrier methods for birth control recommended, report to state public health office, if appropriate, and the specific following treatments:

GC

- Ceftriaxone 125-250 mg im single dose (Sex Transm Dis 1986;13:199), covers syphilis, and both pharyngeal and resistant gc, or
- Cefixime 400 mg po single dose (Antimicrob Agents Chemother 1990;34:355), or
- Cefpodoxime 200 mg po single dose (Pathology 1995;27:64), or
- Ciprofloxacin 250-500 mg po single dose (Sex Transm Dis 1994;21:345), although no good vs syphilis and resistance appearing, or
- Ofloxacin 400 mg po single dose; norfloxacin 800 mg po single dose (Scand J Infect Dis suppl 1988;56:49); or
- Second-line treatment with spectinomycin 2 gm im single dose (Nejm 1977;296:889)—good if PCN allergy, but no good vs syphilis or vs gc pharyngitis, resistance developing in Army where used as first-line drug in Korea.
- If complications with septicemia or arthritis, hospitalize, and tap joint—irrigate joint if clinically worsens. Give 10 million units aqueous PCN iv over 24 hr or divided bolus every 4 hr until afebrile × 3 d, then 7 d of cefoxitin 1 gm qid iv or spectinomycin 2 gm bid im.

- Ceftriaxone and spectinomycin OK in pregnancy (Obgyn 1993;81:33).

Chlamydia:
- Tetracycline 250-500 mg po qid for 7 d, or doxycycline 100 mg po bid for 7 d (Acta Derm Venereol 1981;61:273); or azithromycin 1 gm po single dose (Eur J Clin Microbiol Infect Dis 1992;11:693); or ofloxacin 300 mg po bid for 7 d (Chemotherapy 1990;36:70); or minocycline 100 mg po once or bid for 7-10 d (Med J Aust 1989;150:483).
- If pregnant, erythromycin 500 mg po qid for 7 d or for 3 wk after treatment failure, non-estolated types OK in pregnancy.

HPV:

Clin Infect Dis 1995;20:S91—No therapy is outstanding.
- Podophyllin soln, leave on 8 hr first time, 24 hr subsequently; or podophyllotoxin 0.5% cream (condylox) (Lancet 1989;1:831); avoid in pregnancy because of fetal damage and even death with only 1-2 cc; use cryotherapy instead.
- Trichloroacetic acid topically (Genitourin Med 1987;63:390)
- 5-fluorouracil, 1% gel intravaginally (Int J STD AIDS 2000;11:371) or topical 5% ointment (Brit J Dermatol 1970;83:218)
- Liquid N_2, although repeated applications at one visit with local reaction (Brit J Vener Dis 1977;53:49).
- Imiquimod (Aldara) 5% cream topically 3 times per wk overnight for 3-4 mon (Arch Dermatol 1998;134:25).
- Topical leukocyte interferon-α (Dermatology 1995;191:129) better than podophyllotoxin cream.
- Interferon injections tid for 3 wk; each d for 1 mon, then tid for 6 mon helps for respiratory papillomas (Am J Obgyn 1990;162:348); consider doing this, if surgery required on papillomas, every 3 mon.

HSV:

- Acyclovir 400 mg po tid or 200 mg po five times per d (Lancet 1982;2:571) for 7-10 d for primary; or for 5 d for recurrent episode, then 400 mg po bid prophylaxis reduces recurrences by > 50% long term (Jama 1991;265:747). Topical treatment is useless.
- Famciclovir 125-250 mg po tid or 250 mg po bid for 5 d at first symptom of recurrence decreases shedding and duration/severity of outbreak (Jama 1998;280:887); or 500 mg po tid for 7 d for primary or severe infection.
- Penciclovir 1% cream five times a d for 7 d speeds healing and end of shedding by 1 d (Int J STD AIDS 2000;11:568).
- Valacyclovir1 gm po tid for 7 d or bid for 5 d (Sex Transm Dis 1997;24:481); 500 mg po qd to suppress transmission long-term (Nejm 2004;350:11) or *Herpes gladiatorum* (Clin J Sport Med 1999;9:86).

Chancroid

- First choice: Erythromycin 500 mg po qid for 7 d, or ceftri-axone 250 mg im single dose, or azithromycin 1 gm po single dose (Clin Infect Dis 1995;21:409).
- Second choice: Ciprofloxacin 500 mg po bid for 3 d (Sex Transm Dis 1998;25:293).
- Consider needle aspiration vs I & D of fluctuant buboes, I & D may be better (Sex Transm Dis 1995;22:217).

8.7 Vaginitis

Clin Obstet Gynaecol 1981;8:241; 1988;31:473; Obgyn 1998;92:757; Am Fam Phys 2004;70:2125

Cause: Infectious with *Gardenerella vaginalis* and other bacteria—aka non-specific bacterial vaginosis; Monilia *(Candida albicans)*; *Torulopsis glabrata; Trichomonas vaginalis;* or foreign body—eg, tampon. Non-infectious, such as atrophic in post-menopausal women, chemical irritant or traumatic. Atopic etiology.

Epidem (Acta Obstet Gynecol Scand 1994;73:802):

Most common are *Gardenerella* and other co-inhabitants such as ureaplasmas and other anaerobes. All are endogenous flora that are not necessarily from a venereal etiology, since they cause vaginitis in 15% of virginal women.

Risk factors for Candidiasis are frequent sexual intercourse, oral contraceptives, spermicide use, previous infection, and black or other race other than white (Am J Pub Hlth 1990;80:329; Epidem 1996;7:182). It is associated with diabetes, antibiotic use, steroids, blood dyscrasias, TPN, various endocrine conditions—hypoparathyroidism, hypothyroidism, and hypoadrenalism.

T. glabrata may commonly be found in asymptomatic females, as well as symptomatic females with vaginitis in approximately 30%—may be coincident finding (Obgyn 1990;90:651).

Trichomonas is considered a venereal disease, 10-25% of adult females carry this asymptomatically, and is present in 30-40% of male partners of infected women.

Gc may be present in girls < 12 yr of age who are Tanner Stage I without history of abuse but have vaginal discharge (Peds 1999;104:e72).

Co-infection with more than one pathogen is not uncommon.

Pathophys: Nonspecific bacterial vaginosis due to diminished presence of lactobacilli, with corresponding increase in pH leading to overgrowth with Gardenerella et al. Local conditions in vagina are influenced by bcp's and IUDs such that anaerobes may predominate—this is not seen with use of barrier methods and condoms (Am J Obgyn 1986;154:520). Candida is an opportunistic invasion.

Sx: Vaginal discharge, dyspareunia except in nonspecific bacterial vaginosis.

Si: Look for foreign body, erythema, evidence of trauma, and the following:

- Candida shows lesions with white centers, erythematous bases, and satellite lesions and a thick white/cheesy discharge.
- Nonspecific bacterial vaginosis shows a watery discharge with a vinegar-like smell, stronger smell with increased pH.
- Trichomonas shows a watery discharge and an erythematous cervix ("strawberry" cervix with erythema and punctate hemorrhages < 2% of those infected).

Crs: Protracted course at times, and consider other etiologies such as *Saccharomyces cerevisiae* (a yeast) (Clin Infect Dis 1993;16:93), which may require a prolonged and different therapy.

Cmplc: Nonspecific bacterial vaginosis with increased incidence of premature labor and low birth weight infant (J Clin Microbiol 1994;32:176).

Diff Dx: Consider above etiologies, consider other STDs if considering Trichomonas.

Lab (Clin Lab Med 1989;9:525):

- Swab should be from vaginal pool, not the vaginal wall or cervix (J Adolesc Hlth 1994;15:245).
- Nonspecific bacterial vaginosis: Vaginal smear shows > 15-20% Clue cells, which is considered 100%; pH > 4.5-5.0; positive amine ("whiff") test, ie, D & C smells of ammonia (70-80%) (Brit J Vener Dis 1983;59:302); few polys; culture positive in 40%.
- *Candida* shows pseudohyphae 20% of the time on 10% KOH exam of vaginal discharge (J Fam Pract 1984;18:549); culture more sensitive but would advocate treat and recheck before going to culture initially; vaginal pH 4-4.5.

- Trichomonas shows a motile 20-μ flagellate with axostyle undulating membrane on wet prep 50-70% sensitivity (Ann EM 1989;18:564); present on Pap smear in 60-70%, but false positives, too; culture possible, rapid DNA and monoclonal antibody test 90% sens and 99.8% specif.; vaginal pH 5-6, with amine smell on "whiff" test (Brit J Vener Dis 1983;59:302).

Emergency Management:

Nonspecific bacterial vaginosis:

- Metronidazole 2 gm po single dose therapy with 75% cure (Lancet 1983;2:1379); or 500 mg po bid for 7 d with 95% cure; 30% recur in 1 mon, at least if partner not treated, although partner treatment not clearly helpful; or try metronidazole vaginal gel 5 gm bid for 5 d (Obgyn 1993;81:963), probably OK in pregnancy, but avoid in first trimester, or
- Clindamycin 300 mg po bid for 7 d (Obgyn 1988;72:799); or as vaginal cream 5 gm qd for 7 d (South Med J 1992;85:1077)— preferred in pregnancy.
- Sulfa and ampicillin are ineffective.
- In pregnancy, advocating treating the cohort of women at high risk for preterm labor, since treatment decreases incidence form 50% to 30%.

Candida:

- Miconazole 2% cream bid intravaginally (Chemotherapy 1982:73), or
- Clotrimazole 100 mg vaginal tab qd for 7 d, 2 tabs qd for 3 d, or 500 mg once (J Fam Pract 1990;31:148), or
- Terconazole 80 mg vaginal tab qd for 3 or 7 d (J Fla Med Assoc 1992;79:693), or
- Nystatin topically (50% effective for vaginal candidiasis) or 5 million units po biweekly for chronic prevention, implicating problem of intestinal reservoir (Am J Obgyn 1986;155:651), or

- Fluconazole 150 mg po single dose therapy (Am J Obgyn 1995;172:1263), or
- Ketoconazole 400 mg po bid for 5 d, or qd for 14 d, then 100 mg po qd as prophylaxis.
- Butoconazole (Femstat) (Mycoses 1993;136:379) and itraconazole (Sporonox) may also be options.
- Perhaps boric acid for recalcitrant cases.
- *Solanum nigrescens,* an ethnobotanical approach, has efficacy (J Ethnopharmacol 1988;22:307).

Trichomonas:
- Metronidazole 2 gm po single dose therapy to patient and partner, 90% cure (J Adolesc Hlth Care 1981;2:41); or 500 mg po bid for 7 d, 85-90% cure; local treatment no good (Sex Transm Dis 1998;25:176), or
- Tinidazole (Tindamax) 2 gm po single dose therapy (Med Lett Drugs Ther 2004;46:70; S Afr Med J 1985;67:455).
- In pregnancy: can use metronidazole after the first trimester; clotrimazole 100 mg vaginally qd for 7 d, is 50% effective (Minerva Ginecol 1975;27:348); Betadine douche to control symptoms no longer used due to suppression of fetal thyroid.

Chapter 9

Hematology/Oncology

9.1 Acute Leukemia

Cause: Lymphocytic and non-lymphocytic varieties. This will focus on acute lymphocytic (blastic) leukemia, or ALL. Two types of ALL, child and adult. Adult type is probably genetic, HLA-linked, autosomal recessive.

Epidem: Adult type represents 15% of adult leukemias. Incidence of childhood type is 32 million per yr. No increased incidence near power lines. Possible hydrocarbon exposure in parents as risk (Cancer Epidem Biomarkers Prev 1999;8:783).

Pathophys: CNS involvement more common (40%) than in AML (7%).
- 78% are B cells; 17% are T-cell types; 5% have no markers using monoclonal antibodies; some also have myeloid antigens that correlate with worse prognosis. Prognostic factors for children not the same for T-cell and B-cell ALL (Leukemia 1999;13:1696).
- Associated with chromosome #9 deletion that has interferon α and interferon β genes.
- Also associated with translocation of chromosome #11 in adult (Blood 1999;94:2072).

Sx: Malaise, fever.

Si: Pallor, white plaque on lateral tongue (oral hairy leukoplakia) (Oral Dis 1999;5:76), hepatosplenomegaly, ecchymoses, petechiae; rarely leukemia cutis, which resembles a viral exanthem type eruption (J Dermatol 1999;26:216).

Crs: In children, now much higher cure rates, 70% 5-yr survivals. In adults, prognosis is much worse than in children; T-cell types have worst prognosis, rest susceptible to treatment; 20-30% cure currently.

Cmplc: Varicella zoster disease with 7% mortality; 6% recurrence in testes, prevent with irradiation, which decreases testosterone later; *Pneumocystis carinii*; CMV; progressive multifocal leukoencephalopathy; AML after chemotherapy in 4%; second primaries in 0.5% of children; sterility; opportunistic infection.

Lab: CBC with diff; metabolic profile including renal function, liver function, calcium, magnesium, phosphorus; UA and urine culture, CXR, and consider LP if looking for secondary infectious focus—consider PCR for specific infections (Ped Infect Dis J 1999;18:395).

Emergency Management:
- Treat secondary infections.
- Order/transfuse appropriate blood products as necessary.
- Consult pt's primary physician or arrange hematology/oncology consult (Med Ped Oncol 1999;32:1; J Clin Oncol 2000; 18:547).

9.2 Primary CNS and Spinal Cord Neoplasms

Am J Med 1978;65:4; Nejm 2001;344:114

Cause: Meningioma, lymphoma (Leuk Lymphoma 1995;19:223), medulloblastoma, gliomas, ependymoma, craniopharyngioma.

Epidem: Recent trends stable except for those > 85 yr of age (J Natl Cancer Inst 1999;91:1382). Environmental risk factors not well-proven (Cancer Epidem Biomarkers Prev 1994;3:197) which includes cell phone use (Nejm 2001;344:79). An increase in

CNS lymphoma in those with AIDS has occurred
(J Natl Cancer Inst 1996;88:675).

Adults: 50% gliomas, 25% meningiomas.

Pediatrics: 50% gliomas; 25% medulloblastoma; 10% ependymoma; 5% craniopharyngioma.

Pathophys: Gliomas incorporate 4 subtypes: (1) Grade 1 is the astrocytoma; (2) Grade 2 is the glioma; (3) Grade 3 is the astroblas-
toma, aka anaplastic astrocytoma; and (4) Grade 4 is the glioblas-
toma. Glioma class of tumors most commonly in cerebellum and
pons in peds; and spinal cord, cerebrum, and cerebellum in
adults.

Sx: Medulloblastoma may present with cerebellar signs, such as ataxia;
all may present with seizures; less likely headache, but possible
including other signs of increased intracranial pressure.

Spinal cord symptoms may be confined to one nerve root or
include "saddle" anesthesia and/or incontinence of bladder
or bowel.

Si: Depends on location; craniopharyngiomas may present with
bitemporal hemianopsia, obesity, diabetes insipidus, growth
failure in children.

Spinal cord findings may include anesthesia, pain, and loss of
patella or Achilles reflexes; consider Cauda Equina syndrome, if
anesthetic in distribution of where one would sit in a saddle,
overflow incontinence, lack of rectal tone, severe pain, and loss
of Achilles and patellar reflexes—usually gradual in onset and
may be asymmetric findings.

Crs:

Meningiomas are benign, yet can be recurrent.

Medulloblastomas are highly malignant with 30-70% 5-yr remis-
sion, 92% 5-yr survival, and perhaps 50% cure.

Glioma class tumors depend on grade; higher the grade, the worse
the prognosis.

Craniopharyngiomas are slow-growing and at least 15-yr survival with treatment.

Cmplc: Panhypopit with post-op patients with craniopharyngiomas.
- *Spinal cord tumors* may present with isolated nerve root findings, but also as Cauda Equina (L1-S5) or Conus Medullaris (S2-5) problems.

Lab: Neuroimaging with CT usually followed by MRI, check electrolytes, cortisol level, and TSH in those with pituitary locations.

N.B. MRI is procedure of choice if considering Cauda Equina or Conus Medullaris process, and should be done emergently. Also procedure of choice for diffuse brainstem glioma diagnosis (Neurosurgery 1993;33:1026,1029).

Emergency Management:
- Treat secondary symptoms of nausea and pain.
- Consider glucocorticoids, such as dexamethasone 4 mg tid for mass effect.
- Consider prophylactic anti-epileptic, such as phenytoin if brain neoplasm, with or without seizures.
- Neurosurgical consult, with arrangements for radiation treatment if Cauda Equina or Conus Medullaris problem.

9.3 Disseminated Intravascular Coagulation (DIC)

Emerg Med Clin N Am 1993;11:465; BMJ 1996;312:683

Cause: Two requirements: (1) reticuloendothelial system blockade by pregnancy, endotoxin, radiation, steroids, colloid, and (2) clotting system activated by:
- Thromboplastin releaser, eg, frozen tissue (hypothermia), placenta, tumors, trypsin, snake venom, open brain trauma, renal transplant rejection; or
- Defibrination agent, eg, amniotic fluid; or
- Platelet factor 3 (phospholipid) release, eg, platelet clot, hemolysis, fat embolism, immune reaction; or
- Activation of factor XII, eg, by endotoxin.

Epidem: More common than TTP. Increased incidence in OB patients especially with septic Ab, abruptio, eclampsia, hydatidiform mole, amniotic fluid embolus, missed Ab, retained dead fetus, fatty liver of pregnancy; leukemia, cancer, and all cases of severe tissue damage; freshwater drownings; Gram-negative sepsis (Jpn J Surg 1977;7:82).

Pathophys: Fibrinogen is low due to consumption and rapid lysis; tissue damage especially in CNS, lung, and kidneys from thrombotic ischemia.

Sx: Bleeding, coma; fever only if a secondary cause, unlike TTP.

Si: Palpable purpuric rash; hypotension; oozing/bleeding at all sites; shock.

Crs: Worse prognosis with extent of PT, PTT, platelet count, and/or thrombin time abnormalities (Thromb Haemost 1978;39:122); usually an acute and fulminant course, rarely chronic.

Cmplc: Renal cortical necrosis, ATN, Sheehan's syndrome, acute cor pulmonale, adrenal insufficiency.

Diff Dx: Vasculitis; implicated infections include "benign" viruses such as varicella (Infection 1998;26:306); cold-induced coagulopathy.

Lab: CBC with diff (microangiopathic anemia with helmet cells and other fragments); metabolic profile including liver and renal markers; ESR = 0 secondary to afibrinogenemia; PT/PTT (PT very sensitive); D-dimer and FDP markedly elevated; fibrinogen < 40 mg% (Am J Hematol 1998;59:65); elevated AT III; UA. Low levels of factors II, VIII, and V (< 50% is diagnostic). Soluble fibrin as a pre-DIC marker (Acta Anaesthesiol Scand 1993;37:125).

Emergency Management:
- Treat underlying cause.
- Replace factors—consider FFP and platelets.

- Perhaps heparinize to break consumptive cycle, LMWH has proponents vs unfractionated heparin (Thromb Res 1993;72:475; 1990;59:37); never do so in the face of liver disease, and only as a last resort if chronic cause and uncontrollable bleeding. Not advocated as a preventative therapy (J Emerg Med 1988;6:277).
- Potential use of dermatan sulfate (Thromb Res 1994;74:65).

9.4   Febrile Neutropenia

Cancer Control 1996;3:366

Cause: Agranulocytosis (absolute neutrophil count < 500/mm^3) due to:
- Allergic directly as with chloramphenicol or via lupus, eg, from procainamide.
- Autoimmune antibodies and occasionally, perhaps, killer T cells; idiopathic usually; ibuprofen-induced is reversible.
- Direct drug toxic effect from chemotherapy, chloramphenicol.

Epidem: Type of opportunistic pathogen changing from Gram-neg to Gram-pos organism (Clin Infect Dis 1999;29:495); autoimmune type associated with rheumatoid Felty's syndrome.

Pathophys:
- *Allergic type:* Delayed hypersensitivity T cells kill in marrow; drugs can act as hapten to induce.
- *Autoimmune type:* Antibodies esp. to HLA surface antigens.

Sx: Fever, rigors, malaise, sore throat, cough.

Si: T > 38.3°C or 101°F (no rectal temperature), pharyngitis, rash, pulmonary findings or other clinical findings of infection (or recurrent infection).

Crs: Idiopathic autoimmune type very benign—rarely progresses to sepsis.

Cmplc: Sepsis.

Diff Dx: Drug fever; pulmonary embolus; genetic cyclic neutropenia.

Lab: CBC with diff; metabolic profile including liver markers; blood cultures × 2 with one from central line if present; UA and urine culture; CXR—those with lower respiratory tract infection fare worse (Infection 1998;26:349); PT/PTT if sepsis suspected; consider LP; cultures of any and all wounds.

Emergency Management:

- Isolation.
- Iv access.
- Treat fever, caution with acetaminophen or with NSAIDs, if liver dysfunction.
- Antibiotic: Imipenem-cilastin 500 mg iv q 6 hr, cefepime 1-2 gm iv q 12 hr, or meropenem 0.5-1 gm q 8 hr alone; or with aminoglycoside [peds (Ped Hematol Oncol 2000;17:93)], eg, gentamicin; combination therapy of qd ceftriaxone 80 mg/kg to 4 gm max or levofloxacin 750 mg iv, if β-Lactam allergy with gentamicin at 5 mg/kg unless creatinine clearance < 20 mL/min (see p236) in which case load at 2 mg/kg (Arch Dis Child 1999;80:125); or aztreonam 1-2 gm iv q 6-8 hr + vancomycin 15 mg/kg iv q 12 hr or 30 mg/kg iv qd; low-risk patients may have oral ciprofloxacin 500 mg bid and amoxicillin-clavulanate 875 mg bid (Nejm 1999;341:305). Use of ceftazidime has become reduced with elucidation of different lactamases.
- Low-risk children may have home therapy with oral ciprofloxacin (20 mg/kg qd divided bid) (Cancer 2000; 88:1710).
- Perhaps GM-CSF for persistent or fungal etiologies in medium to high-risk patients (Eur J Cancer 1999;35:S4).
- Consult medicine, hematology/oncology, or ID service.

9.5 Hemophilia and Replacement Factor Guidelines

Emerg Med Clin N Am 1993;11:337; Nejm 2001;344:1773

Cause: Hemophilia A is factor VIII deficiency and is genetic, sex-linked recessive. Hemophilia B is factor IX deficiency and may be genetic, sex-linked genetic or acquired in nephrotics or those with amyloid. Not covered here is pseudo-hemophilia (Von Willebrand factor deficiency), and other more rare factor deficiencies such as factors I, II, V, VII, X, XI, and XIII.

Epidem: Hemophilia A patients are 80% of all patients with lifelong bleeding diathesis; 1:7000-10,000 male births, only $\frac{1}{3}$ have complete VIII deficiency. Hemophilia B has a prevalence of 1:10,000, and represents 16% of those with lifelong bleeding diathesis. Factor XI deficiency is common in Ashkenazi Jews, with 1:190 people in Israel affected— < 1 per million, all others.

Pathophys: Both with defective intrinsic system, hemophilia A secondary to defective factor VIII protein—thus present in plasma immunologically.

Sx: Possibly chronic bruising, hematuria, no significant bleeding after minor cuts.

Si: Bleeding after trauma, and hemarthroses possible.

Crs: Lifelong, survival nearly comparable to normal population if patients do not acquire HIV, hep B, or hep C.

Cmplc: Hemophilia A with flexion contractures of joints, and intracranial bleeding cause of death in 25%; proteolysis of Factor VIII by IgG antibody during replacement (Nejm 2002;346:662).

Diff Dx: Von Willebrand disease or other factor deficiencies (Nejm 2004;351:683); acquired hemophilia (Haematologica 1994;79:550)—circulating antibody inhibitors due to SLE or multiple myeloma.

Lab: CBC with diff, PT/PTT. Consider fibrinogen, fibrin split products, bleeding time, clotting time, tourniquet test—BP cuff at 100 mm Hg for 5 min with normal response as no petechiae (this tests vessels and platelets). Factor levels and specific antibodies as dictated by screening work-up.

- *Factor VIII* levels: None detectable = severe disease; 1-4% = moderate disease; 5-25% = mild disease.

Emergency Management: *If new and symptomatic diagnosis,* consult hematology. Avoidance of ASA and NSAIDs.

If known hemophiliac, determine desired factor level:

- For bleed of head, throat, neck, eye, abdomen (gi), lower back, groin, or hip—desired factor level for those with Factor VIII deficiency is 80-100%, and those with factor IX deficiency is 60-80%.
- For bleed of joints or muscles in arms and legs—desired Factor VIII and Factor IX levels are both 40%.
- For bleeds of minor abrasions, bruises, minor lacerations, minor epistaxis, and minor mouth or gum bleeding may not require any factor replacement.
- If in doubt, consider infusion and consult hematology.
- Perhaps use of activated recombinant Factor VII (Haemostasis 1998;28:93) in those with hemophilia A or B that have inhibitors in the perioperative period.

If known diagnosis of Factor VIII deficiency:

- Consider desmopressin (DDAVP) (Med Lett Drugs Ther 1984;26:82) 0.3 μgm/kg over 30 min iv or nasal spray (Thromb Res 1979;16:775, J Peds 1983;102:228). This increases Factor VIII transiently for uses, such as post-traumatic or perioperative—probably induces release of factors from endothelium. Adequate alone in 80%.
- Determine desired factor from above, and calculate factor VIII units (The Hemophilia Handbook 1992:59): Weight (lbs) ÷ 4.4 × desired factor level (eg, "80" for 80%) = # units of

Factor VIII needed. Use all factors from opened vials; it is better to infuse too much rather than too little.

- Outpatient treatment may consist of recombinant DNA VIII, goal is to keep level > 15%.
- Follow-up in 24-36 hr if sx still persistent.
  If known diagnosis of Factor IX deficiency:
- Determine desired factor from above, and calculate Factor IX units *needed* (The Hemophilia Handbook 1992:61): Weight (lbs) ÷ 2.2 × desired factor level = # units Factor IX needed. With Factor IX, do not give more than the maximum dosage calculated.
- Outpatient treatment may consist of alphanine; danazol 600 mg qd, which increases endogenous production; goal to keep levels 5-15% at all times, and > 40% for surgery.
- Follow-up in 24-36 hr if still symptomatic.

N.B. *If continued bleeding or known platelet deficiency/dysfunction* (consider ITP, von Willebrand's disease, etc)

- Consider Aminocaproic acid at 50-60 mg/kg q 4-6 hr or tranexamic acid 10-15 mg/kg q 8-12 hr either topically, po, or iv—not universally accepted (Nejm 1998;339:245).

9.6 Sickle Cell Disease (SCD)/Sickle Cell Crisis

Emerg Med Clin N Am 1993;11:365; BMJ 1997;315:656

Cause: Sickle cell anemia is genetic, autosomal.

Epidem: In U.S. blacks, 7% are trait, 0.5% homozygous. Genetic distribution in world correlates with history, geography, and malaria.

Pathophys (Am J Epidem 2000;151:839) Val substituted for Glut in β chain leading to Hgb S, which is unstable at low O_2, leading to precipitation and sickling red cells. Sickled cells stick to vessel walls causing clots and infarctions. Splenic infarcts produce diminished antibody formation, which leads to increased infections. Hgb F ($\alpha_2\gamma_2$) may persist as survival mechanism into adult life. Heterozygous cells sickle only in severe hypoxia or if Hgb C or D present. Renal damage to medulla causes decreased concentration ability, K^+ loss, papillary necrosis, and ongoing renal disease. α-Thalassemia trait protects and vice versa.

Sx: Painful crises arise in 60%; frequency correlates with worse prognosis.

Si: Retarded growth and sexual maturation; frontal bossing; skin ulcers, especially lower legs; angioid streaking of fundi indicates neovascularization; pain may occur anywhere; pericarditis with rub; pleurisy with pleural rub; peritonitis with peritoneal signs.

Crs: 50% live to age 45 yr, longer if fetal Hgb > 8.6%; more severe disease in those with dactylitis, leukocytosis, and anemia < 7 gm/dL (Nejm 2000;342:83).

Cmplc:

- Aplastic crises with severe pain most commonly secondary to infection with human parvovirus B19.
- Infections: *Pneumococcal* infections in younger age groups; *Salmonella* infections, especially osteomyelitis, which can be difficult to differentiate form bony infarcts/necrosis (J Ped Orthop 1996;16:540); increased infections because essentially auto-splenectomized by 3-4 yr of age.
- CVAs (Ann IM 1972;76:643), which may be predictable by intracranial Doppler studies.
- 25% have proteinuria that may progress to renal failure.
- Gout
- Gallstones
- Sudden death rate with heavy exertion increased to 32:10,000 in heterozygotes in contrast to 1:100,000 in whites.
- Myonecrosis and myofibrosis
- Priapism; impotence

Lab: Most labs not helpful in established patient who finds the crisis as a reminiscent episode, all others may want to consider the following: CBC with diff, reticulocyte count, ESR low, sickled cells in peripheral smear; Hgb electrophoresis shows Hgb S + increased Hgb F.

- *X-ray:* Long bone infarcts/necrosis; "hair on end" skull; step fractures of vertebrae; acute chest syndrome (new pulmonary infiltrate) cannot be predicted on physical exam and CXR for all with this disease who are febrile (Ann EM 1999;34:64).

  Perhaps US to help differentiate osteomyelitis from bony infarcts (J Ped Orthop 1998;18:552).

  Abdominal CT for those with peritonitis.

Emergency Management:

- Iv access; rehydration; O_2 (Nejm 1984;311:291).
- Parenteral narcotics and/or benzodiazepines; avoid using nitric oxide [potential neuropathy perhaps secondary to B_{12} deficiency (J Intern Med 1995;237:551)] (Clin Lab Haematol 1999;21:409).
- Possibly steroids (Nejm 1994;330:733).
- Consider antibiotics; ceftriaxone OK in low-risk children (Nejm 1993;329:472) and adults.
- Transfusions, but treatment limited by sensitization, less with black blood donors.
- Prevention with vit E 450 IU each day potentially helpful (Am J Hematol 1992;41:227); hydroxyurea 10-25 mg/kg qd gradually increased to just start suppressing polys—stimulates Hgb F production, but if used with erythropoietin, no benefit (Nejm 1990;323:366); erythropoietin (Blood 1993;81:9; Nejm 1993;328:73).

9.7 Transfusion Guidelines

Transfus Med 1994;4:63; 1997;7:153

Cause: Whole blood, red cells, platelets, FFP or cryoprecipitate needed for replacement due to consumption or external loss.

Component therapy (the preceding list less whole blood) is preferred to maximize resources.

Epidem: Use of these practices is common.

Pathophys: Lack of or abnormal hematologic components may necessitate emergent replacement—the etiologies may be myriad. None of these products can be made completely pure, and especially platelets may be prone to bacterial contamination because they are stored at room temperature.

Sx: Bleeding; shock.

Si: Obvious bleeding source; shock; except for trauma, therapy guided by laboratory testing.

Crs: Use of component therapy listed here usually necessitates admission.

Cmplc: Febrile and allergic reactions may occur with use of these agents, as well as CMV and other viral transmission.

Lab: CBC with diff; metabolic profile; PT/PTT; blood bank tubes for appropriate agent replacement.

Emergency Management with Component Therapy:

- *Fresh frozen plasma* (J Emerg Med 1998;16:239): One mL of FFP contains one unit of coagulation factor activity. Use FFP for those who need replacement of multiple factor deficiencies—as seen in DIC, liver failure, massive blood or volume replacement—either due to symptomatic bleeding or those about to undergo an invasive procedure. Using an INR of 1.6 or higher may help guide the decision on those who may need FFP. The usual dose is 10-20 cc/kg, which is approximately 4 U in an adult (220cc/U). A lesser dose may be used—2 U—if supplementing the replacement of a vit K deficiency.
- *Platelets* (Transfus Med 1992;2:311): Composed of $> 5.5 \times 10^{10}$/U with some red cells and white cells and plasma unless leukocyte reduced where the final WBC is $< 5 \times 10^6$ for final

dose—less febrile reactions and CMV transmission with leukocyte reduced; May have HLA matched, which is a pheresis pack. One U raises platelet count ~5,000/μL in a 70 kg person, usual order is for a six-pack. Transfuse for bleeding due to thrombocytopenia or abnormal platelets, or consider empirically for platelet count < 10,000/μL. Consider argatroban (direct thrombin inhibitor) if heparin-induced (2 μg/kg/min) or lepirudin (Refludan), which is a recombinant hirudin derivative, or danaproid sodium (Orgaran), which is a heparinoid (Med Lett Drugs Ther 2001;43:11).

- *Packed red blood cells* (J Emerg Med 1998;16:129): Composed of red cells at a hematocrit of approximately 75% with some plasma, WBCs, and platelets. May come prepared in different fashions to reduce allergic reactions, febrile reactions, and CMV transmission (Transfus Med 1998;8:59). Use in normovolemic patients with chronic anemia who may require increased oxygen carrying capacity, such as those with symptomatic ischemia to any organ. In trauma, if patient not responding to a fluid bolus of 20 cc/kg of crystalloid, then should move to blood products if suspect hemorrhagic cause. Whole blood may be used, but the hypervolemia caused by rapid infusion and other fluid infusion has made packed RBCs the preferred replacement agent. Infusion of one U of packed RBCs in an adult will increase the hematocrit by approximately 3%.

- *Cryoprecipitate* (Ann IM 1983;98:484): It contains Factor VIII, fibrinogen, von Willebrand factor, and Factor XIII. When Hemophilia A and von Willebrand's disease concentrates are not available, cryoprecipitate may be used. Fibrinogen will increase approximately 5 mg/dL for each U, and an adult needs a level of > 100 mg/dL to be hemostatic. For Factor VIII replacement, the total number of bags required is the # of Factor VIII U needed divided by 80—at least 80 IU are in each bag (See Hemophilia and Replacement Factor guidelines on p172 to calculate number of Factor VIII U needed).

9.8   Venous Thromboembolism (VTE)

Arch IM 1998;158:2315; Nejm 2001;344:1222; 2004;351:268

Cause: Venous stasis as seen in long plane or car rides, immobilization post fracture, or post-surgical; intimal injury; coagulation abnormalities, eg as seen in some cancers; ivs are an occasional cause—⅔ due to particulates in iv, ⅓ chemical and/or needle irritation, < 1% bacterial; and trauma pts have a 69% incidence; 18% is proximal DVT. Usually lower extremity although upper extremity DVT becoming more common and with similar causes (Contraception 1998;57:211).

- *Inherited protein deficiencies:* One of these 4 deficiencies is present in 31% of outpatients with lower and 9% with upper extremity DVT; a h/o DVT in the family or at a young age does not increase the likelihood.
- Protein C deficiency or resistance; autosomal dominant, vit K dependent. Factor V (Leiden) mutation in 25-40% of pts with DVT, a heterozygous point mutation, causing resistance to protein C is a separate inherited condition—possibly conferring higher risk of CVA. Screening asymptomatic population not cost effective since annual incidence of DVT is < 1%.
- Protein S deficiency is autosomal dominant, vit K dependent. Protein S is a Protein C co-factor and is associated with nephrotic syndrome. Can also occur as acquired autoimmune deficiency.
- Antithrombin III deficiency; autosomal dominant.
- Antiphospholipid antibodies—anticardiolipin, lupus anticoagulant. Seen in SLE, ITP, or primary antiphospholipid syndrome. Look for elevated PTT, manifest by arterial thrombi or DVT of any organ system (Ann EM 1992;21:207).

Epidem: Associated with major surgery, especially hip (Am J Roentgenol 1996;166:659) or abdominal surgery (Brit J Surg 1977;64:709) and previous thromboembolism (Arch IM

HEMATOLOGY/ONCOLOGY

2000;160:769). Also associated with atherosclerosis but the exact connection (whether atherosclerosis induces venous thrombosis or simply shared risk factors) is not clear (Nejm 2003;348:1435). Use of estrogen plus progesterone doubles the risk for venous thrombosis (Jama 2004;292:1573), with an even higher risk seen in older women, those who are obese, or with Factor V Leiden. Association is high in hospitalized ICU patients (33%), who may be asymptomatic and despite > 60% of patients receiving prophylactic treatment (Jama 1995;274:335). Association with occult cancer after one episode is equivocal (Arch IM 1987;147:1907), although if cancer diagnosed within 1 yr of DVT, prognosis is poor (Nejm 2000;343:1846). Children (J Vasc Surg 1996;24:46) and Asian/Pacific Islander ethnic groups (Ann IM 1998;128:737, Am J Cardiol 2000;85:1334) appear to have protective traits to avoid DVT.

Pathophys: As under Cause.

Sx: Calf pain; unilateral edema.

Si: None; or Homan's sign, increased calf circumference or warmth, which can be equivocal findings (Arch Surg 1976;111:34).

Crs: 75% 5-yr survival; 25% recurrence over 5 yr.

Cmplc:

- Pulmonary embolus (14%), but incidence is decreased to < 0.4 % with treatment.
- Chronic post-phlebitic syndrome (edema, pain, stasis dermatitis, and ulcers) (Int J Dermatol 1987;26:14) in 30% after 5 yr; incidence can be decreased by half with use of compression stockings for 2-3 wk; treat symptoms with herbal venastat 1 po bid, avoid in pregnancy.
- Thrombotic skin necrosis, especially of penis with protein C deficiency and warfarin treatment; treat with vit K, avoid by using heparin treatment.

Diff Dx:

- *Superficial phlebitis:* Treat with local heat, ASA, NSAIDs [perhaps the same for upper extremity DVT, although some advocate same treatment as with DVT of lower extremity (J Vasc Surg 1997;26:853)].

Scoring System: A risk assessment initially proposed by Wells with major and minor criteria with a multifactorial risk score (Lancet 1995;345:1326) that has been honed to a point scale that, when used with a negative d-dimer, may be used to safely exclude low risk people from further testing if their pretest probability is low risk [this study split the moderate risk group (Nejm 2003; 349:1227)]. In reality, the d-dimer functions no better than a clinical score of low risk, which still conveys a risk for DVT of somewhere between 2-3%. To reduce the risk to < 2% in low risk patients, an imaging study will be needed (but would not heparinize pending the study with a negative d-dimer).

Table 9.1   Well's Criteria

Criteria	Points
Active cancer (Rx or palliation within 6 mon)	+1
Paralysis, paresis or recent (4 wks) immobilization of extremity	+1
Recently bedridden for > 3 d and/or major surgery within 4 wks	+1
Localized tenderness along the distribution of the deep venous system	+1
Thigh and calf swollen	+1
Calf swelling 3 cm > asymptomatic side measured 10 cm below tibial tuberosity	+1
Pitting edema—symptomatic leg only	+1
Dilated superficial veins (nonvaricose) in symptomatic leg only	+1
Alternative diagnosis as or more likely than DVT	−2

Risk Calculation

Greater than or equal to 3 points	High Risk
1 or 2 points	Moderate Risk
0 points or less	Low Risk

Lab: CBC with diff; PT/PTT; d-dimer (ELISA); fibrin split products.
5-min bedside d-dimer is 90-93% sensitive and 80-90% specific for proximal DVT compared to ELISA (Thromb Res 1997;86:93), may be helpful if negative in identifying people who do not need an acute imaging study and/or prophylactic heparinization who have low risk although risk stratifies them the same as a low risk score, thus increased number of false pos— (Thromb Haemost 2000;83:191) vs (Ann EM 2000;349:121). Is probably more helpful in those with moderate risk to see if further acute work-up is needed (Nejm 2003:1227); ie, negative d-dimer in moderate risk patient does not need an acute imaging study nor prophylactic heparinization. Hypercoaguable blood test may need delayed work-up if concerned about influence of clot and/or heparin on results, although Factor V Leiden is a DNA test. Also, theoretical concern of hypercoaguability increase with warfarin use if Factor C or Factor S deficiency without a couple days of heparin use, so these may be appropriate acute tests.

Non-invasive testing:
- US: simple compressibility or duplex: noncompressibility with probe 91% sensitivity and 99% specificity or better (J Clin Ultrasound 1999;27:415); 6-10% of positives may be missed with single test, but no data showing that one week follow-up with repeat US testing as an effective strategy to find those who may have been missed. ER physicians may be able to do this if so trained with one study showing good concordance with non-invasive laboratory evaluation (Acad Emerg Med 2000;7:120).
- Impedance plethysmography (IPG) is not as good or as frequently used as US; valid in pregnancy if done in the decubitus position.

Invasive: Venography, but 2% of the time it causes DVT—can trust a negative exam as true (Circ 1981;64:622). Fibrinogen scans may diagnose the rare miss on venography (Jama 1977;237:2195).

Emergency Management:

- Low molecular weight heparin (LMWH) protocol (Ann IM 1998;129:299), as effective as iv unfractionated heparin (Haemostasis 1996;26 suppl 4:189): enoxaparin (Lovenox) 1 mg/kg sc q 12 hr or 1.5 mg/kg sc q 24 hr (Ann IM 2001; 134:191; Thromb Res 1997;86:349); all LMWHs are not the same! Begin warfarin on Day 1 at 5-10 mg po per d. Oral heparins are on the horizon (Circ 2000;101:2658).
- Unfractionated heparin option is iv dosing × 5 d + warfarin started on Day 1.
- Overlap heparin and warfarin with therapeutic INR of 2-3 at least for 2 d to avoid theoretical warfarin induced hypercoagulable state—lack of critical clinical data exists about this theory.
- Continue warfarin for 6 mon if no specific cause; for 1-2 mon, if specific transient cause; for 4 wk with enoxaparin after cancer surgery (yet not trialed against warfarin) (Nejm 2002;346:975), lifelong if recurrent idiopathic type or if due to hypercoagulable state but may decrease the INR goal to 1.5 to 2 (Nejm 2003;348:1425). Risk of recurrent thrombus does not change if treatment is 3 mon or one year (Nejm 2001; 345:165).
- Low molecular weight dalteparin 200 IU/kg subcutaneous qd for 6 mon was superior to dalteparin initiation (5-7 d) with warfarin for 6 mon in those with cancer—dalteparin alone for 6 mon with less recurrence of VTE and no increased bleeding risk (Nejm 2003;349:146).
- Direct thrombin inhibitor ximelagatran (Exanta) 36 mg bid post surgical for prevention of VTE was superior to warfarin (Nejm 2003;349:1703); and ximelagatran (Exanta) 24 mg bid as extended treatment to prevent VTE is superior to placebo (Nejm 2003;349:1713); and ximelagatran at a dose of 36 mg bid for treatment of VTE is as effective as initial treatment

HEMATOLOGY/ONCOLOGY

with enoxaparin followed by warfarin but may increase liver function tests (approximately 9.6% of the time) (Jama 2005;293:681).

- Not thrombolysis, risk of systemic thrombolysis, or procedural complications if catheter directed has not been shown to out-weigh conservative treatment with anticoagulants, despite some literature (Can J Surg 1993;36:359).
- IVC filter to reduce pulmonary embolus rate from 4% to 1.5%, but subsequent recurrent DVT is 20⁺% vs 11%, and short- and long-term mortality is the same.

Chapter 10
Infectious Disease

Med Lett Drugs Ther 2001;43:69; 2002;44:9

10.1 Fournier Gangrene

Cause: Polymicrobial infection of scrotum from skin, urethral or perianal nidus.

Epidem: Uncommon; mortality rate from 20-42% in adults; increased risk in older age and those with chronic alcoholism (Eur Urol 1998;34:411).

Pathophys: Most commonly seen in those with diabetes mellitus or other immunocompromised states, the scrotal area is at risk for secondary or rapidly progressing infections.

Sx: Scrotal pain, rectal pain, dysuria.

Si: Hard and erythematous scrotum, diffuse tenderness, fever.

Crs: May be protracted and lead to death; less ominous course in children (Urology 1990;35:439).

Cmplc: May progress to abscess formation or necrotizing fasciitis; acute renal failure; adult respiratory distress syndrome (Brit J Urol 1989;64:310).

Diff Dx: May arise from intra-abdominal processes (Urology 1994;44:779).

Lab: Glucoscan with serum glucose if elevated, HgbA1C if undiagnosed diabetic, UA, metabolic profile—metabolic abnormalities correspond with severity of disease (J Urol 1995;154:89).

- *X-ray:* Consider scrotal US to r/o abscess or delineate extent of disease (Radiology 1988;169:387).

Emergency Management:
- IVF and parenteral antiemetics and/or pain medications, if needed.
- Iv ampicillin/sulbactam, second generation cephalosporin or antibiotic combination to give coverage for Gram-pos, Gram-neg, and anaerobes.
- Treat underlying metabolic disorders, such as hyperglycemia.
- Topical unprocessed honey (Surgery 1993;113:200).
- Hyperbaric oxygen is controversial (J Urol 1984;132:918).
- Urologic consult.

10.2 HIV

N.B. This is a dynamic field; identify local experts and resources.

Adv IM 2000;45:1; AIDS Read 2000;10:133 and the entire issue of *The AIDS Reader,* Ped Clin N Am 2000;47:155

Cause: Human immunodeficiency virus (HIV) type 1; rarely in U.S., but commonly found in Africa is HIV type 2; a retrovirus.

Epidem: Spread via sexual intercourse; dirty shared needles; blood products, eg, screened blood transfusion 1996 risk = 1:500,000, factor VIII concentrates, and probably breast milk; rarely by casual or nonsexual familial contact, and percutaneous inoculation in health care workers—0.3% incident that increases with volume and HIV titer. Transmission enhanced by the presence of chancroid or other genital ulcers.

Prevalence increased in men who have sex with men, drug users, hemophiliacs, female partners of infected males.

90% of persons transfused with HIV-pos blood convert to pos themselves; 30% of babies from HIV-pos mothers who are untreated are pos at 6 mon of age.

Pathophys: AIDS defined by HIV infection and T4 count < 200 (Semin Thorac Cardiovasc Surg 2000;12:130).

Increased suppressor T8 and decreased helper T4 cells (CD4); deficient production of interferon γ. Conversion rate of HIV pos to AIDS is approximately 2% per yr in hemophiliacs, but is age-dependent so that 7% of HIV-pos young hemophiliacs have AIDS after 8 yr, but 50% of those who are age 35-70 yr will have AIDS after 8 yr, and this is a similar pattern in homosexuals.

Billions of virons produced daily from infection with high viral RNA mutation rate that allows rapid selection of resistant organism in the face of treatment. Also sequestration of virus in lymphoid tissue (J Infect Dis 2000;181:354). Oxidative stress of illness appears to be reversed with effective therapy (J Acquir Immune Defic Syndr 2000;23:321).

Sx: *Primary HIV infection:* mono-like syndrome 5-30 d after exposure, lasting approx. 2 wk; fever (95%), sore throat (70%), weight loss (70%), myalgias (60%), headache (60%), cervical adenopathy (50%).

AIDS: Diarrhea (60%), malaise, weight loss, fever adenopathy, dyspnea.

Si: *Early:* lymphadenopathy; oral monilia/thrush (exudative, chelosis or erythematous diffuse rash types) precedes overt disease often; dermatoses including warts and shingles; chronic fatigue syndrome.

Later: wasting syndromes; chronic diarrhea, Kaposi sarcoma, hairy leukoplakia corrugations on sides of tongue due to reactivation of EBV.

Crs: Variable RNA viral loads in first 4 mon, but worse course predicted by levels at 5-12 mon from infection and by severity of primary infection symptoms.

Of HIV infection: evolution to AIDS 10-yr post-seroconversion varies from 0-72% inversely with RNA copies (viral load) at 12-18 mon after seroconversion.

Of AIDS: 1997 mortality figures markedly improving with aggressive multi-drug treatment based on viral loads, eg, from 29 to 9:100 person yr in pts with CD4 counts < 100; older data were 50% 1-yr, 15% 5-yr survival, 5% 10^+-yr survival because of some viral attenuated pathogenicity; in pts with AIDS on AZT, 50% 1-yr survival after CD4 count < $50/mm^3$; increased time to clinical AIDS and opportunistic infections (AIDS 2000;14:561). Prognosis (survival) worse with increasing age, but not associated with gender, iv drug use, race, or socioeconomic status.

Cmplc:

- *Infections* with common bacterial pathogens, as well as opportunistic organism, especially when CD4 count < 50 include the following [less since highly active anti-retroviral therapy (J Acquir Immune Defic Syndr 2000;23:145)]:

  Pneumocystis or other pneumonias (J Infect Dis 2000;181:158)

  TB, and as a marker for HIV risk based on CD4 and CD8 ratio (AIDS Patient Care STDS 2000;14:79).

  Atypical mycobacterium, especially M. *avium* M. *intracellulare*, rarely M. *haemophilum* or M. *fortuitum* (Am J Med Sci 1998;315:50).

  Herpes infections including tongue fissures: CMV; *Candida; Aspergillosis; Strongyloides*.

  Hep B and C (Sex Transm Dis 1993;20:220)

  Nocardia

  Mucor

  Cryptococcus, especially meningitis

  Toxoplasma

  Legionella

  Chlamydia, Gonorrhea perhaps as marker for HIV risk (AIDS 2000;14:189), and other STDs (Sex Transm Dis 2000;27:259)

  Monilia and torulopsis

  Cryptosporidiosis (Nejm 2002;346:1723)

Isospora belli

Listeria

Cat scratch *Bartonella (Rochalimaea) henselae* or *B. quintana* causing bacillary angiomatosis and peliosis hepatitis.

Syphilis with rapid ($<$ 4 yr) appearance of neurosyphilis manifest by strokes, meningitis, and cranial nerve palsies and that is only transiently suppressed by penicillin regimens.

- *Tumors* including the following (Jama 2001;285:1736):

Kaposi sarcoma—HHV-8 coinfection, venerally spread among gay males

　　Sx/Si: Violaceous skin eruptions, ulcers on legs.

　　Crs: 80% mortality.

　　Diff Dx: bacillary angiomatosis.

　　Emergency Management: ID or HIV specialist referral, to consider intralesional HCG, interferon, vinblastine.

Non-Hodgkins lymphoma, in 15% after 3 yr of AZT treatment.

Burkitt's lymphoma, EBV-associated, in adults.

Leiomyosarcomas, EBV-associated, in children.

Cervical cancer due to higher prevalence of HPV infection— Pap q 6 mon.

- *Gastrointestinal:* upper gi hemorrhage, protease inhibitors helpful (Am J Gastroenterol 1999;94:358).

- *Hematologic:* ITP and aplastic anemia—both of these from parvovirus infection and diminished half-life and megakaryocyte infection.

- *Metabolic:* insulin resistance with protease inhibitor therapy (J Biol Chem 2000) and elevated lipid levels (AIDS Read; 2000;10:162,171).

- *Myocardiopathy*

- *Neurologic* includes the following:

CNS degeneration leading to dementia.

Progressive multifocal leukoencephalopathy (J Neurol 2000;247:134) associated with papovavirus, seen in transplant pts, as well.

Cord lesions

Meningitis (Arch IM 1995;155:2231), lower risk with fluconazole use.

Peripheral neuropathy

Cerebral toxoplasmosis

Cerebral lymphomas

- *Nephropathy.*
- *Rhematologic* including Reiter's without conjunctivitis, and psoriasis with arthritis.
- *Psychiatric* includes depression and suicide.
- *Treatment* may confer hyperglycemia and/or hyperlipidemia, but this does not limit treatment usefulness with concerns of increased vascular disease (CVA/ACS) in a preliminary study (Nejm 2003;348:702)

Diff Dx:

- HTLV I infection, associated with paraparesis.
- HTLV II infection, no disease association.
- CD4 cell lymphopenia syndrome—rare and idiopathic disease.

Lab: *Immunology:*

- Viral load, most important test; RNA by PCR, peripheral mononuclear cell viral m-RNA levels predict prognosis and treatment success; indicates rapidity of disease progression; < 10,000/cc, good; 10,000-100,000/cc, moderately OK; > 100,000/cc, bad. Consider genotyping/resistance testing of strain to guide therapy.
- T4 (CD4) < 200/cc defines AIDS now and predicts opportunistic pneumonias; 200-500 = intermediate risk; a form of mile marker in disease progression.
- ELISA with Western blot test, only 1.5% false pos in low-risk military population; if indeterminant, repeat in 1 mon and

should become pos if really HIV; if persistently equivocal, get PCR and viral culture. Tests neg for 4+ mon incubation period. Peds with more variables (Ped Clin N Am 2000;47:39), peds referral.

- Ora-Sure HIV-1 test from 2-min swab between cheek and gum as specific as serum by ELISA/Western blot.
- p24 nuclear antigen detection either of free antigen or disso-ciated form IgG antibody-antigen complexes pos usually in early disease or in primary infection when ELISA still neg in 50%.

Routine: If newly diagnosed, CBC with diff, metabolic profile, hep B status, syphilis serology, baseline toxoplasmosis and CMV titers, PPD plus controls, UA warranted in that 10% have nephrotic syndrome. If known to be HIV positive, check other tests as war-ranted if evaluating secondary complaints. CXR if hypoxic or TB contacts (J Epidem Community Hlth 2000;54:64).

Emergency Management:

Immediate *Public Health, Social Service* (Am J Publ Hlth 2000;90:699) and *Medical AIDS* specialist referral, if AIDS-defining diagnosis is present.

> *If new diagnosis,* consider the following:

- Prevention: Condom use, AZT possibly with nevirapine (Nejm 2004;351:217) if pregnant—pre and post partum use decreases infant HIV positivity by one third. Protease inhibitors may predispose to low birth weight infants (Inf Dis Ob/Gyn 2000;8:94); this is a dynamic field
- *Haemophilus influenzae* vaccine, Pneumovax, flu shot.
- VZIG, if exposed to chickenpox.
- Fluconazole 200 mg po q wk, if local mucosal or systemic can-didal infections.

N.B. Treatment of disease a dynamic field (thus the guidelines are routinely updated) and saves lives (Lancet 2000;355:

1131)—review article of HIV counseling, testing and referral (Am Fam Phys 2004;70:295). Most would treat with CD4 < 200 or if symptomatic. If CD4 is > 350 and viral load < 55 most would monitor. Thus, significant "grey area" zone. Consultative resources for treating can be reached via the "Warm Line" 8 am to 8 pm Pacific Standard Time at 1-800-933-3413 (at University of California, San Francisco). Post-exposure prophylaxis guidance for HIV concerns can be reached at 1-800-448-4911. Classes of drugs that may be considered are the following:

- Nucleoside reverse transcriptase inhibitors: Zidovudine (AZT, ZDV; Retrovir), didanosine (ddI; Videx, Videx EC), zalcitabine (ddC; Hivid), stavudine (d4T; Zerit, Serit XR), lamivudine (3TC; Epivir), AZT/3TC (Combivir), abacavir (1592, ABC; Ziagen), AZT/3TC/ABC (Trizivir), emtricitabine (FTC; Emtriva)
- Nucleotide reverse transcriptase inhibitor: tenofovir (TFV, TDF, PMPA; Viread).
- Non-nucleoside reverse transcriptase inhibitors: nevirapine (NVP; Viramune), delavirdine (DLV; Rescriptor), efavirenz (EFV; Sustiva).
- Protease inhibitors: HGC-saquinavir (SQV; Invirase), SGC-saquinavir (SQV; Fortovase), indinavir (IDV; Crixivan), ritonavir (RTV; Norvir), nelfinavir (NFV; Viracept), amprenavir (APV; Agenerase), lopinavir/ritonavir (ABT-378, LPV/r; Kaletra), atazanavir (ATV, Reyataz), fosamprenavir (f-APV; Lexiva).
- Fusion inhibitor: enfuvirtide (T-20; Fuzeon).

Listing of available medications in *The Medical Letter: Drugs for HIV Infection* (Med Lett Drugs Ther 2001;43:103).

N.B. Avoid combinations of d4T + AZT; or ddC with ddI, d4t, or 3TC. Failure of treatment usually due to compliance and therapy potency (Jama 2000;283:205).

Specific Preventions:

- Multivitamins delay disease progression (Nejm 2004;351:23).
- Pneumocystis prophylaxis with CD4 counts 100-200 all 3 equally good so once a month pentamidine best since least toxic, but with CD4 counts < 100, TMP/SMX better than dapsone, which is better than pentamidine.
- TB prevention for those tuberculin pos with either 1 yr of isoniazid or 2 mon of rifampin/pyrazinamide (Jama 2000; 283:1445).
- M. *avium* (MAI) prophylaxis if CD4 counts < 100 with clarithromycin, azithromycin, or rifabutin.
- Toxoplasmosis after encephalitis with sulfadiazine and pyrimethoamine folate po qd or 3 times per week (Eur J Clin Microbiol Infect Dis 2000;19:89); or if pos titer and CD4 < 100 with TMP/SMX DS qd.
- CMV infections with ganciclovir 1 gm po tid if CD4 < 50-100 decreases rate by half.
- Cryptococcal with fluconazole, but no prolongation of survival.
- Aphthous stomatitis with equal parts elixir of Mylanta: Benadryl: Tetracycline: Nystatin with 1 tsp qid swish and spit. Persistent cases—thalidomide 50-200 mg po qd × 2-4 wk (Clin Infect Dis 1995;20:250); or topical granulocyte-macrophage colony-stimulating factor (Br J Dermatol 2000;142:171).
- Wasting syndromes may be treated with megestrol (Megace) 40 mg po qid, or marijuana, androgens growth hormones or thalidomide.
- Diarrhea should be treated by finding the primary cause with consideration of the following: octreotide 50 mg sc q 8 hr, opiates, loperamide (Imodium), or diphenoxylate-atropine (Lomotil). Endoscopy for refractory cases with negative stool studies (Gastrointest Endosc 2000;51:427).

- Those responding to highly active anti-retroviral therapies may be considered for discontinuation of secondary prophylaxis for opportunistic infections (AIDS 2000;14:383; Nejm 2001; 344:472).
- Influenza vaccination, may require repeat boosters or prophylaxis with antiviral therapy (Ann IM 1988;109:383).

10.3 Influenza

Nejm 2000;343:1778; Emerg Med Clin N Am 2003;21:353; Hlth Technol Assess 2003;7:iii,xi,1.

Cause: An orthomyxovirus; viral infection with types A, B, and C (rare); the surface glycoproteins include those that contain hemagglutinin (H) or neuraminidase (N); the differences in H and N convey the different strains of influenza.

Epidem: Worldwide infection that usually occurs in the winter; attack rates as low as 20% and as high as 50%; variable course in children, with immunocompetence and age as partially determining factors.

Pathophys: Respiratory droplets spread (Nejm 1978;298:587); 2-d incubation with viral shedding beginning 1 d before symptoms and lasting about 1 wk.

Sx: Rigors, fever, sweating, cough, nasal congestion, inability to cope with daily activities, confined to bed (J Am Board Fam Pract 2004;17:1).

Si: Fever, adenopathy, wheezing or rhonchi, muscle tenderness.

Crs: Fever is up to 4 d, recovery from myalgias and fatigue may take weeks.

Complc: review article (BMJ 1966;5481:217)—anosmia, COPD exacerbation, encephalitis, Guillian-Barre, myocarditis, pericarditis, parotitis (Nejm 1977;296:1391); Reye syndrome, pneumonitis, pneumonia [synergism between influenza virus and *Streptococcus pneumoniae* (J Infect Dis 2003;187:1000)].

Diff Dx: Rhinovirus, parainfluenza virus, adenovirus, respiratory syncytial virus, *Mycoplasma pneumoniae* (Am Rv Respir Dis 1963; 88:73); this upper respiratory syndrome may be also seen in those who inhale metals or polymers (Jama 1965;191:375).

Lab: (Med Lett Drugs Ther 1999;41:121) Consider point of care testing, such as Directigen Flu A Test with a 70% sensitivity and 92% specificity (J Clin Microbiol 2000;38:1161); Directigen Flu A + B test with sensitivities of 96% for type A, 88% for type B, and specificities of 99% for type A, 97% for type B (J Clin Microbiol 2002;74:1675); or ZstatFlu with a 65-77% sensitivity and 77-98% specificity (J Med Virol 2004;74:127). Review article for rapid testing—(Curr Opin Peds 2003;15:77). Confirmatory tests if needed may be agglutination-inhibition test (uncommon now) (Public Hlth Rep 1951;66:1195) culture, direct immunofluorescence, and/or PCR. Once influenza is known to be in your community for the season, empiric treatment for outpts based on symptoms is OK (Ann IM 2003;139:321). May want to test those in whom the therapy may be considered somewhat difficult, or if the patient is to be an inpatient.

Emergency Management:
- Vaccines may benefit all, including healthy, working adults (Nejm 1995;333:889). As a rule, they reduce post-influenza complications and may halve the incidence in the elderly (Jama 1994;272:1661, J Infect Dis 1997;175:1); also in the elderly, reduces the risk for hospitalization for heart disease, cerebrovascular disease, and pneumonia and reduces the risk of overall death (Nejm 2003;348:1322). May consider live attenuated intranasal A vaccine; OK in peds (Nejm 1998; 338:1405); or live-attenuated intranasal influenza A and influenza B vaccine (FluMist) in patients 5-49 yr of age (Med Lett Drugs Ther 2003;45:65).
- Neuraminidase inhibitors (active against A and B strains) (Curr Drug Targets 2004;5:119; Drug Saf 2003;26:787; Jama

1999;282:1240)(Med Lett Drugs Ther 2004;46:85)—review (J Clin Virol 2004;30:115). Start treatment as early as possible and certainly within 48 hr if planning to use as treatment; Zanamivir (Relenza) is an oral inhalation of two 5 mg inhalations q 12 hr for five d (Jama 1999;282:31) or Oseltamivir (Tamiflu) 75 mg capsule q 12 hr for 5 d (Jama 2000;283:1016; Nejm 1999;341:1336)—OK in children with dose of 2 mg/kg bid (Eur J Clin Pharmacol 2003;59:411; Ped Drugs 2003; 5:125); of note, these resemble flavonoids as seen in the seeds of *Aesculus chinensis* (J Nat Prod 2004;67:650); may also use these long-term through a flu season as prophylaxis. These also do work as post-exposure prophylaxis in reducing spread to household contacts (when initial contact is treated) (J Infect Dis 2004;189:440). Ostelamivir appears safe in those with underlying respiratory disease.

- Adamantanes (M2-blockers), such as amantidine and rimantadine (Med Lett Drugs Ther 2004;46:85; Clin Pharmacol Ther 1966;7:38): effective against A strains only, and used for prophyaxis or early treatment—amantadine (Symmetrel) 100 mg capsule bid × 1 wk (may be extended) (Nejm 1990;322:443) or rimantadine (Flumadine), 150 mg capsule bid × 1 wk (may be extended) (Med Lett Drugs Ther 1993;35:109) and rimantidine with less CNS side effect than amantadine (Nejm 1982;307:580); also may use both long-term during a flu season as prophylaxis, although may not be able to tolerate the side effects.
- Treat secondary symptoms of dehydration (IVF), nausea/vomiting (antiemetics) and bronchospasm (nebulized β-agonists).

10.4 Lyme Disease

Ann EM 1999;33:680; Nejm 2001;345:115

Cause: *Borrelia burgdorferi* spread by *Ixodes dammini* tick bite—same tick also spreads babesiosis.

Epidem: Deer tick also infests white-footed deer mice. Northeastern and northwestern U.S. HLA DR4 and DRw2 B-cell allotypes associated with increased CNS, cardiac, and arthritic involvement. Most common tickborne spirochetal disease in U.S.; attack rates up to 66% of people living in a highly endemic area over 7 yr; annual incidence = 20-100 (or more) :100,000 per yr, depending on geographic locale (Jama 1997;278:112); also common in Northern Europe.

Pathophys: Sometimes an immune complex disease, but organisms now identified in joints most of the time. Clinical syndromes very much like primary, secondary, and tertiary syphilis; but much overlap between Stage 1 and 2 symptom complexes.

Sx: Tick bite hx in 80%; disease rare if tick on < 24 hr, usually takes 72 hr and most ticks associated with disease have stayed on 1 wk.
- *Stage 1:* Arthralgias (98%), malaise (80%), headache (64%), fever (60%), stiff neck; rash (77%).
- *Stage 2:* Neurologic and cardiac.
- *Stage 3:* Arthritis; chronic neurologic changes.

Si:
- *Stage 1:* Fever, lymphadenopathy, erythema migrans—a warm "ringworm" around bite with median diameter 15 cm present in 60-80%.
- *Stage 2:* Neurologic: lymphocytic meningitis (15%), and meningoencephalitis, peripheral motor or sensory neuropathies, facial nerve palsies including Bell's palsy. And/or cardiac: myocarditis (8%), like rheumatic fever with heart block but valve disease rare or never; sometimes heart block is only symptom, no fever or even malaise; usually transient, approximately 6 wks after primary infection.
- *Stage 3:* Recurrent polyarthritis at first, then 1-2 large joints; onset up to 4-6 mon after skin rash with decreasing recurrences over years. Late keratitis.

Peds: presentation is variable, and usually diagnosis made with later stage findings (Ped Emerg Care 1998;14:356)

Crs: Stage 1 lasts 3-4 wks. Symptoms and signs of Stages 2 and 3 may be chronic and recurrent over months to years. Even after treatment, especially if given > 3 mon after symptoms, residual arthralgias, fatigue, memory problems may persist. Benign course in children.

Cmplc: Chronic myocardiopathy. Neurologic: chronic encephalopathy in 90% of those who have Stage 2 neurologic symptoms; cerebral vasculitis (Ann EM 1990;19:572); also chronic polyneuropathy and leukoencephalitis. Treatment and testing of those not meeting clinical criteria (Jama 1993;269:979; 1998;279:206).

Diff Dx: Ehrlichiosis, babesiosis as separate or concomitant infection(s).

Lab: CBC with diff and ESR with WBC < 10,000 (92%), hematocrit > 37% (88%), and ESR > 20 mm/hr (53%) in those with disease. Serum IgG and IgM ELISA titer increased and pos Western blot; rare false pos with most occurring in low prevalence populations, in syphilis, and SBE; ≤ 5% false neg especially in late stage, seen if early po antibiotic treatment or early in course or with some labs that run 10-50% false neg and up to 25% false pos. Synovial fluid organisms pos by PCR.
   • Path: pos silver stain or culture of rash edge for organism in 86%.

Emergency Management:

Med Lett Drugs Ther 2000;42:37

Prevention of Tick Bite: with treatment with permethrin (NIX) treatment of clothing and DEET at 23.8% concentration with approximately 301.5 min of protection time and superior to other non-DEET products (Nejm 2002;347:13) and

- Tick checks and removal every 24 hr.
- Prophylaxis after tick bite doubtful, perhaps 2 wks of doxycycline in high prevalence areas (Nejm 1992;327:534).
- Consider vaccination with LYMErix (Med Lett Drugs Ther 1999;41:29) in highly endemic areas, a series of three shots at 0, 1, and 12 mon—long-term safety and effectiveness is unknown (Nejm 1998;339:209; Med Lett Drugs Ther 1999:29).

After tick bite prophylaxis:
- After Ixodes scapularis bite, Doxycycline 200 mg po one time within 72 hr changes risk of Erythema migrans from 3.2% to 0.4% (Nejm 2001;345:79).

Stage 1: Decreases post-rash arthritis and illness.
- Tetracycline 250 mg po qid or doxycycline 100 mg po bid for 21 d; or amoxicillin 250-500 mg po tid for 21 d; or
- Second line with erythromycin 250 mg po qid for 10 d; or penicillin 20 million U each day iv for 10 d; or cefuroxime 500 mg po bid for 21 d.

Stages 2 and 3:
- Doxycycline 200 mg po bid or amoxicillin as above, but for 4-6 wks or ceftriaxone 2 gm iv/im for 14-21 d, especially if bad arthritis or cardiac/neurologic findings, only 1 in 13 failures; or penicillin G 20 million U qd iv for 10-21 d for cardiac or neurologic abnormalities (including meningitis), cures 55% of arthritis.

  N.B. Avoid intra-articular steroids.

For acute non-meningitis disseminated disease:
- Doxycycline 100 mg po bid for 21 d, equally effective as ceftriaxone 2 gm im qd for 14 d.

For heart block: Antibiotics and temporary pacer.

For chronic encephalopathy: 60-85% improve with ceftriaxone treatment given even after several years.

N.B. If pos titers and chronic fatigue or fasciitis syndrome, no treatment.

10.5 Meningitis

Cause: Different infectious causes in neonates, children, young adults, and the elderly.

Neonates: 1st—Group B *Streptococcus*; 2nd—*Listeria*; 3rd—*Pneumococcus*; 4th—*E. coli*, vaginal flora, and *Staphylococcus epidermidis*.

Children 2-24 mon of age (if vaccinated against Haemophilus influenzae): 1st—*Pneumococcus*; 2nd—*Neisseria meningitidis* (serotype Y> C> B> A); 3rd—Group B *Streptococcus*; 4th—*Haemophilus influenzae*.

Children 2-18 yr of age (if vaccinated): 1st—*Meningococcus*; 2nd—*Pneumococcus*; 3rd—*Haemophilus influenzae*.

Adults aged 20-60 yr: 1st—*Pneumococcus*; 2nd—*Meningococcus*, 3rd—*Haemophilus influenzae*; 4th—*Listeria*.

Age > 60 yr: 1st—*Pneumococcus*; 2nd—*Listeria*; 3rd—all others.

Epidem: Increased prevalence of *Meningococcal* meningitis after influenza infection. Children with cochlear implants, especially if they have a positioner, at increased risk (Nejm 2003;349:435).

Pathophys: Primary infection from bacteremia leading to a change/problem with blood-brain barrier. May also occur from direct extension of mastoiditis or otitis media, for example, or as a secondary site from a distant focal infection, such as pyelonephritis.

Additionally, host factors of immune function may play a role, which is why the very young and very old have a different set of pathogens. Immunodeficiency associated with complement problems or generalized decreased immune function from chronic disease or splenic problems may also predispose to meningitis.

Pathogens in these cases may be opportunistic (Lancet 2000:1426).

HIB (*Haemophilus influenzae* type B) vaccine has changed the major pathogens in pediatric meningitis (Lancet 1992; 340:592).

Sx: Headache, fever, change in mental status, stiff neck—usually present with 2 or more of these symptoms (Nejm 2004;351: 1849).

Si: Fever; nuchal rigidity (30% sensitive), Brudzinski sign (5% sensitive)—hip flexion elicited by active neck flexion, Kernig sign (5% sensitive)—neck pain resulting from knee extension (Clin Infect Dis 2002;35:46); focal neurologic deficits, seizures; petechial rash in *Haemophilus influenzae* and meningococcus; joint pain and erythema seen in meningococcal disease as well. Physical exam not helpful for peds < 1 yr of age (Ann EM 1992;21:910).

Crs: Death if bacterial meningitis not treated. High chance of mortality with treatment in those with pneumoccocal disease, especially if decreased level of consciousness (Nejm 2004;351:1849). Worse prognosis with change in mental status, hypotension, or seizure (Ann IM 1998;129:862). Children with partially treated (previous antibiotics) meningitis may have no fever, no mental status change, and more URI si/sx. (Ann EM 1992;21:146).

Cmplc: CNS thrombophlebitis with focal seizures and deficits, cranial nerve neuropathies, communicating hydrocephalus, developmental problems.

Diff Dx: Aseptic meningitis [predominant lymphocytes in CSF; if polys in first LP, re-do in 6-12 hr to look for change to lymphs (Nejm 1973;289:571)]:
- *Treatable:* TB, SBE, fungal (cryptococcosis), tumor, *Listeria*, *H. simplex*, NSAIDs (Ann Pharmacother 1992;26:

813), syphilis, subdural or epidural abscess, cysticercosis (*T. solium*), leptospirosis, partially treated bacterial, RA, rickettsia, Lyme disease, HIV, cat scratch fever, Borrelia (relapsing fever), high-dose immunoglobulin treatment.

- *Untreatable:* Sarcoid, viral including enteroviruses (polio, coxsackie, echo), mumps, mono, rabies, arbovirus, rarely benign recurrent aseptic meningitis (Mollaret's meningitis) (Arch Neurol 1979;36:657), rarely CMV (infants), eosinophilic [such as in *Angiostrongylus cantonensis* (Nejm 2002;346:668)].

  Rarely anaerobic meningitis (in infancy) from source, such as pilonidal cyst abscess (Clin Neurol Neurosurg 1985;87:131).

Lab: CBC with diff although usually of little help (J Emerg Med 1988;6:33), CRP > 1 in children (Ann EM 1991;20:36), Serum procalcitonin level > 0.2 ηg/mL in adults with bacterial meningitis (Clin Infect Dis 1999;28:1313), Metabolic profile, blood cultures, UA and urine culture, CXR if suspected pulmonary component.

- *LP:* CSF has > 10 white cells/mm^3—although children > 6 mon of age usually at low risk if < 30 white cells/mm^3 (Arch Ped Adolesc Med 2001;155:1301)—usually > 200, mostly polys (87%); glucose < 40 mg% (50%); protein > 45 mg% (96%), usually > 100 mg%; *Haemophilus influenzae* may have a paucity of abnormalities (Ped Emerg Care 1990;6:191); Gram stain of CSF may show pathogen—Gram-pos cocci in pairs in pneumococcus, intracellular Gram-neg diplococci in meningococcus, coccobacillus in *Haemophilus influenzae*. Do fluid culture, consider bacterial antigen screen, if bloody tap, do cell counts on tubes 1 and 3 and look for clearing of red cells [xanthochromia is equivocal (Acad Emerg Med 2004;11:131)]. Perhaps PCR for enteroviral meningitis (J Peds 1997;131:393). Perhaps peds 1-3 yr of age may be screened by those with < 6

WBCs/mm^3 only requiring bacterial culture [98% sensitivity, 75% specificity (J Peds 1991;119:363)]. CSF lactate level not much help (J Infect 1983;6:231).

- *X-Ray:* Head CT first before LP, if focal signs including seizure, but do not delay antibiotic treatment; if no focal neuro deficit and normal mentation, head CT usually not necessary in healthy adults (Nejm 2001;345:1727).

Emergency Management:

- Give first dose of iv antibiotics in ER (Ann EM 1986:544; 1989;18:856).
- *Neonates:* Ceftriaxone 100 mg/kg and ampicillin, consider gentamicin or cefotaxime.
- *Age 6 mon to 6 yr:* ceftriaxone and ampicillin.
- *Older children and adults:* Ceftriaxone 2 gm iv q 12 hr, add ampicillin if considering *Haemophilus influenzae* or *Listeria*. Cefotaxime, cefoperazone (Antimicrob Agents Chemother 1982;21:262), or rarely chloramphenicol may be used—if suspect resistance, better to use vancomycin.
- If considering pseudomonas, add ceftazidime, gentamicin, or ciprofloxacin.
- Therapy may be altered depending on culture results.
- Dexamethasone is controversial (J Emerg Med 1996;14:165). Some studies have shown children have better hearing outcomes—[using CSF level of TNF-α > 1000 pg/ml as level for initiation of dexamethasone (J Infect 1999;39:55)] vs (Eur J Peds 1999;158:230; J Antimicrob Chemother 2000;45:315), dose is 0.15 mg/kg iv 20 min before antibiotic, then q 6 hr $\times$ 4. No benefit in most adults (Intensive Care Med 1999;25:475), but may be helpful to adults with the following criteria: the organism is pneumococcus, the dose is given with the antibiotic, and the patient is not septic (it may be as helpful to withhold dexamethasone if penicillin/cephalosporin resistant pneumococcal strain)—dose is 10 mg iv q 6 hr $\times$ 4 d.

N.B. Very limited indication with important caveats (Nejm 2002;347:1549).

   Also consider dexamethasone if the organism is tuberculosis and normal GCS with focal neurologic deficit or abnomal GCS—this improves survival but not preventive re: disability—iv dose of 0.4 mg/kg/d for 1 wk; then 0.3 mg/kg/d for the second wk; then 0.2 mg/kg/d for the third wk; and 0.1 mg/kg/d for the fourth week; and then finally switched to an oral taper (Nejm 2004;351:1741).

- Ketorolac controversial as used to prevent hearing loss (J Infect Dis 1999;179:264).

Prevention: Treat household and day care contacts of those with meningococcus or *Haemophilus influenzae*, using either rifampin or ciprofloxacin.

- For meningococcus, rifampin 600 mg po qid for 2 d or ciprofloxacin 500 mg bid for 2 d if an adult. For children, rifampin 10 mg/kg bid for 2 d.
- For *Haemophilus influenzae*, rifampin 600 mg po qd for 4 d or ciprofloxacin 500 mg po bid for 4 d if an adult. For children, rifampin 20 mg/kg qd for 4 d.

10.6 Periorbital Cellulitis

Head Neck Surg 1987;9:227

Cause: *Staphylococcus influenzae aureus, Pneumococcus,* and *Haemophilus influenzae—Haemophilus influenzae* now rarer with vaccine (Ann EM 1996;28:617). Rarely mucormycosis (Clin Exp Neurol 1994;31:68).

Epidem: Young children have higher risk of periorbital disease, or those who are not immunocompetent (J Rheumatol 1988;15:840).

Pathophys: Extension to periorbital area from underlying sinusitis, from hematogenous spread or from external trauma such as eyebrow plucking (Am J Ophthalmol 1986;102:534).

Sx: Facial pain, fever.

Si: Periorbital tenderness, erythema, sinus tenderness.

Cmplc: Abscess formation or meningitis.

Diff Dx: Allergic reaction, trauma, orbital cellulitis (may present the same but with pain with ocular movement and/or diplopia), conjunctivitis, insect bite, scabies can present here in children less than 1 yr of age.

Lab: CBC with diff, blood culture, ESR if diagnosis somewhat equivocal. TSH if bilateral proptosis in someone adolescent age or greater. LP should be considered in those < 6 mon of age, or in anyone with symptoms of meningeal disease, but not necessary as part of routine evaluation (J Peds 1993;22:355).

- *X-ray:* CT of orbit and sinuses if unilateral proptosis, cranial nerve or visual field/acuity deficit to r/o abscess, osteomyelitis, or tumor.

Emergency Management:

- Iv access, if systemically ill or orbital cellulitis, and consider ceftriaxone 2 gm iv or ampicillin/sulbactam 3 gm iv.
- Outpt treatment of dicloxacillin or cephalexin, with next day follow-up.

10.7 Peritonitis (bacterial)

Cause: Inflammation of peritoneal cavity; the most common bacteria in these settings are bowel flora and *Streptococcus spp.*, but many other pathogens have been found as well.

Epidem: Unknown, no identifiers for localized versus "frank" peritonitis, and definition of localized with negative cultures (if done) is not well characterized.

Pathophys: Inflammation of peritoneal surfaces, specifically the parietal peritoneum from either blood, infectious causes, gastric acid, digestive enzymes, or release of pancreatic enzymes. Free blood in the peritoneal cavity should be suspected if peritoneal si in a traumatic or suspected aneurysmal condition. Infectious causes may be spontaneous as seen with spontaneous bacterial peritonitis (SBP) in those with end-stage liver disease, or as a secondary complication of peritoneal dialysis, intraperitoneal chemotherapy (Am J Med 1985;78:49), hollow viscus perforation such as appendiceal rupture (Peds 1979;63:36), or previously unrecognized intra-abdominal abscess. Rarely due to congenital abnormalities such as infected urachal cysts (Arch Surg 1984;119:1269).

- Pancreatitis may cause release of enzymes into the peritoneum, with resultant tissue self-degradation.
- Peritonitis in those with continuous ambulatory peritoneal dialysis (CAPD) is not uncommonly due to other process other than the dialysis intervention (Ann R Coll Surg Engl 1998; 80:36).

Sx: Abdominal pain, fevers, chills, spasm of abdominal muscles causing inability to straighten up.

Si: Pain with palpation; cough tenderness (pain with coughing) (BMJ 1994;308:1336); peritoneal signs such as rebound, percussion, or heel strike tenderness, as well as involuntary guarding or rigidity of the abdomen.

Crs: Spontaneous bacterial peritonitis and peritonitis from pancreatitis have a high morbidity and mortality. Hemorrhagic causes are variable depending on the degree of hemorrhage and a pt's individual physiologic response.

Cmplc: Sepsis or septic shock. Those with peritoneal dialysis may need to have site changed or go onto hemodialysis.

Diff Dx: Sclerosing peritonitis in those with CAPD (Am J Kidney Dis 1994;24:819); colitis or pseudomembranous colitis such as from C. diff. (Arch Surg 1985;120:1321); ruptured AAA; MI; DKA; hemoperitoneum from any cause, such as ruptured ectopic pregnancy or hemorrhagic ovarian cyst.

Lab: CBC with diff; metabolic profile; amylase; lipase; blood cultures × 2.

Peritoneal fluid for cell count, gram stain, culture, protein, glucose, and LDH, although turbidity most consistent finding if secondary to chronic ambulatory peritoneal dialysis (Perit Dial Int 1989;9:179). If not hemorrhagic issue or malignancy, combine 2 out of the 3 findings to help decide if this is SBP: pH of peritoneal fluid < 7.40, WBC of peritoneal fluid > 1,000/mm^3 or PMN > 500/mm^3, and lactate > 25 mg/dL (Hepatology 1985;5:85) although pH less than 7.31 alone is consistent with SBP (Hepatology 1982;2:408). Finding of candida on ascitic smear in a pt without chronic ambulatory peritoneal dialysis, recent abdominal surgery, or suggestive disseminated candidiasis by medical hx is associated with bowel perforation (Am J Gastroenterol 1980;73:305).

- *X-ray:* Consider CXR for sympathetic effusion or lower lobe pneumonia; plain films rarely show free air with SBP (Jama 1983;249:921), but may show with bowel perforation from any cause; abdominal CT may help delineate anatomy for abscess, or perhaps carcinomatosis vs infectious etiology (Am J Roentgenol 1996;167:743).

Emergency Management:
- Iv access
- Parenteral narcotics and/or antiemetics, as needed.
- *If infectious* etiology, consider paracentesis. iv antibiotics, consider 3rd generation cephalosporin.
- *If hemorrhagic* cause, surgical consult and abdominal CT if pt stable—resuscitate pt if not stable, and consider bedside US.
- *If from pancreatitis,* consider gallbladder US and obtain gi consult.
- *If unknown* cause and pt is stable, consider abdominal CT to elucidate cause.

10.8 Rabies

Ann EM 1983;12:217; Am J Emerg Med 1993;11:279;
Nejm 2004;351:2626

Cause: Rabies virus is a rhabdovirus.

Epidem: From saliva of infected animal, inhaling infected guano in bat caves, or corneal transplant. Bats may be reservoir since not killed by it, whereas uncommon in mice and squirrels as carriers since they probably die quickly. Cats are most commonly affected domestic animal. Most common wild animals affected are foxes, skunks, raccoons; and prey species like woodchucks; and possible in domestic animals such as goats, horses, and cows.

Pathophys: Spread along nerves to CNS.

Sx: H/o animal bite, except in bat rabies where often no bite or contact hx. Pain/paresthesias at site; difficulty swallowing; fever; priapism; nausea; vomiting.

Si: Guillain-Barré like syndrome; tonic contractions, especially on throat with minimal stimulation—thus the presumed hydrophobia.

Crs: Fifteen to 60-d incubation period, rarely up to 6 yr later—depends on nerve length from CNS. Fatal unless treated before sx, usually, although some severe cases now recovering with intensive supportive care. Domestic animals that are behind in their vaccination series may be quarantined for 10 d to detemine if rabies prophylaxis is needed in bite victim—a nonprovoked attack with a bite wound to the head of the victim from a nonimmunized domestic animal is more murky when deciding to opt for a 10-d animal quarantine, as the distance to the CNS is very short.

Complc: Actual disease complications more common in third world countries; in the U.S., tendency to vacillate between under- and over-treat post-exposure scenarios (J Emerg Med 1996;14:287; Public Hlth Rep 1998;113:247).

Diff Dx: Guillain-Barré.

Lab: CSF shows elevated protein after 1 wk—cells are a mix of lymphs and polys, 6-300/mm^3. Serology shows half pos after 1 wk of symptoms, $^2/_3$ after 1$^1/_2$ wks, all pos by 2 wks of symptoms. Brain pathology shows *Negri* bodies.

Emergency Management:

For prevention (Ann EM 1999;33:590): Vaccinate with human diploid cell vaccine—HDCV (Imovax)—OK in children with HIV disease (Clin Infect Dis 2000;30:218):

- Primary series post-exposure: HDCV 1 mL im in deltoid or thigh for young children on day of event, then d 3, 7, 14, and 28.
- Pre-exposure: d 1, 7, 28
- Booster every 2 yr to veterinarians and other high-risk people; chloroquine malaria prophylaxis may prevent adequate immunization.

For acute single exposure: HDCV (as above) + HRIG (immune globulin) 20 IU/kg, half the dose in wound and the other half im deltoid—not gluteal! Perhaps purified chick embryo cell vaccine (Bull World Hlth Organ 2000;78:693) in the future. HRIG not studied in children.

> **N.B.** Use liberally in bat exposures even with no bite.

10.9 Sepsis

Crit Care Med 2004;32:858; Nejm 2003;348:138; 2001;345:588; Ann EM 1993;22:1871; Emerg Med Clin N Am 1996;14:185

Cause: Most commonly Gram-neg shock, but many occur secondary to any infectious etiology (virus, fungus, etc). Postsplenectomy at risk for encapsulated organisms (eg, Pneumococcus) (Brit J Surg 1989;76:1074). Iv drug users may have soft-tissue nidus in descending order of frequency: wrist/forearm, antecubital fossa, fingers/hand, and thigh/groin (Brit J Addict 1990;85:1495).

Epidem: Sepsis is more common in men than women and non-white population than the white population in the U.S.—while the incidence from 1979 to 2000 showed an increase, the mortality did decrease from 27.8% to 17.9% for those hospitalized (Nejm 2003;348:1546); most common organisms were Gram-pos cocci. Septic shock in 25% of those who present with sepsis; septic shock mortality 34% at 28 d and 45% at 5 mon (Jama 1997;278:234). Nasal carriage of S. *aureus* as risk for bacteremia (Nejm 2001;344:11).

Pathophys: Important to differentiate the different levels of infection and their responses (Chest 1992;101:1644). Bacteremia may lead to systemic inflammatory response which is defined by the following: P > 90, RR > 20, T > 36°-38.0°C (96°-99°F), pCO_2 < 32, WBC > 12,000 or < 4,000. Systemic inflammatory response that is due to infection is the sepsis syndrome. This may progress to severe sepsis, which is laboratory evidence of end-organ dysfunction. When hypotension ensues with inadequate end-organ perfusion, this is septic shock. Cytokine and nitric oxide production may be mechanisms that can be treated with inhibitors— exact role in sepsis is controversial (Ann EM 2000;35:26).

Sx: Fever, localized discomfort, dyspnea, mental status changes.

Si: Fever, possible rash [eg, cellulitis (Nejm 2004;350:904)] or other localized findings.

Crs: Severe sepsis identified in ER is difficult to prognosticate, and does not mimic the mortality seen for inpatients with severe sepsis (Acad Emerg Med 1998;5:1169); early aggressive therapy with fluid resuscitation, maintenance of CVP > 8 mm Hg, $SCVO_2$ ≥ 70%, and MAP ≥ 65 mm Hg associated with decreased mortality (Nejm 2001;345:1368). Not influenced by antiseptic central lines—ie, not preventive for line sepsis (Arch Surg 1996;131:986); pre-operative antibiotics and antiseptic prep does prevent wound sepsis in abdominal surgery that carries high risk of peritonitis (Arch Surg 1984;119:909).

Trend toward uncomplicated infections requiring short courses of antibiotics such as levofloxacin 500 mg qd for 5 d for uncomplicated cellulitis (Arch IM 2004;164:1669) or levofloxacin 750 mg qd for 5 d for uncomplicated community acquired pneumonia (Clin Infect Dis 2003;37:752). Other first-line therapies, such as cephalexin for cellulitis or erythromycin for pneumonia, require longer courses of treatment. Lower dose regimens confer a risk of acquiring resistance.

Cmplc: Encephalopathy correlates with severity of sepsis and Glasgow coma scale score; renal failure (Nejm 2004;351:159); ARDS; systemic edema.

Diff Dx: Acute intoxication/overdose such as salicylate or anticholinergic; heat stroke; NMS; AMI; spinal shock.

Lab: ABG; CBC with diff; serum lactate—its trend is prognostic (Crit Care Med 1983;11:449; Circ 1970:989); metabolic profile; ESR if suspect bony origin; blood cultures; UA and urine culture; consider DIC profile if evidence of end-organ damage; tumor necrosis factor α (TNF-α) (Crit Care Med 1999;27:1303) and procalcitonin levels (Crit Care Med 2000;28:950) with persistent elevation may identify those who will do worse; consider LP for CSF evaluation; perhaps tympanocentesis by ENT for infants with sepsis and unknown organism (Laryngoscope 1989;99:1048); consider EKG if hypotensive or if cardiac hx or if age > 60 yr.
- *X-ray:* CXR; specific bone x-ray, if considering osteomyelitis (Am Fam Phys 2001;63:2413); spinal MRI, if suspect disciitis; abdominal CT, if suspect intra-abdominal process.

Emergency Management:
- Airway management, oxygen therapy, and endotracheal intubation if required to resuscitate patient.
- Iv access with fluid bolus should resuscitate approximately 50% of those who present with sepsis (Surg Forum 1971;22:3)— goal of resuscitation is 20-40 cc/kg urgently and aggressive

resuscitation with PRBC's if Hct < 30% (Nejm 2001;345:
1368) or Hgb < 8 g/dL. Try to use Rh neg in females of childbearing age; if more than one volume of blood products given,
give FFP to replace factors (Am J Surg 1996;171:399). Saline
as good as albumin when looking at 28-d outcome (Nejm
2004;350:2247).

- Antibiotic: Imipenem-cilastin 500 mg iv q 6 hr; cefepime
1-2 gm iv q 12 hr; meropenem 0.5-1 gm iv q 8 hr; or flouro-
quinolone (such as levofloxacin 750 mg iv) along with aminoglycoside promptly (ideally within 1 hr, but definitely within
3 hr of ER arrival) to cover for *Staphylococcus* and
Pseudomonas. Dose gentamicin at 5 mg/kg unless creatinine
clearance < 20 ml/min (p236), in which case load at 2 mg/kg.
Use of ceftazidime has become reduced with elucidation of different lactamases.

- Central line for CVP measurement (see Table 10.1) if blood
pressure does not rally to goal. If Swan-Ganz catheter placed
based on clinical need (Crit Care Med 2003;31:2734), the following indicators can be measured to help define the type of
shock. CVP, LVEDP, MAP, and PCWP are in units of mm Hg.
CO is in L/min. CI is in $L/min/m^2$. SVR is in $dynes/cm^2$.
Cardio, sepsis, and neuro headings refer to types of shock.
Remember that those with sepsis may have a fever and those
with neurogenic shock will be paralyzed.

Table 10.1   Central Monitoring Measurements

Indicator	Normal	Cardio	Sepsis
CVP	2 to 8	> 8	< 8
LVEDP	5 to 10	var*	< 5
MAP	70 to 110	var*	< 70
CO	4 to 7	< 4	> 7
CI	2.5 to 4.5	< 2.1	> 4.5
SVR	900 to 1200	var**	< 900
PCWP*	8 to 12	> 18	< 12

*PCWP is greater than LVEDP if mitral stenosis, left atrial myxoma, pulmonary venous obstruction, or high intra-alveolar pressure as seen with continuous positive pressure ventilation; conversely, PCWP may be lower than LVEDP if stiff left ventricle or high LVEDP such as > 25 mm Hg.

**The variability seen in LVEDP, MAP, and SVR with Cardiogenic Shock has to do with the severity of the patient's process. Initially, LVEDP, MAP, and SVR are high and therapy is initiated to return these values to normal. In later stages, LVEDP, MAP, and SVR drop, thus requiring addition of preload, inotropic and pressor support.

- Foley catheter keeping urine output > 0.5 cc/kg/hr.
- Consider pressors and ionotropes if MAP < 65 mm Hg. Consider beginning with dopamine 5-20 μg/kg/min or begin with norepinephrine at 2-20 μg/min if heart rate is not bradycardic (Crit Care Med 1999;27:639); norepinephrine may work better in septic shock (Chest 1993;103:1826). Add dobutamine 2-20 μg/kg/min if central venous oxygen saturation $(S_{CV}O_2)$ < 70% as this may indicate relative failure of resuscitation for those who are hypotensive (Chest 1991;99:1403) or if cardiogenic shock. Add other pressors as needed, including considering phenylephrine 0.5-8 μg/kg/min or 50-180 μg/min iv; may give 50 μg boluses iv (Crit Care Med 1991;19:1395), epinephrine 1-4 μg/min iv (Crit Care Med 2003;31:1659); and/or vasopressin 0.01-0.08 IU/min (Anesthesiology 2002;96:576) drips (p50).

- NSAIDs help fever, but no survival advantage.
- Steroids indicated in those with adrenal suppression, consider hydrocortisone 100 mg iv q 6 hr (Mill Med 1996;161:624) or if using coincident vasopressors and incomplete physiologic response (Crit Care Med 1998;26:645)—empiric steroids may be considered controversial but if decide to use, use physiologic doses, not supratherapeutic doses (Ann IM 2004;141:47).
- Perhaps use of recombinant human activated protein C, may lessen mortality, but increases significant bleeding (Nejm 2001;344:699).
- Isoproterenol (Isuprel), 2-10 µg/min iv (J Oslo City Hosp 1989;39:23); rarely used.
- Experimental monoclonal anti-endotoxins of no help.
- Tumor necrosis factor receptor treatment is of no help.

10.10 Syphilis (Lues)

Clin Microbiol Rv 1999;12:187

Cause: *Treponema pallidum*.

Epidem: Incidence = 20^+:100,000 in U.S., increasing since 1985; spread via direct contact (venereal) with primary or secondary lesion; screening all young adults presenting to ERs for any reason during epidemics will diagnose approximately 4% more cases (Ann EM 1993;22:1286). Strongly associated with HIV positivity (Sex Transm Dis 1990;17:190).

Pathophys: In secondary, marked bacteremia is present. Tertiary (Acta Derm Venereol 1969;49:336): Probably represents a hypersensitivity reaction, since few organisms are present. Gummas from endarteritis obliterans that cause necrosis, eg, in aortic media. Three types of neurosyphilis:
- Tabes dorsalis
- Meningovascular

- General paresis of the insane; primary parenchymal involvement.

All tertiary complications are increased in AIDS (Genitourin Med 1996;72:176).

Sx:

Primary: Painless chancre.

Secondary: Rash, round with pigmented center; fever; headache, alopecia, eye pain from iritis.

Si:

Primary:

- Chancre with edema (looks like a squamous cell CA)
- Non-suppurative lymphadenitis

Secondary:

- Macular/papular/pustular rash with pustules, annular-appearing as ages, on palms and soles and split papules at mouth corners and other moist body areas (condyloma lata) (Brit J Dermatol 1975;93:53).
- Diffuse lymphadenopathy
- Meningitis

Tertiary:

- Neurosyphilis: Argyle-Robertson pupils (small, unequal, reactive to accommodation not light); general paresis dementia; meningovascular, strokes, meningitis, and cranial nerve palsies most commonly seen within 3-4 yr of primary infection especially in AIDS pts, tabes dorsalis with motor long tract and sensory losses in lower extremities.
- Vascular including aortitis with AI and aneurysms in 10%.
- Gummas in 15%; 75% are cutaneous.

Congenital: Onset at age 14+ wks even if seronegative at birth. Look for rash, fever, hepatosplenomegaly, rhinitis, lymphadenopathy, elevated LFTs, CSF cells, and protein; notched permanent

(Hutchinson's) teeth, in 25%; interstitial keratitis in 50%; saddle nose.

Crs:

Primary: 9-90 d; 20-30% develop secondary syphilis.

Secondary: Months, if no treatment.

Cmplc:

Secondary: Obstructive pattern hepatitis; nephrosis from immune complex disease.

Tertiary: Cirrhosis

Diff Dx: Herpes and chancroid—both with painful ulcers. The rash may resemble an allergic reaction, pityriasis rosea, guttate psoriasis, or nummular eczema. The meningitis/encephalitis may resemble those reviewed in meningitis (p200) and encephalitis (p 246).

- Bejel (Brit J Vener Dis 1984;60:293)/Pinta (J Am Acad Dermatol 1993;29:519, 536) from *Treponema carateum*, spread by skin-to-skin contact with lesions, as well as by flies in pinta. Bejel in Arabia, pinta in Central and South America. Primary disease consists of a non-ulcerating papule; secondary, of pigmented skin lesions later becoming depigmented and hyperkeratotis; tertiary of cardiovascular and nervous system involvement. Treat with PCN.
- Yaws (J Am Acad Dermatol 1993;29:519, 536) from *Treponema pertenue*, spread skin to skin in many tropical areas, especially affecting children. Ulcerating papules with "strawberry" scar formation. Treat with PCN.

Lab (J Emerg Med 2000;18:361): VDRL or RPR is pos in 76% of primary cases (if neg, dark field still pos), 100% of secondary cases, and 75% of tertiary cases; false pos ($> 1/16$) in mononucleosis, malaria, collagen vascular diseases, sarcoid, leprosy, yaws, pinta. TPI is pos in 50% of primary, 98% of secondary; and 90% of tertiary cases. FTA is pos in 90% of primary, 98% of secondary, and

98% of tertiary; false pos in only 30% of VDRL pos patients, some with yaws, pinta, or in 10% of those with lupus, but is atypical; remains pos all life.

- Bacteriology may show a dark field exam with bacteria with 8-14 spirals, approximately 7 μm long: false pos in mouth from normal treponema flora.
- CSF: Do LP 1 yr post-treatment of primary and secondary types if VDRL or FTA still pos; in meningovascular syphilis elevated protein and cells are present; VDRL pos in 50%, but can be neg even if bacteremia present, thus FTA better (J Neurol Sci 1988;88:229). Probably best just to treat for 3-4 wks without LP if asymptomatic, except for those with AIDS (do LP) (Genitourin Med 1996;22:176).
- X-ray: congenital type has lytic areas (bites) in long bones, subperiosteal (J Bone Joint Surg [Br] 1989;71:752)

Emergency Management:
Mmwr 1998;47:1

- Partner and public health notification.
- Of early disease (primary, secondary, or latent < 1 yr): first, benzathine PCN (Bicillin) 2.4 million U im single dose; or second, doxycycline 100 mg po bid × 14 d; or third, erythromycin 500 mg po qid × 14 d.
- Of late, short of neurosyphilis: first, benzathine PCN 2.4 million U im weekly × 3; or second, doxycycline 100 mg po bid for 4 wks.
- Of neurosyphilis: PCN G 2-4 million U iv q 4 hr for 10-14 d, or procaine PCN 2.4 million U im + probenecid (Benemid) 500 mg po qid for 10-14 d.
- Of congenital: PCN G 50,000 U/kg im/iv q 8-12 hr for 10-14 d; or procaine PCN 50,000 U/kg im qd for 10-14 d.

- If PCN allergy: Ceftriaxone im qd for 10 d, or tetracycline 2 gm qd or doxycycline 100 mg po bid × 15 d or erythromycin 2 gm qd for 10 d (30 d for tertiary)—12% failure rate for both erythro and doxycycline. Treat for 28 d, if late latent disease. Macrolide resistance has been seen in U.S. and Ireland (Nejm 2004;351:154).
- Less than 1% relapse; follow VDRL, goes neg in 3-6 mon; with CNS lues, follow CSF results; Jarisch-Herxheimer reaction (endotoxin symptoms with fever) within hours after PCN. Longer treatment in AIDS where early neurosyphilis develops and PCN treatment only transiently effective, since long-term cure normally depends on immunity.

10.11 Tetanus

Ann EM 1986;15:1111; 1987;16:1181; Am J Surg 1974;128:616; Bull Am Coll Surg 1992;77:22)

Cause: *Clostridium tetani*, via wound contamination with dirt.

Epidem: Present in most soils; < 120 cases/yr in U.S. (Mmwr CDC Surveill Summ 1992;41:1); mainly in southern states with Texas having 56%; highest incidence in those inadequately immunized, such as born outside of U.S., older age (Ann EM 1990;19:1377), fewer years of formal education, and female gender—hx is not reliable (Am J Emerg Med 1989;7:563); increased incidence in "skin popping" drug addicts.

Pathophys: Exotoxin production and transported both via circulation to CNS (probably most significant in humans), and along motor nerves to CNS (but cannot correlate wound distance from CNS with morbidity and mortality in humans). Meticulous wound care helps prevent exotoxin production.

Sx: Puncture wound or lacerations, or post-partum, post-surgery, or skin ulcers.

Si: Spastic paralysis; tonic convulsive contractions precipitated by intrinsic or extrinsic muscle movement—lockjaw; facial muscles pulled tightly into smile—*rhesus sardonicus*; rarely any fever.

Crs: One to 54-d incubation period, median of 8 d with 88% within 14 d; short incubation period in patients under age 50 is poor prognostic sign. 60% mortality.

Complc: ERs tend to overimmunize, which can lead to toxoid reactions (Ann EM 1985;14:573).

Diff Dx:
(1) Neuroleptic malignant syndrome
(2) "Stiff man syndrome"—autoimmune antibodies against GABA neurons inducing muscle spasms over years, seen with hypopituitarism, IDDM, Graves' and other endocrinopathies; occasionally is an autoimmune paraneoplastic syndrome in breast cancer.

Lab: A clinical diagnosis with laboratory studies usually unhelpful (J Emerg Med 1998;16:705).

Bacteriology studies show smears with Gram-pos bacilli; culture shows fastidious anaerobe, positive in 32% of proven cases.

Protective serum level of antibody is 0.01 IU/ml.

Emergency Management:

Prevent with toxoid vaccine primary series, after 4 or more injections the protection is for at least 12 yr after last injection and too many injections may cause toxoid reaction (Nejm 1969;280:575); some argue that routine dT booster is unnecessary in adults; booster of dT is enough if > 5 yr since last injection for dirty wound (perhaps still too frequent [Arch EM 1988;5:4]) and > 10 yr for clean wound.

For dirty wounds with no primary series completion: Tetanus human immune globulin 250 U im (J Hyg (Lond) 1978;80:267) with coincident vaccine administration in different area.

For clean wounds with no primary series completion: DPT or dT in those < 7 yr of age and Td in all others.

If active tetanus:
- Metronidazole 500 mg iv q 6 hr (J Appl Bacteriol 1968;31:443, BMJ (Clin Res Ed) 1985;291:648);
- Tetanus human immune globulin;
- Intubate and place on ventilator, if inadequate ventilation/respiration.

Chapter 11

Metabolic

11.1 Acidosis

Am J Med Sci 1999;317:38; Post Grad Med J 2000;102:249, 253, 257

Cause: Ketosis from DKA; isopropyl alcohol poisoning; lactic acidosis (Am J Med 1994;97:47)—ethanol intoxication (Hum Exp Toxicol 1996;15:482), septic shock, metformin treatment, hypotension, respiratory failure, liver failure, or short bowel *Lactobacillus* overgrowth; salicylate; acetaminophen (Ann EM 1999;33:452); ethylene glycol, methanol, isopropyl alcohol, paraldehyde or toluene poisoning; severe diarrhea, D-lactate produced by gut flora, pancreatic fistulas; uremia, RTA; ileal conduit. Non-anion gap in those with asthma secondary to prolonged hypocapnia, not lactic acidosis (Crit Care Med 1987;15:1098).

Crs: In trauma, severity of metabolic acidosis correlates with development of acute lung injury (Crit Care Med 2000;28:125).

Lab: Metabolic profile, ABG (venous pH OK if low suspicion, do ABG if pH < 7.3), salicylates, acetaminophen, ketones, ethanol level, measured vs calculated osmoles, lactate level; Wood's lamp evaluation of urine to assess for ethylene glycol of variable utility.

Emergency Management:
- Address the primary disease.
- Treatment with any alkali, even sodium bicarbonate may paradoxically worsen the physiology (Metabolism 1966;15:1011)

METABOLIC

221

even if pH $<$ 7.2 although helpful in "low" (normal) anion gap acidoses, especially if not associated with tissue hypoxia (Brit J Anaesth 1991;67:165).

- Dichloroacetate no help in lactic acidosis (Am J Med 1994; 97:47).
- Tris buffer (Resuscitation 1998;37:161) no help in acidosis, even during CPR.

11.2 Calcium Disorders

Nejm 2000;343:1863; Emerg Med Clin N Am 1989;7:795

Cause:

- *Hypocalcemia* (J Clin Endocrinol Metab 1995;80:1473) seen in hypoparathyroidism due to post-thyroidectomy (Arch Surg 2000;135:142) seen in first 48 hr; spontaneous/sporadic (Am J Med Sci 1989;297:247); acquired through renal failure; pancreatitis; hypomagnesemia—seen post-thyroidectomy (World J Surg 2000;24:722); alcoholism—by hypomagnesemia or direct suppression of PTH; major/minor abdominal surgery (J Clin Endocrinol Metab 1999;84:2654); sepsis (Crit Care Med 2000;28:93); and consuming soft drinks with phosphoric acid, F $>$ M, although this probably has a negligible clinical effect (J Clin Epidem 1999;52:1007).
- *Hypercalcemia* (J Clin Endocrinol Metab 1993;77:1445) seen in hyperparathyroidism via renal calcitriol production (Am Fam Phys 2004;69:333); cancers (Nejm 2005;352:373; Int J Oncol 2000:197)—especially lung, breast, hepatoma; granulomatous diseases—sarcoid, talc granulomas (Chest 2000;117:1195), chronic TB, coccidioidomycosis; Hodgkin's lymphoma; non-Hodgkin's lymphoma; cat scratch disease; vitamin D intoxication—including the milk-alkali syndrome (Yale J Biol Med 1996;69:517); immobilization (Clin Orthop 1976:124);

thyrotoxicosis; thiazides—rarely; vitamin A intoxication; benign familial hypocalciuric hypercalcemia—autosomal dominant; and adrenal insufficiency.

Epidem: Hypoparathyroidism associated with Addison's disease, pernicious anemia, Hashimoto's thyroiditis, DiGeorge syndrome (3rd and 4th pharyngeal pouches).

Pathophys: For parathyroid physiology, PTH is necessary for an osteoclastic response to low calcium, renal tubular calcium resorption, renal tubular phosphate excretion, and vitamin D activation. Lack of parathyroid glands or PTH results in hypocalcemia and hyperphosphatemia. An ensuing alkalosis is due to blocked PTH stimulation of organic acid production in bones in hypoparathyroidism.

Hypercalcemia may be due to excess PTH or PTH-like proteins—as seen in some T-cell leukemias/lymphomas, secretion of other bone-resorbing substances, tumor conversion of 25-OH vitamin D to 1,25-OH vitamin D (calcitriol), local osteolytic mets, or other causes as seen on the list above.

METABOLIC

Sx:

- Hypocalcemia: Circumoral paresthesias, carpal-pedal spasms, stridor, seizures—brief and mild, bronchospasm, gi cramps, anxiety, cataracts.
- Hypercalcemia: Fatigue, weakness, sleepiness, nausea/anorexia, constipation, polyuria/polydipsia, and volume depletion.

Si:

- Hypocalcemia: Tetany (carpal-pedal spasm, Chvostek's sign, which is facial muscle twitching from tapping on the facial nerve, and Trousseau's sign, which is carpal spasm after inflating BP cuff on upper arm), hyperreflexia, cataracts, ophthalmoplegia (Am J Emerg Med 1999;17:105), vascular corneal opacities, psychiatric changes, dystonias, and dyskinesias.
- Hypercalcemia: Confusion, delirium, drowsiness, coma.

Cmplc: Patients with hypoparathyroidism may have pustular psoriasis and dermatitis herpetiformis. Patients with hypercalcemia at increased risk for pancreatitis and digoxin toxicity, commonly untreated in patients with cancer (J Intern Med 2001;250:73).

Lab: Metabolic profile to include calcium, albumin, magnesium and phosphate, TSH, amylase, lipase; consider ABG; EKG—special attention to QT interval (J Peds 2000;136:404; J Clin Psychopharmacol 2000;20:260); urine for calcium in hypocalcemia.

Emergency Management:

Hypocalcemia:

1st: vitamin D_3 50,000-100,000+ U each day; or 1,25-$(OH)_2$ vitamin D (Rocaltrol), expensive; narrow margins of safety for hypercalcemia.

2nd: Calcium po or iv; Calcium gluconate 10% 10 cc iv or calcium chloride 10% 5 cc iv—repeat PRN every 5 min.

3rd: Chlorthalidone 50 mg po qd or other thiazide, with low-salt diet, voids renal stones of vitamin D treatment.

Experimental use of synthetic PTH.

Hypercalcemia:

Acute treatment for Ca > 13 mg%:

• Normal saline 2.5-4 L/24 h iv to ensure intravascular volume adequately replaced (CVP or Swann-Ganz monitoring), avoid furosemide initially, but often needed after volume replaced to prevent volume overload and accelerate renal clearance.

• Pamidronate (Aredia) 60-90 mg iv over 24 hr, or 4-8 mg/hr.

Chronic treatment:

• Biphosphonates, eg, pamidronate (Aredia) 60-90 mg iv infusion over 8-24 hr or 1200 mg po qd × 5 d.

• Steroids primarily for sarcoid patients, eg, prednisone 20 mg po tid or iv 3-4 d.

• Calcitonin 4 U/kg q 6 hr sc or im, relatively weak agent alone.

- Indomethacin (rarely helpful if due to cancer).
- Gallium nitrate iv infusion, experimental 200 mg/M^2 in 1 L continuous infusion qd × 5 d.

11.3 Magnesium Disorders

Emerg Med Clin N Am 1989;7:795; Can Med Assoc J 1985;132:360

Cause:
- *Hypomagnesemia* seen with gi fluid and electrolyte loss treated with Magnesium-free fluids; malnutrition; diabetes mellitus (Arch IM 1996;156:1143); fistulae; burns; diuretics; cisplatinum-induced renal disease; cyclosporine use in transplant recipients (J Am Coll Cardiol 1992;20:806), and commonly associated with hypokalemia (Clin Chem 1983;29:178), hypophosphatemia, hyponatremia, and hypocalcemia (Arch IM 1984;144:1794).
- *Hypermagnesemia* seen in renal failure often parallels potassium; chronic Magnesium containing antacid and laxative use (Ann Emerg Med 1996;28:552). Enemas, especially in megacolon, with Magnesium-containing soaps.

Epidem:
- Hypomagnesemia associated with large gi fluid losses and malnutrition, eg, with ulcerative colitis, regional enteritis, chronic alcoholics, toxemia of pregnancy, primary hypo/hyperparathyroidism, primary hyperaldosteronism, thyrotoxicosis, RTA, diuretic phase of ATN.
- Hypermagnesemia is much less common.

Pathophys: Average daily intake of Magnesium is 20-40 mEq. Total body stores are 2000 mEq, half in bones, half intracellular. Low Magnesium inhibits PTH secretion, which in turn causes hypocalcemic si/sx. Ethanol also inhibits PTH secretion.

METABOLIC

Sx:

- Hypomagnesemia causes cramps.
- Hypermagnesemia causes difficulty with defecation, and urination; nausea; drowsiness at pharmacologic doses only.

Si:

- Hypomagnesemia causes carpal-pedal spasm, Chvostek's sign, Trousseau's sign (p223); delirium, muscle tremor, and bizarre movements, convulsions, hypotension.
- Hypermagnesemia causes depressed DTRs and hypotension.

Crs: Ventricular arrhythmias can be abolished with magnesium supplementation in those with hypomagnesemia (J Intern Med 2000;247:78). Ataxias in hypomagnesemia take months to clear. No correlation of hypomagnesemia with degree of cardiac distress in those with chest pain (Arch IM 1991;151:2185).

Cmplc:

- Hypomagnesemia may have hypocalcemia; and/or hypokalemia in cisplatin type.
- Hypermagnesemia may go onto heart block and respiratory paralysis, and hypocalcemia, as well (Nejm 1984;310:1221).

Lab: Metabolic profile to include magnesium, calcium, albumin, and phosphate; EKG

Emergency Management:

- *Hypomagnesemia* requires 40-80 mEq of $MgSO_4$ (10 cc of a 50% hydrated soln, 1 gm = 8 mEq) iv in 1 L D_5NS or D_5W over 3 hr.
- *Hypermagnesemia* requires calcium gluconate 5-10 mEq (10-20 cc of 10% soln iv) (Nejm 1984;310:1221).

11.4 Phosphorous Disorders

Crit Care Clin 1991;7:201; Endocrinol Metab Clin N Am 1993;22:397

Cause: *Hypophosphatemia* seen in sepsis (Am J Med 1998;104:40); malnutrition (J Peds 1998;133:789) or drugs such as aluminum-binding antacids, iv glucose, catecholmines, β-agonists, $NaHCO_3$, or acetazolamide (Ann Pharmacother 1994;28:626)—think COPD (Chest 1994;105:1392); renal tubular damage from hypokalemia; osmotic diuresis; or rarely Fanconi's anemia or hyperphosphaturia from vitamin D intoxication (Ann IM 1966;64:1066). In types without cell injury like acute DKA, hyperalimentation, or acute respiratory alkalosis, no bad consequences occur because total body PO_4 depletion has not occurred.

   Hyperphosphatemia may be seen in renal failure (Clin Nephrol 1977;7:138), hypoparathyroidism, exogenous phosphate loading via po or enema, ketoacidosis, rhabdomyolysis, and rarer causes such as tumor lysis syndrome.

Epidem: Hyperphosphatemia much more uncommon than hypophosphatemia.

Pathophys: Hypophosphatemia can be classified as follows: mild is 2.3-3 mg/dL, moderate is 1.6-2.2 mg/dL, and severe is < 1.5 mg/dL (Crit Care Med 1995;23:1504).

Sx: Hypo—confusion, weakness.

Si: Both—nothing specific.

Cmplc:
- Hypo—bleeding (impaired platelet function) and infections (impaired granulocyte function) (J Lab Clin Med 1974;84:643); rhabdomyolysis (Am J Med 1992;92:458).
- Hyper—complications secondary to induction of hypocalcemia (p222).

Lab: Metabolic profile with phosphorous, calcium, and magnesium.

Emergency Management:

Hypophosphatemia:
- 2.5 mg elemental phosphorous/kg in NS over 12 hr via iv or po with NeutraPhos.

Hyperphosphatemia:
- Oral phosphate binders to decrease phosphate absorption in the gi tract.

11.5 Potassium Disorders

Hypokalemia

J Am Soc Nephrol 1997;8:1179

Cause: Loop diuretics—most common; gi losses with persistent vomiting, diarrhea, or other drainage; β-agonist medications (Ped Emerg Care 1998;114:145; Ped Pulmonol 1999:27)—such as nebulized meds; renal tubular acidosis—Type I; hyperaldosteronism; ion shifting with $NaHCO_3$ or insulin and glucose administration iv; malnutrition; hypercalcemia; and hypomagnesemia. Rarely thyrotoxic periodic paralysis (Am J Emerg Med 1989;7:584), theophylline overdose (since this overdose is now more uncommon) (Am J Emerg Med 1988;6:214), or acute leukemia; in children IVF resuscitation (Ped Emerg Care 1990;6:13) or head trauma (J Ped Surg 1997;32:88).

Epidem: Common in those using loop diuretics.

Pathophys: K^+ levels < 2.5 mEq/L considered severe; < 2 mEq/L may induce respiratory paralysis.
- Paradoxical aciduria
- Nephrogenic DI with severe dehydration
- Glycosuria
- Increased ammonia production

Sx: Fatigue; nonspecific.

Si: Fatigue; nonspecific.

Crs: Worse with accompanying ventricular ectopy.

Cmplc: Coincident digitalis; use necessitates higher threshold for normal, with K^+ preferably > 4 mEq/L.

Diff Dx: Bartter syndrome; Liddle syndrome (pseudohyperaldosteronism).

Lab: Metabolic profile with calcium, magnesium; EKG—low voltage, flat T-waves, widening QRS, prominent U waves. Urine K^+ levels < 20 mEq/L suggests chronic etiology.

Emergency Management:
- Continuous monitoring
- Iv KCl with no more than 40 mEq/hr, put in 250 cc iv bag.
- KCl 20 mEq po if possible.
- Consider co-incident magnesium correction with 2 gm iv, especially if arrhythmias present.
- Consult for admission if necessitating ongoing iv replacement, serum level severe/critical or symptomatic.

Hyperkalemia

Semin Nephrol 1998;18:46

Cause: Renal failure, hemolysis, rhabdomyolysis, freshwater drownings, Addison's disease, ACE inhibitor use (Nejm 2004;351:585), NSAID use (Am J Kidney Dis 1994;24:578), TMP/SMX use especially in AIDS patients.

Epidem: Unknown.

Pathophys: Worsening or inability of kidneys to excrete K^+, versus overwhelming cell lysis as seen in hemolysis or freshwater drowning.

Sx: Palpitations or nonspecific constitutional complaints.

Si: Nonspecific.

Crs: Variable.

Cmplc: Lethal arrhythmias may manifest.

Diff Dx: "Pseudo"-hyperkalemia due to thrombocythemia, increased white cells, fist-clenching (causing hemolysis) with blood draw or delay in processing blood specimen.

Lab: Metabolic profile.
- EKG shows tall peaked T waves, which may evolve to wide QRS, then evolves to sine wave as K^+ increases—do not base diagnosis on EKG findings (PPV 65% and NPV 69%) (Ann EM 1991;20:1229).

Emergency Management:

Conn Med 1999;63:131
- Iv access.
- Calcium gluconate 10% 10 cc iv or calcium chloride 10% 5 cc iv—repeat prn in 5 min for cardioprotective effects. **N.B.** DO NOT USE CALCIUM IF SUSPECTED DIGITALIS TOXICITY.
- $NaHCO_3$ 1-2 amps iv, lowering plasma H^+ will force H^+ out of cells with tradeoff of K^+ going into cells.
- Regular insulin 10-30 U iv, give along with amp (50 cc, which is 25 gm) of D50 if sugar is normal, low, or unknown—this will drive K^+ into cells.
- Albuterol nebulizer 10-20 mg over 30 min (each U dose is 2.5 mg) (J Intern Med 1990;228:35).
- In children, may consider salbutamol 5 µg/kg iv D_5W over 15 min (Clin Nephrol 1996;46:67), may give nebulized, if iv access a problem.
- K^+-resin binder po such as Kayexalate, may give along with Sorbitol.
- Consider dialysis or hemofiltration (Child Nephrol Urol 1988;9:236).

11.6 Sodium Disorders

Emerg Med Clin N Am 1989;7:749; Clin Lab Med 1993;13:135; Peds (Ped Ann 1995;24:23)

Hyponatremia

Am J Emerg Med 2000;18:264

Cause: Elevated antidiuretic hormone (ADH) from: (1) SIADH or tumor; (2) Drugs such as vincristine, cytoxan, clofibrate, narcotics, nicotine, isoproterenol or tricyclic antidepressants; or (3) Hypovolemia.

- Increased renal ADH sensitivity due to: (1) 1st but not 2nd generation hypoglycemics; (2) NSAIDs; (3) Thiazides; or (4) Carbamazepine.
- Lab error (pseudohyponatremia) due to elevated triglycerides, proteins, glucose, mannitol, or post-TURP glycine.
- Free water replacement of isotonic emesis, diarrhea, blood, serum; or seen as idiopathic cause post-operatively.
- Dehydration in extreme athletes (Clin J Sport Med 2000;10: 52) or prolonged heat exposure with exertion (Am J Emerg Med 1999;17:532).
- Hypothyroidism, Addison's disease.
- Psychiatric patients with polydipsia, SIADH, and decreased renal free water excretion.
- Alcoholics, especially if only nutrition is ethanol (Ann EM 1986;15:745).
- Post-op for 1-3 d, equal sex ratio, 1% incidence; caused by high ADH levels and hypotonic or sometimes even isotonic iv fluids, but respiratory arrest and mortality much higher in menstruating women.

Epidem: F > M.

Pathophys: Free water replacement/conservation without regard for sodium.

Sx: Confusion.

Si: Altered mental status; seizures [especially infants < 6 mon of age (Ann EM 1995;26:42)].

METABOLIC

Crs: Variable based on cause—morbidity/mortality usually based on underlying cause, with hyponatremia usually a poor prognostic sign.

Cmplc: Mortality increased 60 × in hospitalized patients when Na < 130.

Lab: CBC with diff; metabolic profile with Na < 125; uric acid < 5 mg% with ADH-producing tumor or SIADH: if fever, pursue ID eval with blood cultures, urine culture, and consider LP and CXR.

Emergency Management:

Acutely:
- Stop drugs
- Iv NS and furosemide—if developed slowly, correct at < 2.5 mEq/hr, not > 10 mEq/d vs not > 20 mEq/d with isotonic or perhaps hypertonic saline (3% NaCl), and possibly iv furosemide, then go slowly to avoid pontine demyelination; or go slowly over days, no benefit from rushing or using twice NS, even when Na^+ < 110, unless symptomatic or is very acute (Am J Med 1985;78:897); use of hypertonic saline must be considered an exceptional practice.
- Consider dialysis with hypertonic solution and intraperitoneal as first choice.

For chronic cases:
- Restrict water and give liberal salt diet or tablets.
- Consider salt tablets plus loop diuretic.
- Consider demeclocycline (Declomycin, a tetracycline) 0.6-1.2 gm qd.
- Consider lithium 300 mg po tid or qid.
- Possible future use of vasopressin antagonist.

Hypernatremia

Endocrinol Metab Clin N Am 1993;22:411

Cause:
- Central and nephrogenic diabetes insipidus (DI)—see Hyperosmolar States on p73.
- Dehydration from inability to drink, betadine treatment of burns or diminished urine concentration and diminished thirst in elderly especially in the setting of adult onset diabetes mellitus—this may lead to a nonketotic hyperosmolar state.

Epidem: Pregnancy may unmask DI.

Pathophys: See Hyperosmolar States for DI; p73. Dehydration as per etiology.

Sx: Excessive thirst and urination; confusion.

Si: Altered mental status; hypotension; dehydration.

Crs: Infantile dehydration may lead to mental retardation.

Cmplc: Mortality > 40% in elderly; infantile.

Diff Dx: Psychogenic water drinker who can partially concentrate urine with fluid restriction.

Lab: CBC with diff; metabolic profile; serum osmoles; UA; urine osmoles—look for Na > 150.

Emergency Management:
- Acutely replace water but not > 12 mEq/24 hr secondary to cerebral edema.
- Calculate water deficit and treatment for DI—p73 (hyperosmolar states).

Chapter 12

Nephrology

12.1 Acute Renal Failure

Am Fam Phys 2000;61:2077; Jama 2003;289:747

Cause:

- *Pre-renal:* Hypovolemia, anemia.
- *Renal:* Drug toxicity [eg, NSAIDs (Am J Epidem 2000;151: 488)—even topical (BMJ 2000;320:93)] and salicylates and acetaminophen possibly implicated in chronic renal failure (CRF) (Nejm 2001;345:1801); acute tubular necrosis (ATN)—as seen in shock, crush injuries, hypothermia, heavy metal toxicity, snake venom toxicity, organic solvent toxicity, intravascular hemolysis; rhabdomyolysis from drug abuse, such as ethanol, iv heroin, and more recently iv temazepam (Qjm 2000;93:29) or wild mushroom intoxication (Nejm 2001; 345:798); iv dye reaction in those with underlying renal insufficiency; multiple myeloma (Nephron 2000;85:96); HIV with many etiologies such as interstitial nephritis (Am J Kidney Dis 2000;35:557).
- *Post-renal:* Obstruction.

Epidem: Community-acquired is much more common (3×) in the black population compared to whites (Arch IM 2000;160:1309), with possibly higher mortality rates.

Pathophys: Many physiologic effects from cellular death and ATP depletion, many competing theories of most significant mechanism (Semin Nephrol 2000;20:4). Ensuing acidosis, calcium

phosphorus imbalances, hyperkalemia, anemia, HT, peripheral and autonomic neuropathy from PTH; delayed hypersensitivity immune suppression, pruritus probably from histamine.
- Uremia may lead to sallow skin, pericardial effusion.

Sx: Lassitude, pruritus, nausea/vomiting, anorexia, muscle cramps, sleep disturbance.

Si: Uremic breath, increased pigmentation, postural hypotension or hypertension, absent tendon reflexes and other peripheral neuropathies—reversible.

Crs: Variable, even straightforward causes (eg, hypovolemia) may progress to a chronic process; poorer prognosis with increased age, recent MI, CHF, requiring respiratory support, or liver dysfunction (Clin Nephrol 2000;53:10).

Cmplc: Chronic renal failure; secondary infection (Nephrol Dial Transplant 2000;15:212).

Lab: CBC with diff; metabolic profile including calcium, magnesium, phosphorus; UA; urine culture; venous pH/ABG; type and screen; EKG. Screening for renal dysfunction before iv contrast with serum creatinine has been advocated, and may even consider urine dipstick for protein as a screen (Emerg Radiol 2004:319)—obviously, risk benefit decision on the utility of the study vs time for screening of renal dysfunction must be weighed.
- *X-ray:* Renal US.
- Calculating Creatinine Clearance (CrCl or C_{Cr}) (Nephron 1976;16:31):

CrCl = $[(140 - age) \times weight (kg)/ (72 \times serum creatinine)] \times (0.85 for women)$

Emergency Management:
- Hold all potentially offending drugs; place indwelling catheter.
- Consider iv fluid bolus for hypovolemia (Drugs 2000;59:79), correction of anemia.

- Trial of α-blocker Alfuzosin 10 mg/d for 3 d with catheter removal after two doses and one additional dose after catheter removal with an odds ratio for success almost 2, with failures seen with older age (> 65 yr of age) and higher initial retention volumes (> 1000 ml)—this was studied in those with BPH (J Urol 2004;171:2316).
- Treat underlying arrhythmias/hyperkalemia, as warranted.
- Thyroxine of no help in euthyroid patients (Kidney Int 2000;57:293).
- Dialysis to prevent complications and death (Kidney Int 1972;1:190), better with daily treatment (Nejm 2002; 346:305).

Prevention:
- Hydration with 154 mEq/L of sodium bicarbonate with a 3 cc/kg bolus 1 hr before the procedure and follow this with 1 cc/kg per hr for 6 hr after the procedure to decrease the incidence of contrast-induced nephropathy from 13.6% to 1.7% when comparing against NS (same volumes) (Jama 2004; 291:2328)—whether this translates into treatment of actual clinical disease is debatable.
- Acetylcysteine 600 mg po bid × 2 d prior to procedure with iv dye in those with moderate CRF (Jama 2003;289:553)—same caveat as to whether this prevents actual clinical disease.
- Perhaps use iso-osmolar dimeric, nonionic contrast (iodixanol) in those who need iv dye (Nejm 2003;348:491).

12.2 Dialysis Patient Issues

J Emerg Med 1992;10:317

Cause: Patients receiving either peritoneal dialysis or hemodialysis have a time intensive commitment, but those with hemodialysis have less flexibility and more side effects.

Pathophys: Continuous ambulatory peritoneal dialysis (CAPD) with similar biochemical results as hemodialysis (HD) (Arch IM 1986;146:1138).

Adverse Effects: Similar in the two types of dialysis patients:

- Folate deficiency (BMJ 1969;2:18)
- EKG artifacts from fistula/cannula arm
- Pericarditis (Am J Med 1977;63:874)
- Pneumonia, atelectasis, and pleural effusion from CAPD (Lancet 1966;2:75)
- Mortality = 10-20% per yr, 5% per yr from peritonitis in those with CAPD (Perit Dial Int 1997;17:S15)
- Zinc deficiency (Am J Clin Pathol 1971;56:17) causes primary gonadal impairment, reversible with 2.5 mg po qd.
- Amyloidosis (Kidney Int suppl 1993;41:S78)
- Rare antacid Magnesium intoxication
- Rare Cu intoxication from tubing (Nejm 1967;276:1209)
- Iron deficiency
- Increased ASHD (Lancet 1980;1:276)
- Gynecomastia (Plast Reconstr Surg 1982;69:41)
- Hepatitis C (Nephron 1993;65:40)
- $CaPO_4$ deposits in joints (Contrib Nephrol 1984;84:58).
- Catheter displacement in those with CAPD (Clin Nephrol 1999;52:124).
- CVA (Stroke 1974;5:725)
- Secondary hyperparathyroidism with change in bony structure (Kidney Int suppl 1993;41:S116).
- Bleeding complications, secondary to platelet dysfunction and perhaps exacerbated by heparin use in those with hemodialysis (J Am Soc Nephrol 1991;2:961).
- Infection at central catheter or shunt site in hemodialysis; tunnel infection and peritonitis in peritoneal dialysis (Arch Surg 1984;119:1325).

- Scrotal swelling if patent processus vaginalis in those receiving peritoneal dialysis (Brit J Surg 1984;71:477)
- Pure red cell aplasia with recombinant erythropoietin (Nejm 2002;346:469).

12.3 Renal Calculi

Nejm 2004;350:684; Am Fam Phys 2001;63:1329; Emerg Med Clin N Am 1988;6:617

Cause: Calcium oxalate (75%), from hyperparathyroidism (approximately 10%) but probably most idiopathic hypercalciuria (rarely sarcoid)—which is genetic in most cases with autosomal dominant inheritance; struvite (10-15%), from UTIs with urease-producing organisms; urate (5%); hydroxyapatite or brushite (5%); cystine (1%). Protease inhibitor (indinavir) stones possible (Urology 1997;50:508), these are radiolucent.

Epidem: Incidence = 100:100,000 men, 36:100,000 women; 3-5% of U.S. population will get sometime in life; incidence higher in Southeast U.S. Increased risk with vasectomy (Am J Kidney Dis 1997;29:207) and associated with medullary sponge kidney (Clin Radiol 1982;33:435).

Pathophys: 80% of stones are calcium type, associate with a red blood cell and probable renal tubular oxalate excretion defect or a deficit of the calcium/magnesium pump; another 10% are associated with hyperparathyroidism.
- Increased calcium absorption may also play a role, either primary or by bringing out deficits like those above, eg, in sarcoid. Uric acid stones may also precipitate calcium on themselves.
- Calcium oxalate stones are increased in colectomy, blind loop syndrome, and intestinal bypass patients due to bacterial breakdown of bile salts leading to absorption of glycolytic acid.
- Struvite stones are caused by ammonia from urea-splitting proteus in patients with chronic UTIs due to indwelling Foley and/or quadriplegia.

Sx: Pain radiating into groin; urine may appear normal, tea-colored, or bloody.

Si: CVA tenderness; usually non-tender abdomen despite severe pain.

Crs: Recurrence after first stone is 15% at 1 yr; 35% at 5 yr; 50% at 10 yr.

Cmplc: Secondary infection; renal failure.

Diff Dx: AAA in elderly patient, which may also have laboratory evidence of microscopic hematuria; renal artery embolism pain; rarely primary hyperoxaluria with oxalosis as renal failure develops.

Lab: Urine dip for blood, consider formal UA if new diagnosis or if concerns of secondary infection; BUN/Cr; consider CBC with diff and urine culture and sensitivity if febrile or other concerns for complicated UTI; stone analysis; outpatient 24-hr urine 3 wks after stone passage in those with recurrent stones or cystine stones (test for volume, pH, calcium, oxalate, uric acid, phosphate, sodium, citrate creatinine, and sulfate—for those with cystine stones check volume, pH, creatinine, and quantitative measurement of cystine).

- CT without contrast better than IVP (Urol Radiol 1992;14:139; Radiology 1998;207:308); and better than US and plain radiograph (Am J Roentgenol 2002;178:379).

Emergency Management:

- Pain control, usually requires iv access with narcotic/antiemetic
- Consider iv NSAID, such as ketorolac 30 mg iv or 60 mg im administration with possible benefit for acute pain relief (BMJ 2004;328:1401, Brit J Urol 1990;66:602; Am J Emerg Med 1999;17:6)
- IVF bolus may make pain worse.
- Consult for admission if secondary infection or pain control issues.

Outpatient regimen:

- Pain control with po NSAID (all equivalent) and po narcotic; consider po or pr antiemetic for pain control synergism with narcotic and to better tolerate narcotic.
- Primary care follow-up; urology, if high-grade obstruction.
- Strain all urine.
- Increase po fluid intake, may be preventive but can make pain worse. Reduce salt and protein intake with normal calcium intake if calcium oxalate stones and hypercalciuria (Nejm 2002;346:77); avoid phosphoric acid-containing soft drinks (equivocal data).
- Avoid calcium supplements, but further restriction not helpful because calcium decreases oxalate and urate absorption.
- Drug regimens: Depending on 24-hr urine, metabolic evaluation, or stone type in peds (Ped Nephrol 1992;6:54) and adults (J Urol 1989;141:760); thiazide diuretics, allopurinol, polycitra K, sodium cellulose phosphate, acetohydroxamic acid, pyridoxine, or cholestyramine may be prescribed.
- Potential benefit of modest ethanol (beer) intake, low-fat diet, or weight reduction to reduce risk of nephrolithiasis (Am J Kidney Dis 1996;28:195).
- Cystoscopic stone retrieval, lithotripsy, or surgical removal may be required for stones causing persistent problems.

12.4 Urinary Retention

Emerg Med Clin N Am 1988;6:419; Ped Emerg Care 1993;9:205)

Cause: Medications (sympathomimetic agonist); voiding avoidance, such as a long car trip in someone with borderline obstruction; mechanical obstruction due to mass or stricture such as seen in prostatic hypertrophy, bladder carcinoma, or urolithiasis; blocked indwelling catheter; post-operative due to catecholamine release or perhaps due to spinal/epidural anesthesia; infection; systemic disease, such as hypothyroidism; or neurologic etiologies, such as trauma, spina bifida, or multiple sclerosis.

Epidem: Approximately 5% in post-op surgical patients, > 50% in those with genitourinary surgery; suggested that males have a higher incidence coincident with the lunar cycle (on the new moon) (BMJ 1989;299:1560).

Pathophys: As above, either inability to pass urine around a fixed lesion, or due to inability to control bladder neck muscles.

Sx: Lower abdominal pain.

Si: Palpable bladder; assess for obvious mechanical problem such as stenotic urethral opening or imperforate hymen (J Accid Emerg Med 1999;16:232); overflow incontinence.

Crs: Drainage is therapeutic and diagnostic.

Cmplc: Post-obstructive diuresis; secondary infection (if frank pus, pyocystis).

Diff Dx: Rarely due to acute abdominal processes such as ectopic pregnancy (Am J Emerg Med 1999;17:44) or appendiceal abscess (Ann EM 1993;22:857), pathophysiology uncertain.

Lab: Urine for culture, if infection suspected.
- *X-ray:* bladder scan or US with > 500 cc post void residual.

Emergency Management:
- Access with 16F Foley catheter; Coude catheter if necessary.
- If cannot access, filiforms and followers if urethral stenosis or urologic consult.
- If post-operative or secondary to chronic process requiring intermittent catheterization, OK to remove catheter after drainage if urine clears with irrigation.
- Iv access with narcotic analgesic if pain uncontrollable and cannot quickly access bladder. May also consider phenazopyridine (Pyridium) 200 mg po tid for 2-3 d PRN for bladder or urethral pain; turns urine dark orange and prolonged use may lead to methemoglobinemia (Acta Urol Belg 1967;35:465).

- If new acute problem, chronic disease with new manifestation, or urine not clearing with irrigation, leave catheter in place and leg bag for home. Urology follow-up in 2-3 d, if not sooner.
- Consider antibiotics if secondary infection suspected.
- Urologic consult for admission if continuous irrigation necessary secondary to pyocystis or recurrent catheter obstruction secondary to blood clots.
- Also consider admission if symptomatic postobstructive diuresis (Brit J Urol 1989;64:559)—profuse passage of urine, hypotension, dizziness, or tachycardia.

12.5 Urinary Tract Infection

Nejm 2003;349:259; Emerg Med Clin N Am 1988;6:403; Inf Dis Clin N Am 1997;11:551; Ped Clin N Am 1999;46:1111

Cause: Infectious cystitis/urethritis in females due to coliforms 70% of the time, with other pathogens such as *Staphylococcus saprophyticus*, Proteus, or STDs, such as *Chlamydia trachomatis*, *Gonorrhea*, or herpes simplex.

Epidem: Incidence approximately 20% of all women each yr, increased with catheters, sexual activity (Epidemiology 1995;6:162), cervical cap or diaphragm use, and previous UTI (Am J Epidem 1986;124:977; Nejm 1996;335:468). Not prevented by various hygiene habits, except voiding after sex. Unknown rate if children < 2 yr of age, but suspect it is common among females, especially in those with fever without origin, and URI and OM do not exclude this diagnosis (Peds 1998;102:e16).

Nosocomial risks include catheter, which may be placed without clear indication in many elderly patients who are hospitalized (Am J Infect Control 2004;32:196), diabetes mellitus, coincident infection, not free draining catheter, and renal insufficiency (Am J Epidem 1986;124:977).

Recurrence within 6 mon associated with initial *E. coli* infection (Am J Epidem 2000;151:1194).

Pathophys: Most likely ascending disease; thus women are more prone secondary to short urethra. Recurrent disease, due to a possible inherent defect in epithelial cell membrane leading to easier adherence by bacteria.

Sx: Dysuria, urgency, frequency, blood in urine; stuttering onset over many days with Chlamydia; cystitis with internal pain (Arch IM 1978;138:1069) or pain at end of urination. One or more symptom makes the probability of infection at least 50% (Jama 2002;287:2701).

Si: Pain superior to pubis symphysis with cystitis; costovertebral angle tenderness with pyelonephritis; prostadynia with prostatitis.

Crs: Many resolve without treatment; catheter-induced UTIs have 2-4 times the mortality of non-catheter-induced UTIs (suspect may be secondary to overall health of those requiring indwelling catheters) and only $\frac{1}{3}$ resolve after removal without treatment; 90% will resolve with single dose or 10-d antibiotic treatment.

Cmplc:
- Pyelonephritis: possibly secondary to ascending infection, may also be due to hematogenous seeding. Increased incidence in neonates, infants up to 18 mon, females of childbearing age, and those s/p gu instrumentation. Increased cases in papillary necrosis as seen in sickle cell disease and diabetes. Look for fever, flank pain, and CVA tenderness.
- Evaluate for reflux in children with first case with renal US and VCUG—outpatient work-up (Am J Roentgenol 1994;162:1393).
- Emphysematous cystitis, seen usually in those with diabetes mellitus.

Diff Dx: Urolithiasis; vaginitis (Peds 1982;70:299), herpes, and chronic interstitial (idiopathic) cystitis (Curr Opin Obgyn 1990;2:605).

Lab: UA—dipstick nitrite with high false pos; although nitrite and leukocyte esterase are sensitive if the pt is thought to have the disease and tests are pos, otherwise less reliable (Ann IM 1992;117:135); rapid urine catalase test (Uriscreen) with 100% sensitivity and thus, high neg predictive value and could be used to predict those who do not have UTI (Peds 1999;104:e41); number of WBCs per hpf only useful depending on pretest probability—symptomatic and > 5-6 WBCs per hpf as threshold with 10% false neg and 50% false pos; urine Gram stain of unspun urine highly predictive of UTI (Ann EM 1995;25:31; J Clin Microbiol 1982;15:468); hematuria may be present.

- Urine culture if neonate, infant (Peds 1998;101:E1), child or those with potentially complicated UTI (this includes pregnancy)—10^5 organisms only in 50% of infected women; 10^2 better criterion when symptomatic. Consider CBC with diff and blood cultures if considering pyelonephritis, although these data not usually helpful (Acad Emerg Med 1997;4:797; Am J Emerg Med 1997;15:137). Need catheter urine in children < 2 yr of age, and first drops of specimen should be discarded (Ped Emerg Care 2000;16:88). PSA may be used in men with occult disease such as work-up of fever of unknown origin (Prostate 2004;60:282).
- IVP and cystoscopy of no value to work-up recurrent UTIs in adult women.

Emergency Management:

Uncomplicated UTI

N.B. *[in peds, difficult to distinguish upper from lower tract infection so treat all for 7-14 d* (Peds 2002;109:E70)]

- Sulfasoxazole 500 mg po qid, TMP/SMX single or double strength bid (peds—4 TMP/20 SMX per kg per dose bid to a max of 160 TMP/800 SMX), ciprofloxacin 100 mg po bid, ofloxacin 200 mg po bid (Am J Med 1999;106:292), or amoxicillin 250-500 mg po tid for 3-5 d; but consider 5-7 d treatment with nitrofurantoin (Macrobid) 1 bid (J Antimicrob Chemother 1999;43:67).
- Single-dose regimens (Ann EM 1984;13:432): TMP/SMX DS 1-2 pills (Rev Infect Dis 1982;4:444), amoxicillin 2-3 gm po, sulfasoxazole 1-2 gm po, or ciprofloxacin 500 mg po—more frequent recurrence.
- Phenazopyridine (Pyridium) 200 mg po tid for 2-3 d PRN for bladder or urethral pain; turns urine dark orange and prolonged use may lead to methemoglobinemia (Acta Urol Belg 1967;35:465).
- Encourage fluids, specifically cranberry juice in women (Epidemiology 1995;6:162; BMJ 2001;322:1571; Can J Urol 2002;9:1558)—complexes with E. coli so that bacteria does not "stick" to bladder epithelium.
- Asymptomatic bacteriuria is not an indication for treatment (J Am Ger Soc 1996;44:293), and is generally not improved with treatment.
- Infants should be treated if any suspicion and follow-up then based on urine culture.

Catheter-related:
- Remove catheter if possible, treat if symptomatic—will not clear UTI with persistent indwelling catheterization.

Prophylaxis:
- Post-menopausal women may benefit from estriol 0.5 mg cream (Ovestin) qd for 2 wks, then biweekly if no contraindications.
- TMP/SMX half single-strength pill each night or post-coital is cost effective if ≥ 3 UTIs/yr.

Complicated UTI (includes UTI in pregnancy, upper tract infection, young children, prostatitis, etc)

- Consider first dose of antibiotics iv/im, such as ceftriaxone 1-2 gm iv; oral ciprofloxacin 500 mg po as expedient as iv medication, and effective (Can Med Assoc J 1994;150:669). Cefazolin 1-2 gm iv and ampicillin 1 gm iv safe in pregnancy.
- Control pain, vomiting, and dehydration issues.
- If outpatient, 10-14 d course of treatment with TMP/SMX DS bid or ciprofloxacin 250-500 mg po bid; if allergic to the former, use amoxicillin 500 mg po tid or cephalexin 500 mg tid.
- Pregnancy (Ann Pharmacother 1994;28:248): simple bacteriuria with single dose amoxicillin or cephalexin; symptomatic UTI with 3 d of amoxicillin or cephalexin at above doses; upper tract infection with 10-14 d of amoxicillin or cephalexin. All with repeat culture 1 wk after finishing therapy.
- If septic or cannot control secondary symptoms (such as vomiting), consult for admission.

Chapter 13

Neurology/Neurosurgery

13.1 Acute Serotonin Syndrome

Nejm 2005;352:1112; J Psychopharm 1999;13:100

Cause: MAO inhibitors (*Hypericum perforatum*, aka St. John's Wort, is a weak MAO inhibitor), SSRIs (selective serotonin reuptake inhibitors), and non-selective 5-HT receptor agonist/antagonist, specifically *meta*-Chlorophenylpiperazine (*m*-CPP) (Psychiatry Res 1998;79:207) as leading causes, with increased likelihood when combined with meperidine (Acad Emerg Med 1999;6:156), dextromethorphan, venlafaxine (Neurol 1998;51:274), bromocriptine, levodopa, buspirone, lithium, cocaine, amphetamines, ecstacy (Ann EM 1998;32:377), tramadol (J R Soc Med 1999;92:474), or other serotonergic drugs (Med J Aust 1998; 169:523). Equivocal data for combination with sumatriptan (Ann Pharmacother 1998;32:33).

Epidem: Not uncommon, with symptoms occurring within hours or days when increasing the dose of or adding a serotonergic drug; in approximately 14-16% of pts who are seen for SSRI overdose (J Toxicol Clin Toxicol 2004;42:277).

Pathophys: Increased activity at the post-synaptic serotonin receptors in the brain (Ped Emerg Care 1999;15:440).

Sx: Agitation, anxiety, shakiness, nausea.

Si: Mental status changes; tremors; seizures; autonomic instability with tachycardia or dysrhythmias, diaphoresis, hyperthermia,

HT, diarrhea, salivation, rigidity, dysarthria, ataxia, myoclonus, hyperreflexia, or localized neuro signs or deficits.

Crs: Most recover within 24 hr; this may be a difficult diagnosis when confounded with drugs of abuse—have a high index of suspicion.

Cmplc: Rhabdomyolysis with subsequent myoglobinuria; fatalities rare but possible.

Diff Dx: NMS, drug abuse, or withdrawal (including serotonin withdrawal syndrome), malignant hyperthermia, meningitis, encephalitis, heat stroke, MAO inhibitor interactions, acute lethal catatonia, central anticholinergic crisis that responds to iv physostigmine, thyroid storm.

Lab: Clinical diagnosis when other etiologies excluded—CBC with diff; metabolic profile with Calcium and Magnesium; UA with myoglobin; CPK; aldolase; panculture if suspect infectious etiology; TSH if suspect endocrine source; consider LP.

- *X-ray:* Head CT or MRI if suspect bleed, focal deficit, or other CNS concerns.

Emergency Management:

- Hold all meds, especially serotonergic agonists—listed above, also avoid codeine.
- Iv fluids; sodium bicarbonate drip, if rhabdomyolysis (p484). Consider norepinephrine (p 51) if persistent hypotension.
- Consider serotonin antagonists such as cyproheptadine 0.5 mg/kg per day divided into q 4-6 hr dosing at a maximum dose of 32 mg/d—usually 4-8 mg po each dose (Ped Emerg Care 1999;15:325; J Emerg Med 1998;16:615); may elect to try olanzapine 10 mg sl (J Toxicol Clin Toxicol 2004:725) or chlorpromazine 50-100 mg im (J Psychopharm 1999:100).
- Benzodiazepines may be used to lessen discomfort or for mild hyperthermia—non-selective serotonin antagonists. Severe

hyperthermia may necessitate non-depolarizing paralysis (such as vecuronium or rocuronium).

13.2 Acute Stroke Syndrome/Cerebral Vascular Accident (CVA)

Nejm 2001;344:1450; Ann EM 2001;37:202; 1999;34:244; Am J Epidem 1999;150:1266; Stroke 1996;27:1711

Cause: Cerebrovascular accident classified according to 3 groups, and all types associated with HT and smoking (Jama 1999; 281:1112)

1) Thrombotic CVA due to atherosclerosis (Cerebrovasc Dis 2000;10:102), which can be thought of to have the same risk factors for atherosclerosis as seen in those with coronary artery disease (for risks, Acute Coronary Syndrome see p7); hypotension—this may be transient and physiologic as seen in sleep; homocystinuria; crack cocaine abuse; migraine; high-dose estrogen birth control pills; arteritis caused by radiation, collagen vascular diseases (Lupus 1997;6:420; Arthritis Rheum 1998;41:1497), drug use, including ethanol in males (Alcohol 1999;19:119); infection leading to venous thrombosis or carotid occlusion; trauma to carotid or head that may cause spasm—associated with hx migraines; hematologic causes such as polycythemia, sickle cell disease (Blood 1998;91:288), TTP, DIC, dysproteinemias. Associated with homocystinuria, crack cocaine use, anabolic steroids (Neurology 1994;44:2405) and immediate post-partum period.

2) Embolic CVA due to proximal arterial atherosclerotic plaque; left-sided cardiac lesion as seen in SBE, left atrial myxoma, or clot (mitral stenosis or mitral valve billowing, prosthetic valve, sustained or intermittent atrial fibrillation (J Am Coll

Cardiol 2000;35:183), post-MI mural thrombus); paradoxical embolus from right heart, fat emboli, or venous system if patent intracardiac (foramen ovale—40% of pts < 55 yr of age with CVA have this open) right-to-left shunt. Associated with homocystinuria.

3) Hemorrhagic CVA is further subdivided into intra-parenchymal vs subarachnoid:

Subarachnoid CVAs due to aneurysm or AV malformation; associated with ethanol use in females (Alcohol 1999;19:119).

Intraparenchymal CVAs are 50% due to HT, 17% from amyloid angiopathy, 10% from anticoagulation treatment, 5-10% from brain tumors, 5% from smoking, 5% from crack cocaine use.

Epidem:

- Thrombotic CVAs comprise 34% of all CVAs in large vessel type, and 19% of all CVAs in lacunar CVAs; 3% are pts < 40 yr of age.

- Embolic CVAs comprise 31% of all CVAs, with 5 times increased incidence in atherosclerotic Afib, and 17 times increase in rheumatic Afib. 35% lifetime increased incidence in Afib, ¾ are embolic. For those with non-valvular Afib, use of warfarin with INR of 2 or greater leads to beneficial pt impact on frequency of ischemic CVA and the morbidity and mortality associated with ischemic CVA episodes (Nejm 2003;349:1019).

- Subarachnoid hemorrhages comprise 7% of all CVAs and 1% of all adults have aneurysm. 2% of all with subarachnoid bleed and aneurysm have polycystic kidneys; associated with iv cocaine use; sometimes familial; sometimes with Ehler-Danlos syndrome, Marfan syndrome, and Type I neuro-fibromatosis.

- Intraparenchymal bleeds comprise 9% of all CVAs.

- Increased risk of hemorrhagic CVA (both types—subarachnoid and intraparenchymal) with use of phenylpropanolamine (Nejm 2000;343:1826).
- Higher risk if previous CVA, especially if patent foramen ovale or atrial septal aneurysm (Nejm 2001;345:1740)
- Increased risk of CVA with white matter lesions on MRI and increased more if coincident retinopathy (Jama 2002;288:67).
- Black Americans with 2 times risk for intracerebral hemorrhage compared to whites (Neurol 1999;52:1617).
- Neurologic syncope of any cause associated with approximately 3 times higher risk for CVA (Nejm 2002;347:878)
- Possible Southeastern U.S. stroke belt (Am J Med Sci 1999;317:160).
- Increased risk with either surgical or radiotherapy of pituitary adenoma (Int J Radiat Oncol Biol Phys 1999;45:693).
- Livedo reticularis may be noted on physical exam in those with CVA who have antiphospholipid syndrome (Sneddon's syndrome) (J Eur Acad Dermatol Venereol 1999;12:157).
- Systemic respiratory infections associated with an increase in vascular events in the first 3 d of illness—this is not seen with immunizations (Nejm 2004;351:2611).

Pathophys: Thrombotic CVAs usually affect a watershed area in anterior circulation or vertebral basilar syndrome. Hypertension is a marker for stroke risk, but CVAs in these patients is a multifactorial issue, genetically determined (Cardiologia 1999;44:433). Hyperglycemia linked to delay in calcium recovery in ischemic stroke (J Cereb Blood Flow Metab 1992;12:469), and degree of hyperglycemia linked to size of infarct (Schweiz Arch Neurol Psychiatr 1993;144:233) and worse outcome (Stroke 1993; 24:1129). Increase in superoxide dismutase (Life Sci 1994; 54:711) in ischemic stroke, perhaps secondary to oxygen radicals causing problems.

Sx:

Thrombotic: TIA hx in 80%; nocturnal onset in 60%.

Embolic: Very abrupt onset; seizures occasionally.

Subarachnoid bleed: Severe headache of sudden onset which is frequently preceded by milder sentinel headache, nausea, vomiting, possible loss of consciousness, possible neck and back pain.

Intraparenchymal bleed:
- Cerebellar with ataxia, headache, vomiting, nausea.
- Cerebral with decreased level of consciousness, sudden onset headache, nausea, vomiting.

Si: Lateralized neurologic findings (see Table 13.1).

Carotid occlusion or significant stenosis may be elucidated with flow reversal through the supraorbital artery that one feels, and then occludes the facial artery as it wraps anterior to the inferior border of the mandible just anterior to the angle of the jaw—if lose pulse, then flow is reversed.

Thrombotic and Embolic with specific occlusion patterns:
- Middle cerebral: Face and arm motor; expressive aphasia (Broca's).
- Carotid watershed: Parietal aphasias, weakness arm > face > leg.
- Posterior cerebral: Homonymous hemianopsia, hemisensory loss, memory loss.
- Lateral medullary plate syndrome—posterior inferior cerebellar artery: Ipsilateral pain and temperature loss on face, contralateral for rest of body, hoarseness, swallowing dysfunction, Horner's, singultus (hiccups/hiccoughs), ipsilateral cerebellar signs.

Subarachnoid bleed: HT, stiff neck, Parinaud's sign—upward gaze paralysis; subhyaloid retinal hemorrhage.

Intraparenchymal bleed:
- Cerebellar: Awake, alert even with ophthalmoplegias; acute hypotonia; conjugate gaze paresis, skew deviation.
- Cerebral: Motor and always sensory deficits; 13% have seizure within 48 hr.
- Brain stem: Early loss of consciousness; brain stem signs including involvement of cranial nerves V, VII, VIII, IX, X, XI, XII; quadriplegia.

Crs: Non-hemorrhagic CVAs with 15% 30-d mortality; hemorrhagic CVAs with worse prognosis if large putaminal or thalamic bleed with HT, whereas subcortical, cerebellar, and pontine bleeds without correlation to blood pressure (Stroke 1997;28:1185). Separate risk factors for those treated with TPA for ischemic strokes, with worse in-hospital mortality corresponding with increasing age and altered mental status (Jama 2004;292:1831); also increased risk for worse outcome in those with elevated blood glucose, later time in administration of thrombolytic within the 3-hr window, and in those with cortical involvement (Jama 2004;292:1839).

Cmplc: Pulmonary emboli, aspiration pneumonia, UTIs, post-stroke depression, possible conversion of non-hemorrhagic CVA to hemorrhagic CVA; increased ICP.

Diff Dx:
- Transient ischemic attack (TIA) (Ann EM 2004;43:592)— CVA symptoms that last less than 24 hours, with anterior circulation symptoms including amaurosis fugax; and posterior circulation symptoms including bilateral blindness, diplopia, and quadriplegia. Carotid bruit correlates poorly with symptomatic disease. Risk of subsequent CVA is 8% in first mon, 5% per yr for 3 yr, 3% per yr thereafter. 41% will die of MI. Risk factors of (1) patient age > 60 years; (2) diabetes mellitus; (3) episode lasting > 10 min; (4) weakness during the episode;

and (5) speech impairment during the episode convey a prognostic risk of CVA within 90 days by the following conversion (Jama 2000;284:2901):

0 risk factors with 0% risk

1 risk factor with 3% risk

2 risk factors with 7% risk

3 risk factors with 11% risk

4 risk factors with 15% risk

All 5 risk factors with 34% risk

- Reversible ischemic neurologic deficit (RIND)—lasts longer than 24 hr, but less than 72 hr.
- Migraine headache
- Metabolic abnormality, such as hypoglycemia
- Seizure, with Todd's paralysis
- Multiple sclerosis
- Benign vertigo
- Tumor
- Carotid artery dissection or vertebral artery dissection (Nejm 2001;344:898)
- Segmental mediolytic arteriopathy in young patients with CVA (Cardiovasc Surg 1994;2:350).

Table 13.1 NIHSS Scoring System

Item	Name	Response
1a	Level of Consciousness	0 = Alert 1 = Not alert, arousable 2 = Not alert, obtunded 3 = Unresponsive
1b	Questions	0 = Answers both correctly 1 = Answers one correctly 2 = Answers neither correctly
1c	Commands	0 = Performs both tasks correctly 1 = Performs one task correctly 2 = Performs neither task
2	Gaze	0 = Normal 1 = Partial gaze palsy 2 = Total gaze palsy
3	Visual fields	0 = No visual loss 1 = Partial hemianopsia 2 = Complete hemianopsia 3 = Bilateral hemianopsia
4	Facial palsy	0 = Normal 1 = Minor paralysis 2 = Partial paralysis 3 = Complete paralysis
5a	Left motor arm	0 = No drift 1 = Drift before 10 seconds 2 = Falls before 10 seconds 3 = No effort against gravity 4 = No movement
5b	Right motor arm	0 = No drift 1 = Drift before 10 seconds 2 = Falls before 10 seconds 3 = No effort against gravity 4 = No movement
6a	Left motor leg	0 = No drift 1 = Drift before 5 seconds 2 = Falls before 5 seconds 3 = No effort against gravity 4 = No movement

Table 13.1   continued

Item	Name	Response
6b	Right motor leg	0 = No drift
		1 = Drift before 5 seconds
		2 = Falls before 5 seconds
		3 = No effort against gravity
		4 = No movement
7	Ataxia	0 = Absent
		1 = One limb
		2 = Two limbs
8	Sensory	0 = Normal
		1 = Mild loss
		2 = Severe loss
9	Language	0 = Normal
		1 = Mild aphasia
		2 = Severe aphasia
		3 = Mute or global aphasia
10	Dysarthria	0 = Normal
		1 = Mild
		2 = Severe
11	Extinction/inattention	0 = Normal
		1 = Mild
		2 = Severe

Lyden, P; Lu, M; Jackson, C; Marler, J; Kothari, R; Brott, T; Zivin, J; Underlying Structure of the National Institutes of Health Stroke Scale: results of a factor analysis, *Stroke*, November 1999;30(11):2347-54. Reprinted with permission from Lippincott Williams & Wilkins.)

Scoring System:

Median score of those treated in NINDS trial was 14, with low of 1 and high of 37—would suggest treating those with moderate deficits (score of 10-20), and not those with mild or severe deficits based on this trial.

Lab: CBC with diff; PT/PTT; metabolic profile including immediate glucoscan; EKG—cardiac markers if abnormal:

- *X-ray:* Consider CXR; head CT without contrast—contrast given if lesion noted, except bleed because may elect to do angiography if bleed noted; although, may elect to perform CT angiography source images to offer prognostic data for regional blood flow and thus may determine risk of infarct growth (Stroke 2002;33:2426). CT has traditionally held the provence of better for acute bleeds, but MRI almost as good—MRI better for chronic bleeds or strokes that are undergoing transformation to hemorrhagic, but may miss a SAH (Jama 2004;292:1823). CT ability and readings moving toward delineating area and size of ischemia to correlate thrombotic vs embolic—still being developed (Stroke 1992;23:1748) and perhaps no significance of early ischemic changes in re: TPA use (Jama 2001;1:2830). MRI will determine ischemic CVAs within hours whereas CT will show in days. MRI or MRA for AVM evaluation.
- *US:* Consider emergent carotid studies. Echocardiogram, if embolic source entertained. Leg studies, if paradoxical embolus suspected.
- *LP:* LP if not anticoagulated and high suspicion for subarachnoid bleed, CT will miss up to 3-10% of these (Acad Emerg Med 1996;3:16; Ann EM 1998;32:297).

Emergency Management:
- Airway; O_2, only if hypoxia—is widely overused (Arch IM 2002;162:49).
- Control/resuscitate blood pressure (Stroke 1998;29:1504); this is controversial and a "double-edged sword"—if hypertensive, get systolic BP around 180 mm Hg, since the hypertensive response is to maintain flow to the brain, which may be experiencing local edema, but even relative hypotension may decrease cerebral perfusion; if hypotensive, get systolic BP > 110 mm Hg to maintain flow to brain.
- Iv meds for pain/nausea/vomiting.

Non-hemorrhagic CVAs (Drugs Aging 1999;14:11). Consider ASA, heparin, and thrombolytics.

- Four baby ASA chew and swallow (Stroke 2000;31:1240); no benefit of warfarin over ASA (Nejm 2001;345:1444).
- Unfractionated heparin iv with weight-based protocol or low molecular weight heparin (LMWH) sc, no help for CVA in progress, but perhaps help in 6-mon survival—*when* to anticoagulate is the difficult decision— (Cochrane Database Syst Rv 2000;2) vs (Cochrane Database Syst Rv 2000;2). With Afib, controversy of ASA vs LMWH (Lancet 2000;355:1205).
- Limit blood draws/procedures if possible if considering thrombolytics (Nejm 1995;333:1581). Complete NIHSS stroke scale as outlined under "Scoring System" in this chapter (Stroke 1999;30:2347).
- The decision to perform thrombolysis should be made within 3 hr of symptom onset, BP < 185/110 with minimal pharmacologic help, no mild or dense deficits, and moderate deficits should not be improving. Should have no recent major surgery or dental work within 2 wk, no recent trauma, no gi bleed, and no history of cancer. Relative contraindications are those associated with embolic phenomenon, such as Afib, carotid stenosis, prosthetic valve, DVT with suspected patent foramen ovale, etc. Use TPA, not other agents—TPA 0.9 mg/kg give as a 10% bolus, and 90% over next 60 min, approximately 6% chance of bleed into CVA (Stroke 1997;28:2109).
- If suspect increased ICP because of large CVA, supine was the best position for cerebral blood flow knowing that this does increase the ICP (Stroke 2002;33:497).
- Equivocal data of Glucose-Insulin-Potassium (GIK) for those with mild to moderate hyperglycemia (Stroke 1999;30:793).
- Permissive hypothermia is currently investigational (Stroke 1998;29:2461; Neurol 1997;48:762; Lancet 1996;347:422;

J Neurosurg 2000;92:91) and has numerous side effects (Int J Dev Neurosci 2003;21:353). *See Head Trauma* (p269).

- Transcranial Doppler US augmentation with TPA use for those with ischemic strokes is investigational (Nejm 2004;351:2170).
- Neither treating hyperhomocysteinemia with folic acid, pyridoxine (vitamin B6) and cobalamin (vitamin B12) (Jama 2004;291:565) nor screening for antiphopholipid syndromes for prognostic information (including response to ASA or warfarin) (Jama 2004;291:576) is warranted at this time.
- Magnesium does not change morbidity/mortality (Lancet 2004;363:439)—positive EMS FAST-MAG study with many limitations (Stroke 2004;35:e106).
- Consult primary physician/neurologist.

Hemorrhagic CVAs:
- Consult neurosurgery.
- Control of systemic HT does not influence cerebral flow unless pt made hypotensive (Crit Care Med 1999;27:965), but better BP control with better morbidity and mortality outcomes (Stroke 1995;26:21). Consider use of nitroprusside, clonidine, labetalol, or ACE inhibitors.
- Consider recombinant activated factor VII (rFVIIa) at 40 µg/kg, 80 µg/kg or 160 µg/kg dose—given within 4 hr of onset of intracerebral bleed, may reduce morbidity/mortality from 69% to approximately 50% in the first 24 hr and at 90 d reduce the mortality from 29% to 18%—this is at the expense of increased (from 2% to 7%) rate of serious thromboembolic disease (Nejm 2005;352:777).
- Consider nimodipine 60 mg po q 4 hr for 21 d—prevents arterial spasm.
- Hypertonic saline as effective as mannitol, and neither influences cerebral blood flow (Neurosurgery 1999;44:1055, 1063).
- EACA (ε-aminocaproic acid) equivocal, but may reverse TPA.
- Dexamethasone no help, although is still tried.

- Hemodilution to hematocrit of 32% with colloid after phlebotomy helps limit damage in spasm. This is controversial.

TIA:

- ER work-up of neuroimaging and EKG for arrhythmia.
- Admit for heparinization if high-risk factors such as recurrent TIA while on antiplatelet treatment that is maximized, presumed embolic source from heart (Afib or Aflut that is new onset or patient is not anticoagulated), symptoms are waxing and waning but worsening with each presentation or occurring more frequently, or
- ER or outpatient vascular work-up of neck vessels with duplex US, CT angiogram, or MRA. Initiate or maximize antiplatelet therapy if no bleed on neuroimaging.
- Perhaps 3 or more risk factors as noted above with a risk of CVA within 90 d of 11% is an appropriate cutoff to admit pts to pursue aggressive evaluation.
- OK for home, if above studies and risk factors OK. Initiate ASA or clopidogrel (Plavix) (Lancet 2004;364:331; Cerebrovasc Dis 2004;17:253; Stroke 2000;31:1779) if needed, and arrange primary care follow-up. Neurology consult in these patients is recommended.

13.3 Bell's Palsy

Nejm 2004;351:1323

Cause: Controversial and many proposed etiologies—idiopathic peripheral seventh cranial nerve (CN VII) palsy is prototypical Bell's Palsy; diagnosis of exclusion after considering differential diagnosis.

Epidem: Possibly increased in diabetics, or possibly due to diabetic nerve infarcts. Seen in all ages with congenital in children

(J Otolaryngol 1997;26:80), sarcoid as most common cause of seventh cranial nerve palsy in young adults (Sarcoidosis Vasc Diffuse Lung Dis 1997;14:115), and a myriad of etiologies with increasing age. Isolated risk for those in Switzerland that used an intranasal influenza vaccine that is now not available (Nejm 2004;350:896).

Pathophys: Peripheral cranial nerve VII dysfunction with drooling and inability to completely close eye as possible consequences.

Sx: Facial weakness; pain; increased noise sensitivity from lack of stapedial muscle tone.

Si: Cranial nerve VII weakness (sparing the forehead in central CN VII lesions, since nerve fibers cross from the contralateral side); absence of taste on the anterior $^2/_3$ of the tongue if lesion proximal to chorda tympani.

Crs: 90% recover completely. If residual motion on affected side, pt always recovers.

Cmplc: Corneal ulceration—treatment is to tape lid. Errors in nerve regeneration: 1) jaw wrinkling; 2) orbicularis oculi with ori, and vice versa; 3) parasympathetic nerve problem with eye tearing when good food tasted, aka "Crocodile tears."

Bilateral Bell's Palsy is considered an encephalitis, such as Lyme encephalitis.

Diff Dx (Otolaryngol Clin N Am 1991;24:613): *Herpes zoster* (Ramsay-Hunt syndrome)—only 50% recover; EBV; sarcoid; Lyme disease; tumor; basilar skull fracture; otitis media; birth; syphilis; HIV, but most likely multiple cranial nerve palsies; central (supra-nuclear) palsy with relative sparing of frontalis and orbicularis oculi.

Lab: Consider Lyme titer; EMG at 2 wk, if ongoing muscular fibrillation; MRI in 6 wk, if not resolving.

Emergency Management:
- Protect eyes with Lacrilube gtts and taping—especially hs.
- Consider prednisone 60 mg taper over 10 d, data equivocal (Ped Neurol 1999;21:814). Perhaps high dose steroids in those with complete paralysis (J Accid Emerg Med 1999;16:445).
- Consider treatment for Lyme disease, if in endemic area or pos titer.
- Consider Acyclovir (Ann Otol Rhinol Laryngol 1996;105: 371) vs (J Neurol Sci 1999;170:19).
- Surgery initially no help, consider surgery if EMG flat at 2 wks, if persistently abnormal electroneurographic pattern (Otolaryngol Head Neck Surg 2000;122:290), or if MRI at 6 wks with lesion—rare consequences (Am J Otol 2000;21: 139) vs (Arch Otolaryngol Head Neck Surg 1998;124:824).

13.4 Encephalitis

Adv Neurol 1978;19:197; Neuroimaging Clin N Am 2000;10:333; Flaviviruses Nejm 2004;351:370

Cause:

Arbo viruses:

(1) St. Louis (Arch Neurol 2000;57:114). (2) Eastern equine, (3) Western equine, (4) La Crosse (Ped Infect Dis J 2000;19:77), (5) West Nile (Emerg Infect Dis 2000;6:370).

Herpes viruses:

(a) HSV type I, (b) HSV type II, (c) Varicella, (d) EBV (Mononucleosis), (e) Cytomegalovirus (CMV).

Paramyxovirus:

Rubeola (measles); Rubella virus (German measles); *Mycoplasma pneumoniae* (Ann EM 1994;23:1375); rarely paramyxovirus (Am J Neuroradiol 2000;21:455).

Epidem: Tick-borne encephalitis is usually a milder illness in children vs adults (Infection 2000;28:74). Regional epidemics may be predicted by estimating snow melt water run-off, since this has some relation to mosquito population (J Am Mosq Control Assoc 2000;16:22). Previous Dengue virus infection conveys some protection against St. Louis and West Nile encephalitis (Proc Soc Exp Biol Med 1970;135:573).

St. Louis: Urban culex mosquito from birds [including birds that may be domestic (J Wildl Dis 2000;36:13)] and invertebrates. Incidence increased in adults > 40 yr of age, many cases unapparent.

Eastern Equine: Mosquitoes [including *Aedes albopictus* (Science 1992;257:526)] or ticks from wild birds, and possibly snakes. In eastern U.S., incidence up after rainy winter; < 100 cases in literature; kills horses by the thousands and children age < 10 yr.

Western Equine: Rural culex mosquito, from birds and snake reservoirs. Incidence in infants and adults > 50 yr of age is 3,000 cases in 1959; endemic in Columbia River basin; many cases unapparent.

La Crosse: Spread by *Aedes triseriatus* mosquitos, usually causes mild disease in children, although severe illness has occurred (Nejm 2001;344:801).

West Nile: 1999 U.S. epidemic, exact transmission unsure, although birds, mosquitoes, and ticks hypothesized (Mmwr 1999;48:845) and originating in Israel (Science 1999;286:2333); 1996 epidemic in Europe (Lancet 1998;352:767).

Herpes Simplex Types I and II: Occurs in babies under age 3 mon born of mothers with active disease or to asymptomatic, but viral shedding mothers; or those who are immunosuppressed or atopic—such as those with eczema.

Varicella: A complication of chickenpox or Zoster. Chickenpox with 14-d incubation period, may return to school/day care when lesions are crusted. Zoster is more common in the elderly or those with HIV or cancer, but not a sign of occult malignancy.

EBV: 18% of adults are asymptomatic; spread by intimate contact with carrier.

CMV: Congenital via transplacental acquisition; newborn via vaginal infection at birth; blood products; organ transplantation; increased in homosexual males.

Rubeola: Spread via direct contact with pt in d 2 or more of incubation period with 12- to 14-d incubation period; common worldwide, higher in vitamin A deficient patients. Encephalitis in 0.1% with 65% of these having neurologic residue—subclinical in 15-20%.

Rubella: Carrier is newborn infant.

Pathophys:

Arbo viruses: Men and horses do not develop enough viremia to transmit these diseases.

HSV Types I and II: See STDs p153.

Varicella: Same organism first causes chickenpox, and then zoster.

EBV: Lives only in B-lymphocytes and oral epithelial cells, only replicates in epithelial cells of mouth.

CMV: Ubiquitous, may be congenital or acquired and found in all body fluids, if carrier.

Rubeola: Respiratory tract involved, viremia within 2 d of contact; Koplik's spots and skin lesions are areas of local intracellular viral replication. Encephalitis is a hypersensitivity reaction, not infectious.

Rubella: A mild virus, damages without killing the fetus.

Sx: Fever, severe headache, nausea, vomiting.
Herpes viruses may also have herpetic rash, gingivostomatitis.
Rubeola, Rubella and *West Nile* with maculopapular rash.

Si: Change in mental status, meningismus, adenopathy, frontal lobe release signs, cranial nerve palsies, seizures. May resemble anticholinergic crisis (J Toxicol Clin Toxicol 1997;35:627).

Varicella: Chickenpox with herpetic rash of various ages, Zoster (shingles) with dermatomal eruption.

EBV: Tonsillitis, posterior adenopathy.

CMV: Mild hepatitis and splenomegaly.

Rubeola: Koplik's spots on buccal mucosa—white on red base opposite molars; palpebral conjunctivitis; vascular spiders on soft palate; the rash is "brown paint spilled over head and neck," starts around ears and can be on palms and soles when severe.

Rubella: Conjunctivitis, splenomegaly, and sore gums; rash is face first and spreads in 3 d.

Crs:

All arbovirus encephalitis patients with moderate to high neurologic morbidity risk and the following mortality risks—St. Louis with 16% mortality, 66% if seize; Eastern equine with 36% mortality; Western equine with 10% mortality.

Herpes encephalitis with about 70% mortality.

Rubeola with a 2-10% mortality in developing countries.

Rubella with severe neurologic sequelae including mental retardation and deafness.

Cmplc: A myriad of problems possible, including multiorgan secondary infections or some degree of failure.

Diff Dx: Meningitis, human granulocytic ehrlichiosis (J Infect 2000;40:55), syphilis, anticholinergic crisis.

Other childhood exanthems—Roseola, scarlet fever, erythema infectiosum (Fifth Disease).

Lab: CBC with diff; blood cultures; metabolic profile; UA and urine culture; CSF with specific viral serologies and look for increased protein, white cells, and red cells, PCR may be helpful (J Neurol Sci 1993;118:213; J Clin Microbiol 2000;38:1527; J Clin Virol 2000;17:31)—If neuro deficit, do CT scan first to look for mass lesion or bleed. MRI may show more abnormalities consistent with encephalitis (J Neurol Sci 2000;174:3). EEG may be helpful in subacute encephalitis (Clin Electroencephalogr 1989;20:1).

Emergency Management: Give co-incident meningitis treatment as diagnosis is developing, and specifically the following:
- *Arbovirus* infections require supportive care.
- *Herpes virus* infections, use Acyclovir 5 mg/kg q 8 hr iv for 5-7 d (Brain Inj 1999;13:935), Foscarnet or Vidarabine. Corticosteroids of equivocal efficacy, but at least not detrimental (J Neurovirol 2000;6:25).
- *Rubella* patients should have contacts immunized or titers tested, if immunization status not up-to-date.
- Rubeola with vitamin A 200,000 IU × 2 increases survival in developing countries.

Prevention:
- Cochrane Database of available vaccines (Cochrane Database Syst Rv 2000;2).

13.5 Epidural Abscess

Neuroimaging Clin N Am 2000;10:333; Rev Inf Dis 1987; 9:265

Cause: Infection of epidural space after surgery or invasive procedure such as epidural catheter for analgesic or other medicine infusion (J Neurol 1999;246:815), from remote or contiguous primary site with extension, or spontaneous. Skin pathogens such as *Staphylococcus spp.* or *Streptococcus spp.* most likely, but also possibly *E. coli* or TB. Less likely intracranial.

Epidem: Uncommon, approximately 0.2-1.2:10,000 admissions to tertiary care centers (Nejm 1975;293:463).

Pathophys: Causes compression of cord with long tract signs below level of lesion.

Sx: Fever, pain, paresthesias.

Si: Hyperreflexia, bladder and rectal sphincter incontinence, paraplegia or quadriplegia, percussion tenderness.

Crs: Usual presenting progression is spinal ache, followed by neuropathic pain, followed by neurologic deficit.

Cmplc: Paralysis.

Diff Dx: Epidural hematoma, Cauda Equina syndrome, Conus Medullaris syndrome, possibly meningitis or vertebral osteomyelitis if no neurologic deficits.

Lab: CBC with diff; ESR; blood cultures.
- *X-ray:* CT, MRI better (Scand J Infect Dis 1988;20:323; Arch Neurol 1992;49:743), of suspected level; if myelogram performed, do not violate infected area.

Emergency Management:
- Removal of catheter, if necessary.
- CSF sampling, if possible not through inflamed site.
- Iv antibiotics, consider third generation cephalosporin with vancomycin.
- Immediate neurosurgical consult (Neurosurgery 1990;27:185).
- Steroids equivocal.

13.6 Head Trauma

Curr Opin Peds 1998;10:350; Emerg Med Clin N Am 1999;17:9

Cause: Myriad of adult causes, consider Shaken Baby Syndrome in infants.

Epidem: Helmets prevent brain morbidity and overall mortality, and do not increase the risk of C-spine injury (Eur J Emerg Med 1998;5:207). Half the deaths due to trauma are from head trauma in those < 44 yr of age, where trauma is the leading cause of death, such as car accidents, assault, bicycle, and motorcycle accidents. Height > 3 feet is significant in those < 2 yr of age

(Arch Ped Adolesc Med 1999;153:15). Falls in the elderly can cause significant damage even from a standing height, although more significant if falling down stairs (J Emerg Med 1998; 16:709).

Pathophys: Our concern is skull fractures and intracranial injuries, although significant scalp lacerations and facial trauma can also be concerns. Primary brain injury is when we speak of neuronal and axonal injury at time of injury, and secondary brain injury is due to delayed physiologic changes that may be treatable—hypoxia, cerebral edema, intracranial hemorrhage, hypercarbia, etc.

Minor head trauma may be classified as those with a normal neurologic exam, no evidence of CNS penetration on physical exam, and with no or fleeting loss of consciousness, and a normal head CT, if one was performed.

A concussion is a closed head injury where loss of consciousness may have occurred, the neurologic exam is normal, a head CT does not show a subarachnoid or other bleed, but a clinically insignificant subarachnoid bleed has probably occurred, especially in those who go onto a post-concussive syndrome where the headaches can last for weeks to months. Different grading scales exist, but a useful one is by Cantu (Sports Med 1992;14:64), and outlines the following: Mild (Grade 1)—no LOC, and amnesia less than 30 min; Moderate (Grade 2)—< 5 min LOC or amnesia > 30 min; and Severe (Grade 3)—> 5 min LOC or amnesia > 24 hr.

Severe head injuries may be seen with skull fractures from blunt or penetrating trauma, cerebral contusions, subarachnoid bleeds, intraparenchymal bleeds, epidural hematomas (arterial bleed, usually middle meningeal artery), and subdural hematomas. Subdural hematomas can be acute or chronic, and are venous in nature due to tearing of bridging vessels between the subarachnoid space and dural sinuses. These are more common in the elderly, and some data that this may be an increased risk with the use of anticoagulants (warfarin) even with seemingly minor trauma— (J Trauma 2004;56:802; 2002;53:668; Am Surg 2001;67:1098; Lancet 2001;357:771; J Accid Emerg Med 1998;15:159), vs (Acad Emerg Med 1999;6:121).

Sx: Change in mental status; nausea; vomiting; headache; neck pain.

Si: Obvious skull trauma; periorbital ecchymosis (Raccoon eyes); postauricular ecchymosis (Battle's sign); focal neurologic deficit; seizure; decreased mental status; Cushing reflex—HT and bradycardia.

Crs: Severe head trauma with only approximately 40% functional recovery. Adults and peds > 2 years of age with minor head trauma, normal neuro exam, no seizure, normal mental status, GCS of 15, and lack of headache, nausea, vomiting, and depressed skull fracture do not need head CT (J Emerg Med 1997;15:453)—for peds who have non-trivial head trauma, then include absence of scalp findings if < 2 years of age, along with any positive previous findings to determine who needs a head CT (Ann EM 2003;42:492). Loss of consciousness is an equivocal finding for predicting a positive head CT (Am Surg 1994:533). Evaluating those who are intoxicated is difficult, and our clinical hx, GCS, and neuro exam criteria will not predict those who have intracranial pathology who present with minor head trauma (Acad Emerg Med 1994;1:227).

Cmplc: Severe head trauma with 35% mortality. Long-term psychological disability in adults (Ann EM 1989;18:9).

Children with minor head trauma rarely have long-term physical disability—parental reassurance is key (Peds 1986;78:497).

Children with severe head trauma present difficulties in evaluating the abdomen—CT OK and useful (J Ped Surg 1987; 22:1117).

Adults with severe head trauma can have abdominal CT or diagnostic peritoneal lavage (Lancet 1980;2:759) as options to evaluate for intra-abdominal injuries.

Lab: CBC with diff; PT/PTT; metabolic profile—transient and mild hypokalemia in children (J Ped Surg 1997;32:88); ABG; ethanol and urine toxic screen to help figure if other reason for altered mental stauts; serum τ^C level greater than 0—this is a CNS structural protein (Ann EM 2002;39:254); EKG to screen for acute injury or arrhythmia as contributing to decreased CNS perfusion.

X-ray: Image C-spine if severe head/neck injury or if clinically suspect injury in the conscious and alert adult pt based on exam, since in these circumstances it is rarely an occult injury—plain film historically touted (Am J Surg 1986;152:643), but CT better (Ann EM 1985;14:973); chest and pelvis x-rays in severe trauma; head CT without contrast for all but minor head trauma—many decision rules exist and are being trialed, but no convincing benefit on either patient safety, ability to affect pretest selection of those with significant CNS disease, or ability to appropriately influence resource allocation; consider CT of C-spine if C-spine imaging needed and intending to CT head, as this would be most effective use of resources and time (J Trauma 2004;56:1022). Plain skull x-rays with no benefit, and does not miss intracranial lesions in low-risk patients because they probably did not need imaging (Nejm 1987;316:84). Facial fractures are not uncommon in even minor head trauma (Injury 1994;25:47).

Emergency Management:

Minor head trauma may go home after period of observation if appropriate, and with reliable observers. First time concussions of Grades 1 or 2 may return to sports after 1 wk of no symptoms, all others should follow-up with their primary physicians in 1 wk before returning to sports.

Moderate head trauma will deserve a prolonged interval of observation at the very least, and should consider neurosurgical consult for observation/admission.

Severe head trauma deserves the following:

- Maintain airway, consider rapid sequence intubation (see p400) (Arch Surg 1997;132:592; Crit Care Med 1994; 22:1471). Avoid hypoxia (J Trauma 1996;40:764).
- Hyperventilate to $PaCO_2$ of 34-38 (about 20 breaths per min)—avoid overaggressive hyperventilation because this decreases cerebral oxygenation (Neurol Res 1997;19:233; J Neurosurg 1992;76:212; Neurosurgery 1991;29:743). This is best done if markers of cerebral edema are noted, such as decreasing neurologic score (such as GCS), signs of herniation (uncal or otherwise) and including either decorticate or decerebrate posturing. These recommendations based on consensus, trying to avoid alkalotic seizures. The national consensus for traumatic brain injury does not advocate using the GCS as a marker, but the critical study is yet to be performed—the study looking at GCS was looking at the motor portion of the scale only and hyperventilation values of the $PaCO_2$ were $25 + 2$ mm Hg, whereas the goal now is approximately 35 mm Hg (J Neurosurg 1991;75:731). Again, avoid aggressive hyperventilation!
- If other co-morbid conditions, address those first—even prior to head CT. The co-morbid conditions/injuries [usually intra-abdominal hemorrhage (J Trauma 1993;34:40)] are usually more significant than the intracranial problems (J Trauma 1995;176:154; Surg Gynecol Obstet 1993;38:327).
- Avoid hypotension—maintain iv fluids for shock (Brit J Neurosurg 1993;7:267; J Ped Surg 1993;28:310); hypertonic saline trialed as a 250 cc bolus with no appreciable change in outcome—not recommended here (Jama 2004;291:1350).

- Consider mannitol 1 gm/kg, although as effective as hypertonic saline, with no change in cerebral blood flow in those with intracerebral hemorrhage (Neurosurgery 1999;44:1055; Acta Neurochir suppl (Wien) 1990;51:320).
- Phenytoin (or fosphenytoin in phenytoin equivalents) 20 mg/kg iv bolus for seizures—fosphenytoin is loaded faster, if this is a consideration. Attempt primary control with Lorazepam (Ativan) at 0.03 mg/kg iv, with usual adult dose 2-4 mg iv (Nejm 2001;345:631) or midazolam (Versed) (J Paediatr Child Health 2002;38:582) and dose at 0.2 mg/kg iv or im (Ped Emerg Care 1997;13:92), but would advocate for a ceiling dose, which would be the same as an adult dose of 2-4 mg iv, which may be repeated. Seizure control medications are not intended to be prophylactic.
- Permissive hypothermia to 32°-34°C is experimental— (J Neurotrauma 1995;12:923) vs (Nejm 2001;344:556); whether a cooling helmet is an appropriate therapy also needs further study (J Neurosurg 2004;100:272).
- Meningitis can occur despite prophylactic antibiotics for basilar skull fracture (Am J Emerg Med 1983;1:295).
- Neurosurgery consult for patients with fractures, and for those with moderate head trauma or worse; and for those with mild head injuries, but who cannot be safely monitored at home.

13.7 Increased Intracerebral Pressure

Cause: Tumor (see CNS neoplasms, p166), infection (see encephalitis, p264), bleed (see Head trauma, p269), cerebral venous sinus thrombosis (Lancet 1996;248:1623), or idiopathic— *Pseudotumor cerebri* (Am J Emerg Med 1999;17:517).

Epidem: *Pseudotumor cerebri* associated with anemia; vitamin deficiencies, and intoxications—especially vitamin A; chronic hypoxia;

post-concussive state; post-otitis media, hypoparathyroidism; start of thyroid replacement in myxedematous patients; steroid replacement and withdrawal (Addisons); lateral sinus thrombosis. Mostly in young, overweight women, and bcp's implicated.

Pathophys: Unknown.

Sx: Headache; nausea; vomiting; visual field losses; no impairment of consciousness.

Si: Enlarged blind spot; central vision losses; later, inferior quadrantic defects/visual field constrictions. Papilledema without hemorrhages or exudates.

Crs: Variable, but concern of intracranial HT necessitates ICP monitoring (Surg Neurol 1978;10:371); worse prognosis with initial unconsciousness, subarachnoid bleed, shift of midline structures, elevated BP, elevated serum glucose, and vomiting (Stroke 1997;28:1396).

Cmplc: Visual loss, monitor with quantitative visual perimetry.

Lab: LP is diagnostic—high pressures of > 20 cm, normal CSF otherwise—neuroimaging to r/o lesion, will see small or normal ventricles.

Emergency Management:

Pseudotumor Cerebri:
- Iv access for pain and nausea control, if necessary.
- Take off CSF to get pressure to 20 cm, may need to repeat in approximately 1 wk.
- Consider 2-6 wks of steroids.
- Consider diuretics, acetazolamide (Diamox) used to be favored, but loop diuretics, such as furosemide OK.
- Surgical shunt rarely needed.

Increased intracranial pressure with mass effect (abnormal neuroimaging):
- Keep head of bed elevated.

- Avoid iv fluid overload, but also avoid hypotension. Maintain iv fluids for shock (Brit J Neurosurg 1993;7:267; J Ped Surg 1993;28:310).
- Maintain airway, consider rapid sequence intubation (p400) (Arch Surg 1997;132:592; Crit Care Med 1994;22:1471). Avoid hypoxia (J Trauma 1996;40:764).
- Hyperventilate to $PaCO_2$ of 34-38 (about 20 breaths per min)—avoid overaggressive hyperventilation because this decreases cerebral oxygenation (Neurol Res 1997;19:233; J Neurosurg 1992;76:212; Neurosurgery 1991;29:743). This is best done if markers of cerebral edema are noted, such as decreasing neurologic score (such as GCS), signs of herniation (uncal or otherwise), and including either decorticate or decerebrate posturing. These recommendations are based on consensus, trying to avoid alkalotic seizures. The national consensus for traumatic brain injury does not advocate using the GCS as a marker, but the critical study is yet to be performed—the study looking at GCS was looking at the motor portion of the scale only and hyperventilation values of the $PaCO_2$ were $25 + 2$ mm Hg, whereas the goal now is approximately 35 mm Hg (J Neurosurg 1991;75:731). Again, avoid aggressive hyperventilation!
- Consider mannitol 1 gm/kg, although as effective as hypertonic saline with no change in cerebral blood flow in those with intracerebral hemorrhage (Neurosurgery 1999;44:1055, 1063; Acta Neurochir suppl (Wien) 1990;51:320).
- Consider high dose steroid of dexamethasone 1 mg/kg or methylprednisolone 10 mg/kg; efficacy equivocal (Neurol 1972;22:56).
- May treat HT with labetalol 20 mg iv every 10-20 min, PRN; or nitroprusside drip 5-20 μg/kg/min; avoid overtreatment, since systemic HT is a response to maintain cerebral blood

flow, and relative hypotension will adversely affect this (Neurol Res 1997;19:169).

- Neurosurgical consult for consideration of ICP monitor or shunting.

13.8 Low Back Pain

Nejm 2001;344:363; Spine 1997;22:2128; Ann EM 1996;27:454; Emerg Med Clin N Am 1999;17:877; Curr Opin Rheumatol 1999;11:151

Cause: Ruptured herniated intervertebral disc; musculo-ligamentous strains/trauma; osteoarthritis of facet joints; perhaps leg length discrepancies; in elderly, vertebral compression fractures (Pain 1984;19:105) or multiple myeloma if no trauma.

Epidem: 65% of the population have low back pain symptoms within lifetime.

Pathophys: Myofascial, skeletal, disc, or ligamentous entrapment/compression of nerve conduction or vascular flow; this causes secondary edema, spasm and contracture, hypersensitivity or paresthesias.

Sx: Segmental pain with distal radiation of burning or shooting pain, or perhaps paresthesias; decreased range of motion due to pain or muscular restriction.

Si: Abnormalities of the following gives approximate level—Patellar reflex is L4 root; Achilles reflex is S1 root; Extensor hallucis longus and first web sensation is L5 root.
    Leg length discrepancy is ≥ 5 mm for significance in literature, most use 1 cm.

Crs: Over 90% improve with conservative therapy over several days to weeks, and no workup is required unless motor loss is present and does not improve or actually worsens. Two-thirds have recurrence within 1 yr, and pain lasts 2 mon on average.

Cmplc: Workman's compensation—those with this as part of the hx have an extended course (Spine 1997;22:2016).

Diff Dx: AAA in elderly; spinal stenosis—pain, pseudoclaudication, numbness, worse with hips extended such as walking downhill, bilateral in ⅔; fibromyalgia; myofascial syndromes; anorectal abscess (Ann EM 1994;23:132); duodenal ulcer (Arch Phys Med Rehab 1998;79:1137); retroperitoneal hemorrhage (Arch Phys Med Rehab 1997;78:664).

Lab: CBC with diff looking for anemia and metabolic profile & UA for renal insufficiency if considering multiple myeloma.

X-ray: Consider plain films empirically in those ≤ 18 yr of age or ≥ 50 yr of age, if no h/o minor trauma; most do not require x-ray evaluation (Ann EM 1986;15:245; Spine 1995;20:1839). CT/MRI is good if observed abnormality correlates with clinical exam, but ⅓ of CTs have abnormal finding, and in normal and asymptomatic people bulges (50%) and protrusions (25%) are found on MRI.

Scanograms for leg length are only accurate measurement—rarely needed. Tape measuring is inaccurate.

Emergency Management:

- Appropriate level of pain management with acetaminophen, NSAIDs, and narcotics as scheduled (not as needed) and time-limited (Drugs 1994;48:189; Spine 1996;21:2840); antiemetics prn. Ibuprofen po as efficacious as ketorolac im (Ann Pharmacother 1994;28:309; Acad Emerg Med 1998;5:118).
- Consider muscle relaxant if crampy or spasm component in hx (Spine 1989;14:438); may not be appropriate if oversedation is an issue.
- Consider calcitonin if osteoporotic compression fracture.
- Resume normal daily activities with pain limited caution for lifting (Nejm 1995;332:351).

- Consider manipulative therapy through osteopaths (Nejm 1999;341:1426), physical therapy or chiropractors—physical therapy (Phys Ther 1988;68:199) and chiropractic data show higher pt satisfaction with no difference in clinical outcome.
- Hard bed/mattress.
- Prolonged bed rest unhelpful (Nejm 1986;315:1064); steroid of no help.
- Exercise not helpful for acute, but good for chronic back pain.
- Consider MRI or primary care consult if persistence > 2 wks; neurosurgical consult if abnormal MRI or exam.

13.9 Migraine Headache

Nejm 2002;346:257; Ann EM 1996;27:448

Cause: Possibly genetic.

Epidem: In U.S. 17.6% of females and 5.7% of males with migraine headache each year, associated with lower income household in females (Jama 1992;267:64).

Possibly autosomal dominant with incomplete penetrance; 80% have pos family hx. Higher incidence in obsessive/compulsives, patients with family history of epilepsy, after psychological trauma, and patients who had motion sickness as children.

Common and Classic: F:M ratio = 3-4:1; women on oral contraceptives have a 9 × increased incidence, 10% have each yr, 15% lifetime risk.

Cluster: M:F ratio = 10:1.

Pathophys: Angiographically documented cerebrovascular constriction, shunting; perhaps form 5-HT induced vascular changes, perhaps sludging leads to brain ischemia, which causes vasodilatation and pain especially in external carotid distribution.

Sx:

Common (80%): Slow onset over 4 hr, no scotomata or other aura; prodrome of yawning, euphoria, depression; usually bilateral; lasts 4-72 hr.

Classic (10%): Precipitated by bright light, sound, or idiopathic; usually unilateral headache follows 20-30 min scotomata, which spread then recede, or other sensory, speech, or motor aura. Headache lasts 4-72 hr; associated with nausea, vomiting, diarrhea, polyuria, and hemiplegias—hemiplegias all on opposite side of headache and scotomata. Consistently on one side 90% of the time.

Cluster (10%): "A migraine packed into 1 hour." Clusters of several/wk for approximately 1 mon; precipitated by vasodilators like alcohol, nitroglycerin during cluster period only; sweating, tearing, flush, salivation, rhinorrhea; nocturnal; severe episodes may precipitate suicide.

Si: Ergotamine trials help most, but not all.

Common: Eye tearing, face and neck muscle stiffness.

Classic: On affected side, small pupil, external carotid pain; carotid sinus pressure temporarily relieves headache.

Cluster: Horner's syndrome.

Crs:

Classic: After attack, approximately 1 wk immunity from recurrence.

Cmplc: CVA.

Diff Dx: Tension headache (may mimic common migraine signs) (Am Fam Phys 2002;66:797); subarachnoid hemorrhage; meningitis/encephalitis; glaucoma—distinguished by cupped discs; epilepsy—scotomata last longer with migraine; trauma/tumor—in migraine no permanent scotomata except in very old, varies to opposite side 10% of the time, headache no worse with Valsalva; Carotid artery (face pain) or vertebral artery (neck pain) dissection.

Lab: Serum tests not necessary if considering headache of migraine or tension physiology; CT/MRI not necessary if classic symptoms, although CT abnormalities have been noted in previous case reports (Headache 1987;27:578); EEG shows spike patterns (Clin Electroencephalogr 2000;31:76).

Emergency Management:

Common or Classic:

- Rest in a quiet and dark room.
- Prochlorperazine (Compazine) 5-10 mg iv, or droperidol 0.625 mg iv or 2.5 mg im (Am J Emerg Med 1999;17:398), or chlorpromazine 25 mg iv (Ann EM 1989;18:360; 1990;19:1079); metoclopramide 10 mg iv is second line therapy (Acad Emerg Med 1995;2:597; Ann EM 1995;26:541).
- Diphenhydramine iv (eg, 25 mg) to prevent akathisia (Ann EM 2001;37:125).
- ASA 900 mg + metoclopramide 10 mg po as effective as po sumatriptan.
- Caffeine/ergotamine 1 mg po or 2 mg pr up to 6 mg/24 hr or 10 mg/wk; overdose can cause vascular occlusion, especially when on β-blockers or erythromycin.
- Dihydroergotamine 0.5-1.0 mg iv/im/sc (Ann EM 1998;32:129); nasal spray (Novartis) 1 inhalation each nostril and may repeat in 15 min.
- Sumatriptan (Imitrex—5-HT analog) 6 mg sc × 1 helps 90% within 2 hr; or 100 mg po × 1 helps 50% within 2 hr; or as nasal spray 5-20 mg/dose helps within 15 min like sc dose (Cephalalgia 1998;18:532); may precipitate coronary artery disease. Similarly zolmitriptan (Zomig) 2.5 mg po, can repeat in 1 hr; rizatriptan (Maxalt); and naratriptan (Amerge) 1-2.5 mg, may repeat × 1 after 4 hr and takes 4 hr to work.

Almotriptan 6.25-12.5 mg po only bid or frovatriptan 2.5 mg po only 3 times daily (Med Lett Drugs Ther 2002;44:19). With all of these, beware drug interactions with MAO inhibitors, SSRIs, ergots, bcp's, and cimetidine.

- Narcotics to "break the cycle," and these should not be considered taboo as patients may have tried many of the aforementioned therapies before presenting to the ER (Ann EM 1998;32:129).
- Butorphanol (Stadol) 1 nasal spray, may repeat × 1 in 4 hr (Am J Emerg Med 1997;15:57).
- Lidocaine 4% intranasally, decreases headache by 50% in 50% of pts in 15 min (Jama 1996;276:319).
- All NSAIDs equal, no benefit of parenteral ketorolac (Ann Pharmacother 1994;28:309; Acad Emerg Med 1998;276:118).
- Nitrous oxide, 50:50 over 20 min (Am J Emerg Med 1999;17:252).
- Dexamethasone, 10 mg iv, data are anecdotal (Headache 1994;34:366).

Cluster:
- Prednisone, 40-60 mg po qd for 7 d; chlorpromazine 100-700 mg qd; indomethacin; sumatriptan as above.

Prevention for frequent repeat attacks:
- *Common and Classic* patients should stop BCPs, and may have prophylaxis with 1 ASA qd, β-blockers, methysergide, calcium channel blockers, valproate, or riboflavin (Headache 2000;40:30).
- *Cluster* patients should avoid vasodilators and may be maintained on lithium.

13.10 Neuroleptic Malignant Syndrome (NMS)

J Clin Psych 1980;41:79; 1987;48:328

Cause: Use of neuroleptic drugs (major tranquilizers) including phenothiazines, butyrophenones, thioxanthenes, loxapine, and rarely clozapine; or withdraw of dopamine agonist, such as bromocriptine or levodopa.

Epidem: Approximately 0.5% of pts given these drugs will develop NMS, unrelated to dose; 96% of cases within one mon of starting drug. Incidence increased with dehydration, exhaustion, and organic brain syndrome.

Pathophys: Diminished CNS dopamine.

Sx: 1- to 3-d onset, up to 5-10 d after drug has stopped, or 10-30 d after im deposited doses. Agitation, confusion, disorganization, and catatonia as risk factors for developing NMS (Biol Psych 1998;44:748).

Si: Fever in 87%; rigidity; hypertonia; mental status changes; autonomic instability such as pallor, diaphoresis, hypotension, HT, tachycardia, arrhythmia; akinesia; tremor; perhaps choreoathetoid type movements.

Crs: 10% mortality in 3-30 d.

Cmplc: Respiratory failure, myoglobinuric renal failure, cardiovascular collapse, arrhythmias, pulmonary embolus.

Diff Dx: Heat stroke, malignant hyperthermia, acute serotonin syndrome, antibiotic (aminoglycoside) induced neuromuscular blockade—usually post-operative, idiopathic acute lethal catatonia (Am J Psych 1989;146:324), drug interactions with MAO inhibitors, central anticholinergic crisis that responds to iv physostigmine, tetanus, tick paralysis, stiff man syndrome, myotonia, meningitis, encephalitis, thyroid storm.

Lab: CBC with diff; metabolic profile including calcium, magnesium, and phosphorous; CPK; aldolase; UA with myoglobin—67% have myoglobinuria; consider panculture if infectious etiology; consider LP if considering meningitis or encephalitis.

X-ray: Head CT or MRI if bleed suspected, focal deficit, or other CNS concerns.

Emergency Management:

Am J Emerg Med 1991;9:360

- Hold all neuroleptics.
- Dantrolene (Dantrium) 1-2 mg/kg iv initial dose, then up to 10 mg/kg qd iv or po divided in doses q 6 hr—beware of concomitant calcium-channel blocker use. Controversial (Brit J Psych 1991;159:709), as is bromocriptine.
- Bromocriptine 2.5-10 mg po tid (J Clin Psych 1987;48:69) or amantidine 100 mg po bid.
- Consider L-dopa.
- Nitroprusside iv (Ann IM 1986;104:56) and minoxidil po is a case report success.
- Treat myoglobinuria with iv fluids most important (Ren Fail 1997;19:283); $NaHCO_3$ iv may prevent damage by myoglobin (J Biol Chem 1998;273:31731), so consider drip (see p484); mannitol of equivocal efficacy.

13.11 Grand Mal Seizure/Status Epilepticus

Emerg Med Clin N Am 1994;12:1027; 1999;17:203

Cause: 20% idiopathic; 80% due to organic disease; trauma (subdural, scar), infection, neoplasia, vascular (AV malformation, CVA), degenerative disease (MS, Alzheimer's), metabolic [intoxications including cocaine (Ann EM 1989;18:774), anoxia, hypoglycemia, fever, hyponatremia, alkalosis, hypomagnesemia, hypocalcemia]. Neonates/infants include congenital malformations and drug withdrawal. Pregnancy includes eclampsia (Emerg Med Clin N Am 1994;12:1013). Failure to take antiepileptic medications.

Epidem: Not a significant cause of car accidents, but clinically more serious if they occur as a result of a head injury (Ann EM 1983;12:543).

Pathophys: Crosses midline; functional brain transection at midbrain (decerebrate), yet our knowledge of epilepsy is poor (Nejm 2003;340:1257).

Sx: Aura or prodrome (96% specificity), bedwetting (96% specificity), blue color observed by witnesses (94% specificity) (J Am Coll Cardiol 2002;40:142); Jacksonian progression, and post-ictal Todd's paralysis all indicate focal onset/origin.

Si: Tonic decerebrate posturing evolving to clonic phase after 1-2 min; cut tongue (97% specificity), head turning (97% specificity), unusual posturing (97% specifity) post-ictal amnesia, post-ictal confusion (94% sensitivity, 69% specificity) (J Am Coll Cardiol 2002;40:142); often Todd's paralysis.

Crs: No decrease in IQ due to seizures unless complicated by status epilepticus.

Cmplc: Status epilepticus—seizures >10-20 min in duration or failure to awaken between tonic-clonic seizures causes brain damage after 1 hr even with normal vital signs; death hypothesized as due to cardiac arrhythmias as the terminal event (Epilepsia 1984;25:84).

Diff Dx: Cardiac etiology with syncope—arrhythmias including prolonged Q-T syndrome (Ann EM 1996;28:556).

Febrile seizures—ages 6 mon to 6 yr; recurrence risk factors include first seizure at young age, febrile seizure hx in first degree relative, low grade fever in ER, and short time interval between onset of fever and seizure (Arch Ped Adolesc Med 1997;151:371); no increased risk for bacteremia or UTIs, and rare to have bacterial meningitis if not evident on initial laboratory tests (LP results) (Ped Emerg Care 1999;15:9).

Hysterical seizures—longer and less precise onset, more pelvic thrusting, side-to-side head movement, eyes tightly shut, and alternating movements of limbs; Lennox-Gastaut syndrome in children.

Lab: Immediate glucoscan; CBC with diff; metabolic profile, including magnesium and calcium—rarely helpful in pediatric (Ped Emerg Care 1992;8:65; 1992;8:13) or adult pts (Ann EM 1985;14:416), unless clinically suspect metabolic abnormalities; PT/PTT if likely intracranial bleed; consider ethanol level; urine toxic screen; EEG abnormal in 30-50% and increases to 60-90% with repeated studies.

X-ray: Head CT to check for bleed emergently, even consider in those with "other" cause for seizure such as alcohol intoxication/withdraw (Epilepsia 1980;21:459) or cocaine use (Ann EM 1992;21:772) if pt not recovering from seizures or other evidence of abnormal neurologic exam; MRI to assess for organic cause.

Children with simple febrile seizures or fever with new onset seizure that does not fit the definition of simple febrile seizure rarely have significant lesion on head CT if non-focal seizure and non-focal neuro exam after post-ictal state (J Peds 1998;133:664); children at higher risk for intracranial lesion if < 6 mon of age, seizure > 15 min long, h/o malignancy, neurocutaneous syndrome, recent closed head injury, recent shunt surgery or abnormal neuro exam post recovery (Ann EM 1997;29:518).

Emergency Management:

If actively seizing/status epilepticus:

Epilepsia 1989;30:S33; J Child Neurol 1998;13:S23, S30)
- Protect patient from self-injury.
- Maintain airway, intubate if necessary. Suction.
- Empiric benzodiazepine (see next bullet), thiamine 100 mg iv, and glucose bolus, if glucoscan not immediately available.
- Intravenous benzodiazepine dosing: lorazepam at 0.03 mg/kg iv with usual adult dose 2-4 mg iv (Nejm 2001;345:631);

midazolam with less respiratory depression (J Paediatr Child Hlth 2002;38:582) and dose at 0.2 mg/kg iv or im (Ped Emerg Care 1997;13:92), but would advocate for a ceiling dose, which would be the same as an adult dose of 2-4 mg iv; and third choice here of diazepam 0.1 mg/kg iv, with a usual adult dose of 5-10 mg iv. These may be repeated.

- Alternate route benzodiazepine dosing: lorazepam 0.04 mg/kg im to a maximum dose of 4 mg or lorazepam 0.05-0.15 mg/kg per buccal; midazolam 0.2 mg/kg im to a maximum dose of 10 mg [im midazolam just as effective in regards to time of seizure cessation as iv diazepam, since no iv needs to be established (Ped Emerg Care 1997;13:92)] or midazolam 10 mg per buccal (may consider 5 mg per buccal midazolam if < 20 kg pt); or intranasal midazolam 0.2-0.3 mg/kg (J Paediatr Child Hlth 2004;40:556; J Child Neurol 2002;17:123; 2000;15:833) or midazolam 0.3 mg/kg pr with a maximum dose of 10 mg pr; diazepam 0.2 mg/kg pr or simply 10 mg pr (Lancet 1999; 353:623).

- First choice: phenytoin iv loading at 20 mg/kg with a rate of 50 mg/min. Second choice: fosphenytoin 20 mg/kg of phenytoin equivalents iv at 150 mg/min—the small differential time in loading that is noted here has not been shown to be clinically significant. Repeat your choice at 10 mg/kg bolus if still seizing. Not effective in ethanol related seizures (Ann EM 1994;23:513).

- If not seizing but need to load phenytoin: oral phenytoin loading 400 mg q 2 hr to reach a load of 20 mg/kg is cost and adverse outcome effective compared to iv dosing (but longer time spent in the ER) (Ann EM 2004;43:386).

- Phenobarbital (first line for children) 10 mg/kg at 100 mg/min with usual adult dose of 0.7-1.5 gm iv—may give an additional 10 mg/kg if not successful—*Be prepared to intubate secondary to respiratory depression.*

- Consider barbiturate coma, such as Pentobarbital 100 mg iv bolus PRN, must be intubated for this.

Patient with AIDS:
- Neuroimaging and lumbar puncture in ER or as inpatient for new onset seizures (Acad Emerg Med 1998;5:905).

If patient with self-limited/easily controlled seizure:
- Consider outpatient treatment with phenytoin—300-400 mg po qd after loading dose; carbamazepine—400-1200 mg po qd; or valproic acid—1-3 gm po qd in divided doses.
- More likely to treat adults than children after first seizure, especially if child has simple febrile seizure or no cause found.
- Phenytoin usually first line for adults, phenobarbital—0.6 mg/kg po qd—first line for children.

13.12 Spinal Cord Injury

Surg Neurol 1978;10:71; 1978;10:60; 1978;10:64; Brit Med J 1990; 301:34; 1990;301:110; J Neurotrauma 1992:S385; Am Fam Phys 2001;64:631

Cause: Usually traumatic, may be due to a transient shock to the cord, prolonged ischemia, cord contusion or direct trauma.

Epidem: Most commonly a male in the 3rd decade of life; usual mechanism of MVA, falls, and firearms in descending order of frequency.

Pathophys: Transient and permanent cord lesions are possible, as well as complete or partial cord syndromes (J Neurosurg 1991;75:15). Cord injury may occur without obvious bony fracture on plain radiograph in children (SCIWORA—see C-spine p480) (J Trauma 1989;29:654) or others with underlying laxity of the vertebral column (Spine 1990;15:466).
- *Spinal shock* is a lower motor neuron problem (areflexia) where a flaccid quadriplegia may last hours to months. If this is tran-

sient, usually turns into a spastic paralysis with return of reflexes in approximately 24 hr. Also manifests with autonomic instability (paralytic ileus and urinary retention, eg) and hypotension with bradycardia in the face of adequate urine output. Important to assess for significant cardiac and hypovolemic event.

- *Anterior spinal cord syndrome* is a problem with motor function (paralysis) and sensory input of temperature and some degree of pain loss distal to the lesion—temperature is lateral columns, whereas pain is lateral columns and posterior columns. The motor loss should show areflexia at the level of the lesion, and hyperreflexia/spasticity (upper motor neuron lesion) distal to the injury. Due to injury or occlusion of the anterior spinal artery, or the cord itself.

- *Central cord syndrome* is another partial cord syndrome where the involved portion affects first the hands, then the upper extremity, and then the legs—this is exactly the anatomic positionings from the center of the cord outward. Usually a hyperextension injury with possibly some degree of predisposition (congenital stenosis, eg); ischemia to the cord center is implicated.

- *Brown-Sequard syndrome* is a cord hemisection with a motor loss and the senses of vibratory, gross proprioception and some pain loss on ipsilateral side at the level of the lesion, and sensory loss of temperature and some pain loss two levels lower on the contralateral side—the lateral columns carry fibers up two levels before they decussate to travel back to the brain, whereas the posterior columns and motor fibers decussate above the spinal cord.

Sx: Back pain; localized weakness; obvious external trauma.

Si: Spinal exam crepitus, ecchymosis, abnormal curvature; paralysis; sensory deficits; loss of sphincter tone; spasticity.

Crs: Variable, "time will tell." Children usually fare well independent of coincident fracture or subluxation (J Neurosurg 1988;68:18).

Cmplc: Permanent dysfunction; syringomyelia.

Diff Dx: Transverse myelitis.

Lab: X-ray with plain films to find obvious fractures—do the whole spine; MRI, if available; CT is an option but less definitive for cord injury. If in shock, do whole trauma evaluation before focusing on the spine—CBC with diff; PT/PTT; type and cross; metabolic profile; ethanol level; liver function tests; UA; urine toxic screen; EKG; plain films of chest and pelvis as well; consider head and abdominal CT.

Emergency Management:

- Treat shock—Airway, iv resuscitation, control bleeding, keep warm.
- Maintain spinal stability, best way to do this has not been elucidated. Whether holding in-line traction conveys any benefit over C-collar and sandbag head immobilization is not clear.
- Iv fluids at 20 cc/kg bolus × 2 if needed; consider cardiac evaluation.
- Pressors (eg, dopamine 5-20 μg/kg/min, or norepinephrine 2-20 μg/min), if still in shock, p49.
- Methylprednisolone 30 mg/kg iv bolus over 15 min followed by 5.4 mg/kg/hr drip if spinal cord injury—data suggest that risk does not outweigh the benefit (Nejm 1990;322:1405; Vet Surg 1995;24:128; J Trauma 1998;45:1088); and this is manifested by increased infection and hospitalization (CJEM 2003;5:9; Ann Surg 1993;2:419)—this treatment is not currently advocated here, but would defer to the trauma surgeon/neurosurgeon caring for the patient.
- Many experimental therapies such as U-50488H, an opioid kappa receptor agonist (Brain Res 1993;626:45).
- Neurosurgery consult.

Chapter 14
Obstetrics

14.1 Abdominal Trauma/Uterine Rupture

Clin Obgyn 1990;33:432; Obgyn Cl N Am 1999;26:419; Am Fam
    Phys 2002;66:823

Cause: Multiple causes, but usually motor vehicle accidents; uterine
rupture may be spontaneous in those with normal labor; as a result
of previous uterine surgery such as myomectomy (Hum Reprod
1995;10:1475) or previous C-section (Am J Obgyn 1991;165:
996)—high risk if previous classical C-section; from cocaine abuse
(Am J Obgyn 1995;173:243); those with Asherman syndrome
(Obgyn 1986;67:864); uterine anomalies; prior invasive molar
surgery; h/o placenta accreta; abnormal fetal presentation; or fetal
anomaly.

Epidem: Most maternal traumas are found to be minor, and fetal
health is directly related to maternal well-being. Even those with
minor maternal trauma, though, may have a problem with significant fetal injury or death. Three-point restraints—low-lying seatbelt with shoulder harness—convey the most protection to
mother and fetus if they were to suffer a motor vehicle accident.

Pathophys: Although uterine rupture can occur with abdominal
trauma, it happens < 1% of the time and it is more common to
get retroperitoneal hemorrhage, splenic lacerations, liver lacerations or kidney lacerations from abdominal trauma in the gravid
patient. Placental abruption may also be a factor in approximately 4% of minor traumas and up to 50% of major traumas.

291

Sx: Uterine rupture presents with a diffusely tender abdomen.

Si: Shock, unable to determine uterine fundus or fetal lie.

Crs: Timely diagnosis of a surgical abdomen is paramount.

Cmplc: Maternal hemorrhage causing shock or fetal distress or death.

Lab: CBC with diff; PT/PTT; medical blood type for consideration of Rhogam; Kleihauer-Betke of limited usefulness despite theoretic considerations in low-risk women (Am J Obgyn 2004;190:1461); consider type and cross; consider DIC profile if significant maternal/fetal transfusion suspected.

- *X-ray:* US for uterine and fetal imaging (Am J Perinatol 1996;13:177), and evaluation of intra-abdominal free fluid, and imaging of kidneys, liver, spleen, and retroperitoneum if possible.
- *Fetal heart:* 10 min with Doppler if < 20 wks gestation, and 20 min of monitoring with contraction monitor if > 20 weeks gestation and pt is stable, longer periods of monitoring for more severely injured pts with 4 hr being the standard of care, if pt is significantly injured.

Emergency Management:
- Iv fluids and O_2.
- Doppler to listen for fetal heart tones.
- Pt on left side if fetal distress.
- Do not limit maternal evaluation during trauma due to pregnancy status—standard of care is the same as for a non-gravid patient.
- Immediate OB consult; general surgical consult, as deemed appropriate.

14.2 Ectopic Pregnancy

Acad Emerg Med 1995;2:1081; 1995;2:1090

Cause: Implantation of embryo other than in uterus.

Epidem: Approximately 2% of all pregnancies with increasing incidence; 95% are tubal, but also can be ovarian, cervical, intra-abdominal (0.5%). Post-tubal ligation rate is 1:1,000 over 10 yr, it is 30:1,000, if electrocoagulation tubal performed. Increased in urban populations due to PID, previous pelvic surgery such as previous ectopic, IUD, and other reasons (Ann EM 1999;33:283); those in rural populations tend to have no risk factors (Fam Med 1996;28:111).

Pathophys: Scarred tubes have a slow transfer rate and the blastocyst implants wherever it is on d 6; of note, efficacy of oral contraceptives not affected by antibiotic use, except for rifampin—reports in past show equivocal findings secondary to bias (J Am Acad Dermatol 2002;46:917).

Sx: Nearly all in first trimester; report of missed period, although withdrawal bleeding may mask this. Abdominal/pelvic discomfort similar to menstrual pains, referred pain to shoulder may be a sign of diaphragmatic irritation from intraperitoneal bleeding.

Si: Nonspecific (Ann EM 1999;33:283), palpable pain or cervical motion tenderness may not be present; check for open cervical os which may be attained by bimanual exam or speculum exam if uncertain (EMJ 2004;21:461); hypotension may be present.

Crs: Without surgery, death in 2:1000 of the population.

Cmplc: Shock, surgical sterility.

Diff Dx: PID, spontaneous abortion (threatened), which has an increased risk in first trimester with caffeine use (Nejm 2000;343:1839), septic abortion, appendicitis, ruptured ovarian corpus luteum or follicle cyst, endometriosis cyst.

Lab: CBC with diff; serum β-HCG, with level < 1,000 mIU/ml with 4-fold higher risk (Ann EM 1996;28:10); type and screen (consider type and cross if in shock); progesterone levels not wholly reliable, but should be < 20-25 nanograms/ml in ectopic (Am J

Obgyn 1989;160:1425); subunit of β-HCG, the core fragment, may be predictive of ectopic if < 100 µg/L in the urine—data dredging (J Clin Endocrinol Metab 1994;78:497). Urine pregnancy test positive when serum level > 50 U, thus 90+% pos at first missed period. Serum CK not helpful (Brit J Obgyn 1995;6:233). Serum amylase is not helpful (Am J Emerg Med 1988:327).

X-ray: US with transvaginal is the gold standard in radiology (Fertil Steril 1998:62) and combined with serum β-HCG shows a sensitivity of 100% and specificity of 99.9% for ectopic pregnancy diagnosis (Obgyn 1994;84:1010)—intrauterine pregnancy (IUP) with an ectopic twin is rare phenomenon. US by US trained ER physicians with 90% sensitivity and 88% specificity for right diagnosis (Ann EM 1997;29:338), but the discriminatory zone was a serum β-HCG of 2000 mIU/ml, whereas other sonographers with discriminatory zone of 1000 mIU/ml or less (J Emerg Med 1998;16:699). Look for thin endometrial stripe (Fertil Steril 1996;66:474); is best when serum β-HCG < 1000 (Acad Emerg Med 1999;6:602), and even indeterminate scans should be subclassified as low, intermediate or high-risk (Acad Emerg Med 1998;5:313).

Emergency Management:

- *If equivocal data,* repeat serum β-HCG in 48 hr—highest risk for ectopic is empty uterus and β-HCG rising <66%, followed by empty uterus and β-HCG decreasing less than 50%; followed by empty uterus and β-HCG rising more than 66%. If β-HCG decreased more than 50%, low-risk for ectopic irrespective of US findings (Ann EM 1999;34:703). Discuss with obstetrician.
- *If pos but stable,* OB consult. Consider methotrexate if fetal tissue < 4 cm in diameter, no fetal heartbeat (Fertil Steril 1989;51:435; Nejm 2000;343:1325) and serum β-HCG < 5,000 mIU/ml (Am J Obstet Gynecol 1996;174:1840) or laparoscopic salpingostomy.

- *If pos and unstable*, 2 large bore ivs, type and cross performed, OB consult for laparotomy.
- Culdocentesis not commonly performed, but will show non-clotting blood from hemoperitoneum along with pos serum β-HCG in 99.2% if ruptured ectopic (Obgyn 1985;65:519). Laparoscopy (diagnosis and therapy) has replaced paracentesis in these cases as well.

14.3 Perimortem Delivery

OBSTETRICS

Cause: Trauma, chronic pulmonary or cardiac conditions, pulmonary embolus, substance abuse [eg, toluene (Obgyn 1991;77:504)] or other etiologies that may cause maternal death.

Epidem: Rare, but increases with increasing maternal age (Obgyn 1983;61:210) and previously higher frequency in adolescents (Clin Obgyn 1978;21:1191).

Pathophys: Fetus at risk with maternal resuscitation, emergent stratification as follows:
- Gestational age
- Length and quality of resuscitation
- Underlying maternal health
- Prenatal problems, such as oligohydramnios, abnormal triple markers or level II US, etc.

Sx/Si: Shock—decreased mentation, hypotension, hypoxia, decreased urine output, abnormal cardiac exam (tachycardia or bradycardia with ectopy or murmur).

Crs: More than 20 min of resuscitation unlikely to have good outcome, with each 5-min increment from 0 to 20 ranging from good to poor prognosis.

Cmplc: Fetal demise.

Lab: None specific since this is a clinical decision—usual trauma labs on mother, remember CBC with diff and glucose on child.

Emergency Management:
- Resuscitate mother.
- Immediate C-section.
- Obstetrics and neonatology consults immediately.

14.4 Placental Abruption

J Perinatol 1988;8:174

Cause: Previous hx, HT, spontaneous, trauma and drug use [cigarette (Am J Epidem 1996;144:881), ethanol, cocaine, amphetamine] are the major causes.

Epidem: Approximately 1% of pregnancies; recurrence rate of approximately 10%; associated with increasing maternal age.

Pathophys: Separation of placenta prior to delivery of fetus, with < 100 cc of blood loss and no other problems as mild; 100-500 cc of blood loss with fetal distress and uterine contractions as moderate, and hemorrhagic shock with imminent fetal demise as severe.

Sx: Painful peripartum third trimester bleeding.

Si: Tender and large uterus; uterine contractions; signs of shock; fetal distress.

Crs: Varies.

Cmplc: Maternal hemorrhage, shock, fetal distress.

Diff Dx: Cervical bleeding, marginal sinus bleeding, uterine rupture, vaginal trauma, bloody show, hematuria.

Lab: CBC with diff; type and cross; PT/PTT.

Emergency Management:
- Iv fluids, O_2, pt on left side, if fetal distress.
- Blood products as appropriate for significant anemia or coagulopathy (p176).
- Delivery, OB consult emergently for anything more than minor bleeding.

14.5 Placenta Previa

J Perinatol 1988;8:174

Cause: Low-lying placenta about the cervical os.

Epidem: 1:150 deliveries; increases with maternal age, h/o previous previa, and with previous uterine scar.

Pathophys: Vessels of placenta will be exposed and prone to bleeding if trying to implant in the cervical region.

Sx: Painless peripartum third trimester bleeding.

Si: US before digital exam—manipulating cervical os region may cause hemorrhage; signs of shock; careful speculum exam with clear speculum (watch as advancing the speculum) is probably OK, as long as it is removed once you confirm bleeding from cervical os.

Crs: Most low-lying placentas found on US during pregnancy migrate from the cervical os by the third trimester.

Cmplc: Maternal hemorrhage.

Diff Dx: As for placental abruption.

Lab: CBC with diff; consider type and cross.
- *X-ray:* US, and transvaginal is OK.

Emergency Management:
- Iv fluids, O_2, patient on left side if fetal distress.
- OB consult for C-section delivery.

14.6 Precipitous Delivery

Cause/Epidem: Uncertain.

Pathophys: Delivery occurs within 3 hr from the onset of true labor.

Sx: Contractions every 2-3 min, urge to defecate, spontaneous rupture of membranes.

Si: Uterine contractions, cervix widely dilated with complete efface-ment, crowning.

Crs: Fast and imminent delivery.

Cmplc: Uterine atony with post-partum hemorrhage.

Lab: Fetal heart monitoring will usually show deep variable decelerations—increased vagal tone from head compression—look/listen for fetal heart rate accelerations that are appropri-ately tachycardic (150-160 bpm) as soon as the contraction eases.

Emergency Management:
- Iv access; OB consult.
- Deliver the neonate (skills to be developed with 1:1 men-toring), but remember to put hands on either side of neonate's head with thumbs toward the nose, bulb suction mouth and then nares; deliver the anterior shoulder with gentle downward pressure, followed by upward pressure delivering the posterior shoulder; slide hand along back and gently grasp the thigh, so that the baby does not slip.
- Hand baby off for warming, drying, and stimulation.
- Anticipate post-partum hemorrhage (Int J Gynaecol Obstet 1998;61:79)—(1) uterine massage or breast feeding, if uterine atony; (2) assess for retained products of conception, and remove if necessary; (3) examination of cervix, vagina and per-ineum for repairs; (4) oxytocin 20-30 U in 1 L IVF and run at 100 cc/hr, if unsuccessful; (5) methergine 0.2 mg im, if unsuc-cessful; (6) prostaglandin 15-methyl PGF_{2a} 0.25 mg im or intrauterine injection (Obgyn 1980;55:665); 7) misoprostol 1000 μg pr (Obgyn 1998;92:212); 8) gemeprost (PGE_1 ana-logue) pessary 1 mg intrauterine (Brit J Obgyn 1993;100:691), intravaginal or pr (J Perinat Med 1999;27:231).

14.7 Abnormal Presentations

J Perinatol 1991;11:297

Cause: Occiput Anterior is the preferred position for presenting fetal portion at perineum. Occiput posterior, transverse, brow presentations, face presentations, and asynclitism (parietal bone presenting) are probably variations that occur as the fetus proceeds through the birth canal. Breech and transverse lie presentations are more common in those with preterm labor and uterine anomalies (eg, fibroids) (Obgyn 1976;47:427).

Emergency Management:
- All deliveries should be performed in a hospital birthing center. Those with known or suspected problems should be encouraged to be checked as soon as labor onset is questioned.
- If the appropriate delivery staff is not available, it may be necessary to perform a delivery in the setting of precipitous delivery or perimortem delivery. This book is not a substitute for appropriate mentoring and training, but as a refresher guide. For breech, limb presentation, and prolapsed cord, please read further.

14.8 Breech Presentation

Curr Opin Obgyn 1992;4:807

Cause: Preterm gestation (fetus did not yet "flip," eg); congenital [eg, associated with torticollis (J Ped Surg 2000;35:1091)] or uterine (eg, bicornuate) anomalies.

Epidem: Approximately 3% of deliveries.

Si: Leopold maneuvers to ascertain fetal lie and locate feet; vaginal exam for same reason. Buttocks presentation with feet about the head is a *Frank breech*, buttocks presentation with feet near bottom is *Complete breech*, and leg presentation is *Footling breech*.

Crs: If breech lie is known, external version may have been performed prior to onset of labor—this is attempted after 37 wks gestation in hospital birthing units.

Cmplc: Entrapment of the fetal head, spinal cord injury, brachial plexus injury, asphyxia, intracranial hemorrhage—with consequent lower APGAR scores and orthopedic or internal organ trauma also possible.

Lab: US if possible to define fetal lie.

Emergency Management:

- OB and anesthesia available for delivery if possible, and they may prefer to perform C-section (Obgyn 1987;69:965). Should be alerted even for precipitous delivery.

- *If delivery is imminent,* let the buttocks and trunk deliver to the midabdominal region, with the fetal back facing the mother's anterior pelvis. A frank breech may need help with leg delivery, and put a finger in the popliteal area behind the fetal knee, fully flex the hip so that the knee delivers followed by the leg and foot. For complete and footling breech, attempt to deliver the legs first—gently direct the feet out. Gently feed out the umbilical cord to have some extra length, wrap the body in a blanket, and when the scapula are seen, sweep your finger across the chest to deliver the arms one at a time—try to hook the volar aspect of the elbow to facilitate arm delivery. Then gently lift so that fetal midscapular region is aiming for mother's superior pubic symphysis region—this gentle lifting should be performed in conjunction with an assistant. While angling the body as above, use one hand and place one finger on the maxilla of the fetal face. Avoid hyperextension of the neck, and use fundal pressure as well to help deliver the head.

- Pitfalls: 1) Be prepared for a neonatal recovery; 2) perform an elective episiotomy if this delivery has to occur in the ER; 3) the head may get trapped at the cervix, and if the cervix is going to tear, you may elect to perform Dursin's incisions to facilitate head delivery and then know where the lacerations are located (which are directed away from the urethra). Dursin's incisions: if the cervix closest to the urethra is 12 o'clock, the incisions are made at 2 o'clock, 6 o'clock, and 10 o'clock; and 4) call OB and anesthesia as soon as it appears that precipitous breech delivery is occurring.

14.9 Limb Presentation

Cause: Seen with vertex, breech, and transverse lie presentations.

Si: Hand or leg presenting.

Crs: Hand and head presentation OK if vertex precedes the limb during delivery.

Cmplc: Leg as with breech (footling breech); transverse lie at risk for umbilical cord prolapse.

Lab: US if possible to delineate anatomy.

Emergency Management:
- To hospital birthing center if possible, OB and anesthesia consults.
- Hand presentations preceding the vertex and transverse lie presentations necessitate C-section and labor does not proceed precipitously.
- Precipitous Footling breech presentations, as above.

14.10 Prolapsed Cord

Lancet 1966;2:1443

Cause: No fetal body part applied to cervix allowing umbilical cord to extrude with rupture of membranes.

Epidem: Incidence of 0.1-0.6%; more common with breech presentation, polyhydramnios, transverse lie. Approximately 47% due to obstetrical intervention (Am J Perinatol 1999;16:479) without increased neonatal morbidity/mortality in these pts.

Sx: Rupture of membranes.

Si: Umbilical cord felt in vaginal vault—check for pulse.

Crs: Poor perinatal outcome even with emergent C-section (J Reprod Med 1998;43:129).

Cmplc: Fetal anoxia.

Lab: None.

Emergency Management:
- Trendelenburg; O_2; iv access; immediate OB consult.
- Place hand in vagina and hold fetal presenting part from compressing the cord between the fetus and the cervix.

14.11 Shoulder Dystocia

Am Fam Phys 2004;69:1707; Obgyn Cl N Am 1995;22:247; Asia Oceania J Obgyn 1994;20:195

Cause: Large fetus/small pelvis but macrosomia with subsequent shoulder dystocia is not predictable (Surg Gynecol Obstet 1992;175:515).

Epidem: Based upon fetal weight, with an increased incidence with an increase in fetal weight; > 5% incidence in fetuses who weigh > 4 kg and > 14% incidence in fetuses who weigh > 4.5 kg—these numbers are higher in mothers who are diabetic (Am J Obgyn 1998;179:476).

Pathophys: A mechanical problem with either the anterior shoulder of the fetus impacted behind the symphysis pubis or less commonly the posterior shoulder of the fetus unable to easily pass by the sacrum/coccyx.

Sx: "Turtle head"—the fetal head partially emerges and then retracts with relaxation without any progress being made.

Si: As under symptoms.

Crs: Varies.

Cmplc: Fetal injury such as fracture or brachial plexus injury (Erb's palsy) (Am J Perinatol 1995;12:44); fetal death.

Lab: None specific.

Emergency Management:
- O$_2$; iv fluid; episiotomy.
- Legs up and out—McRobert's maneuver (most effective intervention) (Am J Obgyn 1997;176:656).
- Fundal pressure, push toward spine with hand just above symphysis pubis.
- Woods screw maneuver or try to push anterior shoulder from behind symphysis pubis by rotating the shoulder either way.
- Deliver posterior shoulder first; fracture clavicle.
- Zavenelli maneuver—push fetal head back into vagina and hold it while C-section performed; 92% successful (Obgyn 1999:312).

14.12 Preeclampsia and Eclampsia (Toxemia)

Clin Obgyn 1984;27:836; Am Fam Phys 2004;70:2317

Cause: Unknown, some association with gestational diabetes mellitus (Diabetes 1991;40:79; J Reproduct Med 1998;43:372) and/or lupus anticoagulant (Nejm 1985;313:1322).

Epidem: Incidence 1.5% of private OB pts, whereas 12% of teaching hospital pts; 20% of urban poor, and approximately 5% in primips, who represent 85% of all pts with PIH/eclampsia; 25% of patients with chronic HT. This is the second most common cause of maternal deaths—pulmonary embolus is number 1. Risk for development increases as pregnancy progresses; if either parent has preeclampsia associated with their birth, then at least double the risk for pregnancy with preeclampsia (Nejm 2001; 344:867).

On the other hand, it has been noted that the risk of preeclampsia lessens with subsequent pregnancies, but this is transient. Over time, the multi-gravid protection lessens (Nejm 2002;346:33).

Pathophys: Preeclampsia is HT in pregnancy associated with edema and/or proteinuria. If this progresses to seizures and/or coma, then the pt has developed eclampsia. Those with isolated HT (excluding proteinuria as well) in pregnancy probably have a mild form of the preeclampsia spectrum (Clin Exp Hypertens [A]1989;11:1565).

Sympathetic vasoconstriction that abates with delivery—this is in contrast to the normal pregnancy reduction in peripheral vascular resistance mediated by an increased resistance to angiotensin; somehow this effect is lost via a trophoblast-dependent process with platelet dysfunction—potential role of hyperaggregation. CNS changes associated with reversible brain edema and leukoencephalopathy.

Preeclampsia with some endothelial dysfunction that is reversible with ascorbic acid 1 gm iv (Jama 2001;285:1607).

Sx: Rapid weight gain; edema; headache; visual changes; epigastric abdominal pain.

Si: HT starting after 20 wks gestation—before this probably due to chronic HT—look for systolic > 140 or diastolic > 90, with diastolic > 110 foreboding eclampsia; edema; proteinuria; hyperreflexia; papilledema if eclampsia—fundoscopic exam somewhat controversial if suspecting eclampsia, since light stimulation may induce seizures.

Crs: All symptoms disappear by 72 hr post-partum in 95% of people. If si/sx occur in first trimester, consider mole or trophoblastic tumor.

Cmplc: Preeclampsia can be severe and these cases are associated with a 1% maternal and 10% prenatal infant mortality—without treatment, 25-50% of those who are severe will evolve to eclampsia.

Eclampsia (Toxemia): Includes seizures, and may be predicted by the same criteria for preeclampsia, as well as renal failure, CHF, CNS bleed; DIC; Sheehan's syndrome; fetal distress or demise; hepatic hemorrhage and rupture; HELLP (hemolysis, elevated liver profile, low platelets) syndrome; newborn neutropenias, which are transient in 50%, but also associated with sepsis.

Diff Dx: Transient HT of pregnancy; chronic HT in pregnancy; pheochromocytoma.

Lab: CBC with diff, look for thrombocytopenia (Am J Perinatol 1989:32); metabolic profile; liver function tests (Am J Perinatol 1988;5:146); uric acid; consider magnesium level; consider calcium level; UA; consider 24 hr urine for calcium—looking for hypocalciuria; consider DIC profile.

Increased levels of soluble fms-like tyrosine kinase 1 (sFlt-1) predates the clinical syndrome of preeclampsia and decreased levels of placental growth factor (PlGF) also predates the clinical syndrome of preeclampsia—these findings confer risk afor development of preeclampsia (Nejm 2004;350:672).

Emergency Management:

Eclampsia:
- Stabilize, protect airway, O_2, iv access.
- $MgSO_4$ 4 gm iv bolus, then 2 gm per hr drip; may use im option of 10 gm loading, then 5 gm every 4 hr (J Reprod Med 1979;23:107). $MgSO_4$ superior to phenytoin (Nejm 1995; 333:201) and nimodipine (Nejm 2003;348:304).
- Immediate OB consult, definitive treatment is delivery.

Preeclampsia:
- OB consult for all decisions on treatment and outpatient options.

- May use hydralazine 5-10 mg iv or labetalol 10-20 mg iv to acutely treat HT; nifedipine 10 mg sl not advocated here.
- Outpatient HT treatment may use α-methyldopa (Aldomet), hydralazine, propranolol, or clonidine. Not ACE Inhibitors—teratogenic.
- Outpatient prevention may include low dose aspirin (Obgyn 1990;76:742)—data are equivocal.
- Treatment of HT does convey some benefit to the mother, not much to the fetus. Definitive treatment is delivery.

Chapter 15

Ophthalmology

15.1 Acute Glaucoma (Angle Closure)

Aust N Z J Ophthalm 1999;27:358

Cause: Genetic predisposition, hyperopia (farsightedness); after
LASIK procedure (J Cataract Refract Surg 2000;26:620);
intranasal cocaine (J Laryngol Otol 1999;113:250).

Epidem: Approximately 0.2% of population; especially in middle-aged
and elderly (> 50 yr of age).

Pathophys: Smaller eye with shallow anterior chamber that impedes
the normal aqueous humor flow, trapping the fluid posteriorly.
Pressure then builds, compressing the optic nerve.

Sx: Rainbow halos; eye pain that is sudden and bilateral; headache;
nausea and vomiting; scotomas in nasal fields; precipitated by
mydriatics, antacids, anesthesia, and darkness.

Si: Red eye, especially circumcorneal; partially dilated fixed pupil;
corneal edema with blistering and haziness; visual field defects
(Graefes Arch Clin Exp Ophthalm 1999;237:908); corneal pressure > 30 mm Hg—pressures > 18 mm Hg have a 65% sensitivity and specificity.

Crs: 3½% of all patients with tonometry reading of 20-30 mm Hg will
go on to glaucoma in 5 yr.

Cmplc: Blindness; other eye affected within 5-10 yr in 40-80%, and
use of pilocarpine does not confer protection.

Lab: Tonometry.

> **N.B.** Anesthetic drops used to facilitate tonometry will not take the discomfort away.

Emergency Management:
- Ophtho consult, with consideration of pilocarpine 1-2% drops every 5-10 min until relieved and systemic carbonic anhydrase inhibitor (acetazolamide 1 gm iv or 0.5 gm po immediately) to lower pressure.
- Definitive treatment is surgical laser iridotomy (Eye 1999;13: 613) or laser iridoplasty if within 48 hr (Eye 1999;13:26).

15.2 Conjunctivitis

Am J Ophthalm 1991;12:2S

Cause: Bacterial 50-80% of the time, mostly pneumococcus in colder climates, consider *Staphylococcus, Corynebacteria, Haemophilus* (including Koch-Weeks bacillus), chlamydia in warmer climates (Arch Ophthalm 1966;75:639); viral 20% of the time—especially adenovirus; allergic, such as giant papillary conjunctivitis, which is associated with soft contact lens use, trauma, and foreign body, but is truly allergic (Acta Ophthalm Scand suppl 1999;228:17).

Epidem: Second most common reason for red eye; if exclude foreign body, is 95% of the reason for a red eye.

Pathophys: Obvious—inflammation of conjunctiva.

Sx: Sand feeling in eye; discharge from eye(s).

Si: Conjunctival injection; PERRLA and with normal vision; allergic types with preponderance of itching.

Crs: Usually clears in 3-4 d, rarely protracted unless secondary problem (foreign body) or if allergic but treating for infectious.

Cmplc: Protracted course.

Diff Dx: Conjunctivitis associated with paraneoplastic syndrome or inflammatory skin disease—Cicatrizing conjunctivitis (Am J

Ophthalm 2000;129:98); hemorrhagic conjunctivitis with enterovirus 70 (Am J Epidem 1975;102:533).

Lab: None, although consider viral and bacterial cultures for atypical or severe cases.

Emergency Management: Recommend fluorescein with Woods lamp exam for all red eyes with pain looking for corneal abrasion; also consider iritis.

Infectious conjunctivitis: With topical treatment qid: sulfacetamide 10% solution or ointment; TMP/SMX (polytrim) drops are bacteriocidal rather than bacteriostatic and sting less than sulfa; bacitracin/polymyxin ointment; bacitracin/neomycin/polymyxin ointment; gramicidin/neomycin/polymyxin solution; erythromycin 0.5% ointment; gentamicin 0.3% ointment or solution; tobramycin 0.3% solution or ointment; not chloramphenicol 0.02% solution or 1% ointment, which can lead to aplastic anemia, although just as efficacious (J Antimicrob Chemother 1989;23:261); or may try the fluoroquinolones (which are more expensive) which include ciprofloxacin 0.3% solution or ointment, gatifloxacin 0.3% solution, levofloxacin 0.5% solution, moxifloxacin 0.5% solution, or ofloxacin 0.3% solution (Med Lett Drugs Ther 2004;46:25).

Allergic conjunctivitis: (Drugs 1992;43:154; Med Lett Drugs Ther 2004;46:35): Consider the following topical options to both eyes: NSAID ketorolac (Acular) 0.5% 1 drop qid; or antihistamine levocabastine (Livostin) 0.05% 1 drop qid or emedastine (Emadine) 0.05% 1 drop qid; or mast cell stabilizers, such as cromolyn (Crolom) 4% 1-2 drops OU qid or lodoxamide (Alomide) 0.1% 1-2 drops qid; or nedocromil (Alocril) 2% 1-2 drops bid; or pemirolast (Alamast) 0.1% 1-2 drops qid; or mast cell stabilizer/H_1 antihistamine olopatadine (Patanol) 0.1% 1-2 drops bid; or azelastine (Optivar) 0.05% 1 drop bid; or epinastine (Elestat) 0.05% 1 drop bid; or ketotifen (Zaditor) 0.1% 1 drop q 6-12 hr.

15.3 Corneal Abrasion/Foreign Body

Optom Clin 1991;1:119; Am Fam Phys 2004;70:123

Cause: Trauma; extended wear contact lens (Optom Clin 1991; 1:123).

Epidem: Most common reason for red eye.

Pathophys: Direct trauma or rubbing causing trauma to cornea for abrasion.

Sx: Teary, red eye.

Si: Usually unilateral conjunctival injection, check under upper and lower eye lids for foreign body. Metallic foreign bodies with more injection.

Crs: Unremarkable if foreign body removed and timely intervention.

Cmplc: Corneal ulcer, with pseudomonas reported after patching (Clao J 1987;13:161); conjunctivitis.

Diff Dx: Occult globe rupture, if significant trauma.

Lab: None.

Emergency Management:
- Topical anesthetic (proparacaine or tetracaine eye drops)—this usually alleviates all the discomfort; if pt still uncomfortable, rethink this working diagnosis. If foreign body known to be under lid, may withhold topical anesthetic so that removal can be confirmed by pt's response to removal.
- Fluorescein with Woods lamp/slit lamp exam; may have to rinse excess fluorescein to see small abrasions.

Foreign body:
- Remove foreign body with soft, cotton applicator that is moistened—touch and lift, do not rub; 25-G needle; or eye spud—remove rust ring if present with drill if available. This is a taught skill. Once removed, follow Corneal Abrasion instructions.

Corneal abrasion:

- Antibiotic eye ointment (such as erythromycin) tid for 3 d.
- Topical Ketorolac 0.5% eye solution qid for 5 d (Ophthalm 1997;104:1353) or Diclofenac 0.1% eye drops 1 drop every 6 hr for 36 hr (Eye 1997;11:79; Ann EM 2000;35:131) for pain relief.
- Consider mydriatic eye drops, such as 2.5% phenylephrine/1% tropicamide (Ophthalm 1995;102:1936).
- Patching is equivocal (Ophthalm 1995:1936; Ann EM 2001;138:129). May provide some comfort.
- Ophtho consult (may be next day), if unable to remove foreign body completely or if not completely better in 3 d.
- Home with narcotic pain meds—manipulation of eye will have significant discomfort.
- Avoid contact lens use, although topical diclofenac with soft lens use (J Refract Corneal Surg 1994;10:640) and a bandage lens (Brit J Ophthalm 1987;71:285) both tried, but not advocated here as an ER procedure secondary to potentiating possible keratitis or ulcer.

15.4 Herpetic Keratitis

Optom Clin 1991;1:45

Cause: Usually *H. simplex*, but consider *H. zoster*, adenovirus, and other viruses.

Epidem: Excluding foreign bodies, 1% of the cause of red eye.

Pathophys: Inflammation of cornea.

Sx: Photophobia; foreign body sensation.

Si: Corneal ulcer; PERRLA; check under lids.

Crs: Usually associated with iritis—look for ciliary flush.

Cmplc: Chronic ulcers; persistent viral presence (Arch Ophthalm 1993;111:522); hypopyon (white cells in anterior chamber);

long-term corneal opacity to some degree (Acta Ophthalm 1970;48:214).

Diff Dx: Overnight contact lens use giving infectious keratitis (Brit J Ophthalm 1998;82:1272); ultraviolet light exposure (Optom Vis Sci 1994;71:125), and UV protective eye drops of no help (Ophthalmic Res 1998;30:286); exanthems; bacterial (Acad Emerg Med 1994;1:391); chronic topical anesthetic use; bacterial and fungal keratitis after corneal transplant (Ophthalm 1988;95:1450).

Lab: Consider bacterial and viral culture; perhaps PCR for HSV DNA (Can J Ophthalm 2000;35:134).

Emergency Management:
- Topical anesthetics will not fully relieve the discomfort.
- Fluorescein with slit lamp exam may show dendrites—consistent with herpetic keratitis.
- Do not patch or instill steroids.
- Immediate Ophtho consult for consideration of the following: Trifluridine (Viroptic) 1 drop 1% solution every 2 hr as first line; second line is Ara A; topical/oral acyclovir (Ophthalmologica 1997;211:29); antibacterials; cycloplegics to relax ciliary spasm such as 1% atropine bid or 5% homatropine tid.

15.5 Iritis

Post Grad Med 1989;86:117

Cause: Idiopathic by far the most common; iatrogenic [many causes, eg, iv cidofovir (Arch Ophthalm 1997;115:733)]; autoimmune diseases (Ann Ophthalm 1978;10:147) [Behcet syndrome, RA, SLE, ankylosing spondylitis, Reiter syndrome, Sjogren syndrome (Arthritis Rheum 1992;35:560), ulcerative colitis (GE 1967; 52:78), Wegener's granulomatosis]; tuberculosis; syphilis; histoplasmosis; sarcoid; coccidioidomycosis; toxoplasmosis; perhaps autoantibody viral-related; *H. simplex; H. zoster*; CMV; candida; hypermature cataract; trauma; intraocular tumor (Cancer 1979;44:1511); Whipple's disease bacterium; Hanson disease; intranasal drug use, such as cocaine (Ann EM 1991;20:192).

Epidem: Excluding foreign body, 2% of the reason for a red eye.

Pathophys: A form of uveitis.

Sx: Pain; photophobia; tearing without exudate.

Si: Tenderness; visual blurring; turbid aqueous humor; low pressure; miosis—constricted pupil with pain on direct and consensual pupillary response to light (Lancet 1981;2:1254); circumcorneal injection—ciliary flush; have the patient accommodate with own finger—a specific (97%) yet not sensitive (74%) test (BMJ (Clin Res Ed) 1987;295:812). Do slit lamp exam with fluorescein to look for other causes; check under lids.

Crs: Variable depending on etiology.

Cmplc: Refractory course; rare renal-ocular syndrome with interstitial nephritis (Am J Med 1984;77:189).

Diff Dx: Acute angle closure glaucoma, keratitis, foreign body.

Lab: None.

Emergency Management:
- Ophtho consult immediately—which will consider topical steroids and cycloplegics.
- Future role of prostaglandin synthetase inhibitors, including NSAIDs (Arch Ophthalm 1980;98:1106; Fortschr Ophthalm 1987;84:353).

15.6 Ruptured Globe

Int Ophthalm Clin 1995;35:71

Cause: Usually traumatic.

Epidem: Uncommon; usually a male in third or fourth decade of life; ethanol use a risk with leisure time activities (Ophthalmologica 1999;213:380).

Pathophys: Usually ruptures at site of muscular insertion, if not readily apparent on exam.

Sx: Eye pain; visual loss.

Si: Complete hyphema; protrusion of globe contents; loss of usual globe contours; perform a careful eye exam without instilling any medicines into eye.

Crs: Visual recovery is usually scant.

Cmplc: Vision loss.

Diff Dx: Foreign body in anterior chamber (Ophthalmic Surg 1985;16:586).

Lab: Facial/head CT (Am J Neuroradiol 1995;16:936).

Emergency Management:
- Metallic or plastic eye shield and keep head of bed elevated; npo.
- Consider broadspectrum iv antibiotics, and update tetanus as in any trauma, if needed.
- Immediate ophthalmology consult.

15.7 Sudden Vision Loss—Traumatic

Acad Emerg Med 1996;3:1056; Neurol Clin 1998;16:323

Cause: Trauma to the optic nerve—laceration, contusion, compression; retinal detachment; retinal hemorrhage. Trauma to the globe or lens (described in previous section).

Epidem: Uncommon, but must be able to recognize.

Pathophys: Optic nerve compression, retinal detachment and retinal hemorrhage can be reversible, if limited involvement. Optic nerve laceration and contusion usually with irreversible vision loss.

Sx: Pain; loss of vision; retinal detachments may simulate flashing lights.

Si: Trauma to the globe either penetrating or blunt; look for abnormality to the retina and vitreous humor.

Crs: As described in Pathophys.

Cmplc: Vision loss.

Diff Dx: Atraumatic causes (much more common): orbital (p204) or sinus (p363) infection (Laryngoscope 1984;94:1050); carotid artery stenosis giving transient monocular findings (Nejm 2001;345:1084); CVA (p251)—eg, amaurosis fugax; migraine (p279); hypertensive crisis (p37); cerebral blindness; ischemic optic neuropathy, central retinal artery or vein occlusion (J Neurol Neurosurg Psychiatry 1993;56:234); optic neuritis; uveitis; ectopia lentis; toxins such as methanol or quinine (Ann EM 1987;16:98); acute cataract formation; rheumatologic disorders such as Giant Cell Arteritis (Semin Ophthalm 1999;14:109) or SLE.

Lab: Facial/head CT; MRI, if available.

Emergency Management:
- Iv pain control if needed; update tetanus if needed; npo.
- Immediate ophthalmology consult for consideration of emergency orbital decompression (Otolaryngol Head Neck Surg 1981;89:252).
- Minor retinal detachments and minor retinal hemorrhages may have next day follow-up after discussion with ophthalmologist.

OPHTHALMOLOGY

Chapter 16

Orthopedics

16.1 Bursitis/Tendonitis

Med Sci Sports Exerc 1998;30:1183

Cause: Inflammation of bursa or tendons; may be infectious in etiology—especially olecranon and prepatellar areas (Septic Arthritis p340).

Epidem: Common.

Pathophys: Overuse or acute stress phenomenon; multifocal bursitis may be associated with homozygous homocystinuria (J Inherit Metab Dis 1999;22:185).

Sx: Pain of specific joint; remember referred pain, such as neck to any location in upper extremity, back to hip, hip to knee, etc.

Si: Pain with palpation in bursitis; pain with range of motion in tendonitis—have pt hold specific position in opposition to your force to isolate specific area; Finkelstein's test in de Quervain's tendonitis.

Crs: Acute with resolution within 2 wks or chronic, if more protracted.

Cmplc: Chronic pain.

Diff Dx: Arthritis; ligamentous sprain; rarely due to sea urchin spines that does not resolve until spines removed (Joint Bone Spine 2000;67:94); consider carpal tunnel syndrome for wrist pain syndromes, which is best treated with corticosteroid injection or splinting, and not NSAIDs (Ann Fam Med 2004;2:267).

Lab: Consider plain radiographs if suspicious for significant fracture. Consider needle aspiration if non-prosthetic joint to ascertain etiology.

Emergency Management:

- Inject with anesthetic agent (lidocaine, bupivicaine) and steroids—pro study of anserine bursitis (South Med J 2000;93:207), equivocal for shoulder tendonitis (Scand J Rheumatol 1985;14:76) and perhaps neg for Achilles tendonitis (Clin J Sport Med 1996;6:245); tendonitis (such as de Quervain's) does not require the injection to be in the tendon sheath to be effective.
- Splinting of shoulder or elbow (tennis elbow) for example—if using sling, be sure to have daily shoulder movements to avoid adhesive capsulitis. Heel cup for plantar fasciitis or Achilles tendonitis (Brit J Sports Med 1981;15:117).
- Ice for 24-48 hr.
- Acetaminophen and NSAIDs about equal efficacy in traumatic situations (Curr Opin Rheumatol 2000;12:150), NSAIDs better in inflammatory realms (RA, gout, etc); im ketorolac as efficacious as po ibuprofen (Acad Emerg Med 1998;5:118; Ann EM 1995;26:117).
- Dimethyl sulfoxide of no help (Med Sci Sports Exerc 1981;13:215).

16.2 Dislocations

Cause: Usually traumatic, although those with joint laxity due to connective tissue disorder may need minimal trauma. Less force needed for recurrent injuries. In peds, remember to consider child abuse. Consider complication of seizure.

Epidem: Variable.

Pathophys: If fracture of joint surface, may go on to arthritis.

Sx: Pain; deformity; swelling.

Si: Tenderness; decreased to no range of motion of affected joint; deformity—palpate location of dislocated part; check distal neurovascular status; intra-articular edema.

Crs: Reduction curative, coincident fracture may prolong rehabilitation.

Cmplc: Fracture, neurovascular damage.

Lab: Plain radiographs—2 pictures 90° from each other. The Y-view in shoulder dislocations is key. Post-reduction views are standard, yet necessity in some areas [shoulder (Ann EM 1996;28: 399)] has been questioned.

Emergency Management:

- Iv access for pain control.
- Local block such as digital, radial nerve, or median nerve, if feasible.
- Ortho consult for all dislocations with neurologic or vascular compromise.
- Procedural sedation with midazolam should be considered for reduction of large joints such as ankle, elbow, shoulder, etc.
- Steady and gradual traction over 2-5 min is more effective than more force attempted quickly.
- Get post-reduction films.

Specific examples:

- *Ankle:* Obvious deformity should be reduced if possible to prevent skin tearing/breakdown—easiest to reduce ankle with both hip and knee flexed (to 90° if possible) so that muscles to the Achilles tendon are relaxed. Most of these have coincident fractures. Most fracture fragments will move during reduction, so patient should be well sedated so that there is minimal muscle tension during the maneuver to avoid injury to the articular cartilage.
- *Digit:* Digital block, being sure to infiltrate the dorsal surface on the hand and the plantar surface on the foot to get a complete block. Reduction should first have outward traction in

the direction of the long axis of the dislocated phalanx. With other hand, move the base of the dislocated bone toward its natural position. Then move the long axis of the phalanx to its natural neutral position, so that the digit is now normally aligned.

- *Elbow:* Five types of elbow dislocations:

  Peds: Nursemaid elbow dislocations are pediatric dislocations of the radial head, and these are uncommon in adults. To reduce a pediatric nursemaid elbow, place your thumb over the radial head, extend the elbow and supinate the forearm, and then flex the forearm. A pop may be felt or heard.

  Adult: The elbow may dislocate posteriorly (most common), anteriorly, laterally, medially, or the radius and ulna may diverge laterally and medially, respectively. Reduction may be accomplished with procedural sedation. Have an assistant anchor the humerus while distracting the elbow and guide the proximal forearm bones around the humeral condyles. Bring the elbow into flexion once the olecranon/radius is felt to re-seat, and apply posterior splint with elbow at 90° flexion. Ligamentous injury is common (Clin Orthop 1987:221), but conservative treatment is usually adequate (Clin Orthop 1987:165).

- *Hip:* Done with Ortho, posterior dislocations are more common.

- *Knee:* A true Ortho emergency, the popliteal artery as at large risk with a knee dislocation. Reduction should be done with ortho involved, splint in position of comfort. Consider arteriogram—perhaps half the patients with vascular injury will require emergent surgery, others with self-resolving spasm or intimal flap, for example, and may be able to advocate for watchful waiting.

  N.B. The ballotable patella or other indications of effusion may not be present (as seen with isolated ligamentous injuries) because the synovial membrane may be torn, and thus traumatic effusion is into the thigh and leg.

- *Patella:* Lateral more common than medial. Completely extend knee which may reduce patella. If not, keep the knee extended while attempting the following. Put thumbs at medial edge if medial dislocation and lateral edge if lateral dislocation, and gently push toward anatomic alignment, may need to lift leading edge with fingers just a little.

- *Shoulder* (Med Sci Sports Exerc 1984;16:444; Am J Emerg Med 1999;17:288): May dislocate anterior, inferior, or posterior. Associated compression fracture of the humeral head is called a Hill-Sachs deformity. Some general reduction principles:
  1) The pt needs to be relaxed;
  2) Distract the humerus so that the humeral head can slip past the glenoid rim;
  3) Sometimes guiding the humeral head directly is needed as distraction is being applied;
  4) Twenty milliliters of 1% lidocaine in the affected shoulder joint can bring about significant relief (sterile prep and injection) and decreases the need for intravenous sedation (J Bone Joint Surg [Am] 2002;84-A:2135);
  5) Bring the arm to the pt's side, elbow 90° of flexion, and immobilize in this position once reduction completed.

- *Anterior dislocation* (Am J Emerg Med 1991;9:180): Methods include:
  (1) Weight (aka Stimson or Wait)—pt prone with 10 lbs. of weight wrapped to freely hanging arm, reduction accomplished over time—this is a good wilderness rescue technique. One variation is with pt sitting in chair with arm draped over backrest and hanging straight down (Injury 1992;23:479).
  (2) Hippocratic variation: patient supine and anchored with one sheet wrapped around affected axilla for countertraction and reducer grasps elbow, which is flexed to 90° with

forearm pointing to ceiling. Distract the humerus—original method was with physician's heel in pt's axilla as countertraction, but can either put other sheet around you and tie off to pt's elbow and lean back, or just hold elbow in antecubital fossa firmly. Walk the humerus into abduction, and gently externally and internally rotate.

(3) Scapular rotation (Ann EM 1992;21:1349): Pt prone (supine if necessary) (Ann EM 1996;27:92), weights in hand, rotate the inferior scapular pole medially and superiorly until reduced.

(4) External rotation (Jacep 1979;8:528): Pt is supine, humerus is completely adducted, elbow at 90° with forearm pointing to ceiling, slowly and gently externally rotate the shoulder.

(5) Walk (Milch) (J Trauma 1992;32:801): Pt supine, bring the arm from adduction with 90° elbow flexion to full abduction with external rotation, while gently walking it to this position.

(6) The backstroke: Begin with pt supine, arm in adduction with elbow at 0°, gently walk the arm to 180° of forward flexion, as if doing a swimming backstroke.

- *Inferior dislocation* (Instr Course Lect 1985;34:232): Significant trauma. Pt is supine; place the sheet over the shoulder for countertraction; the arm vector for reduction is approximately 180° abduction. May be truly irreducible with closed technique.

- *Posterior dislocation*: Pt supine; vector for reduction is the long axis of humerus with arm adducted.

16.3 Fracture Management

Emerg Med Clin N Am 2000;18:85

Cause: Usually traumatic, possibly due to child abuse in children, or osteogenesis imperfecta (OI) as underlying cause in children with multiple fractures and low intensity trauma, pathologic fractures in people with either neoplastic or other chronic diseases, such as TB in which the bone is abnormal, and more common in the elderly or in those with impaired mobility due to osteoporosis; a difficult diagnosis is that of stress fractures where repetitive forces may cause x-ray negative fractures. Be sure to screen the whole patient in the setting of multisytem trauma, and look for syncope or other co-morbid illnesses in the elderly or those with chronic diseases.

Epidem: Common; perhaps increased osteoporosis risk in women with increased vitamin A intake based on hip fracture study (Nejm 2003;348:287, Jama 2002;287:47)

Pathophys: Bony anatomy core knowledge includes bony landmarks (the trochanteric area in the hip is the basis for our hip fracture descriptions, eg) and remembering that pediatric bones will a have growth plate (physis)—with regards to the physis, the segment at the end of the bone with the joint cartilage is called the epiphysis, and the segment toward the major portion of the bone mass is called the metaphysis. Transverse or oblique fractures usually due to uniform load without rotation, whereas spiral fractures associated with a rotational force to the bone. Children may have fractures involving the physis that are called Salter-Harris (SH) fractures (Am Fam Phys 1992;46:1180):

- (<u>S</u>lip) SH I is a fracture through the complete physis and may not show on initial x-ray or may show as a slipping of the epiphysis relative to the metaphysis
- (<u>A</u>ground) SH II is the physis with a portion of the metaphysis, in our picture is the bone on the bottom (aground) relative to the physis
- (<u>L</u>esser) SH III is a portion of the epiphysis and physis, in our picture is the bone with the lesser mass (epiphysis compared to metaphysis)

- (Two) SH IV is an oblique fracture through the physis so that the fracture segment has both metaphysis and epiphysis—two (both) are involved
- (Ram) SH V is a compression injury of the physis and may not show on initial x-ray, or may appear as the epiphysis rammed into the metaphysis.

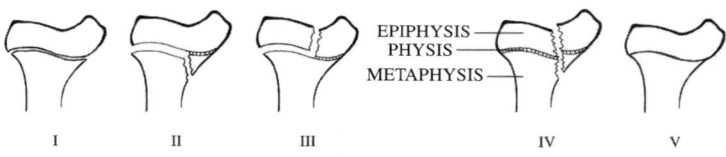

Figure 16.1 Pediatric Fractures

When *describing fractures*, we need to be specific in the following areas:
- Bone(s) involved
- Displacement of bones from their usual anatomic location
- Angulation from their normal anatomic angle
- Secondary dislocation
- Amount of skin tension or breach in skin overlying the fracture
- Status of distal peripheral vascular and neurologic function

Specific Considerations:

Ottawa ankle rules (Jama 1993;269:1127)

Pts aged 16 years or older (Ped Emerg Care 2003;19:73; Acad Emerg Med 1999;6:1005) may have ankle or foot radiographs based on some basic triage criteria (100% sensitive for significant fracture), which are the following:
- Injury < 10 d
- Not a reassessment

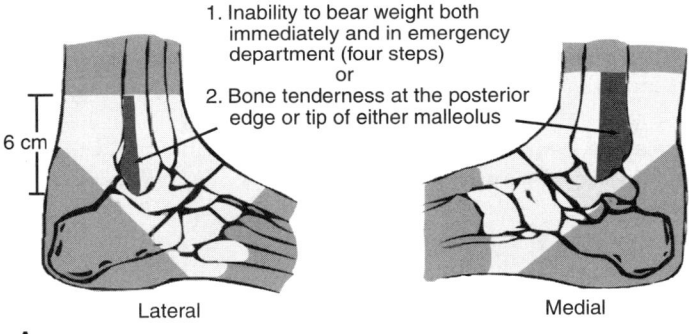

An ankle x-ray series is only necessary if there is pain near the malleoli and any of these findings:

1. Inability to bear weight both immediately and in emergency department (four steps)
   or
2. Bone tenderness at the posterior edge or tip of either malleolus

6 cm

Lateral   Medial

A.

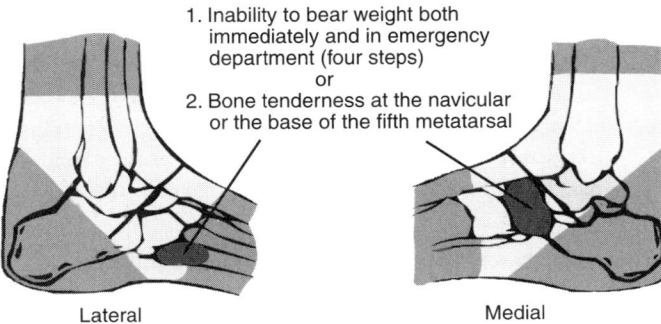

A foot x-ray series is only necessary if there is pain in the midfoot and any of these findings:

1. Inability to bear weight both immediately and in emergency department (four steps)
   or
2. Bone tenderness at the navicular or the base of the fifth metatarsal

Lateral   Medial

B.

Figure 16.2 Ottawa Ankle Rules: **A.** Refined clinical decision rule for ankle radiographic series in ankle injury patients. **B.** Refined clinical decision rule for foot radiographic series in ankle injury patients. (Reproduced with permission from Stiell IG, et al., Decision rules for the use of radiography in acute ankle injuries. Jama 1993;269:1130.)

16.3 Fracture Management **325**

<u>Ottawa knee rule</u> (Ann EM 1995;26:405; 2001;38:364)

Pts > 5 yr of age should have plain x-rays of the knee for acute knee injury for any of the following indications—in comparing these two rules (knee and ankle), knee injuries are unlike ankle injuries in that ligament injury and avulsion fractures may necessitate surgical intervention and thus, x-rays will usually be needed—and provides 95% sensitivity and specificity for detecting clinically significant fractures in adults (Jama 1996;275:611) and 100% sensitivity and approximately 43% specificity in children 5-16 yr of age (Ann EM 2003; 42:48):

- Age ≥ 55 yr old
- Tenderness at head of fibula
- Isolated patella tenderness
- Inability to flex knee to 90°
- Inability to bear weight for 4 steps immediately and in the ER.

Sx: H/o trauma; pain, usually with pinpoint location to affected bone; obvious deformity.

Referred pain—knee pain in hip fractures is common (Ann EM 1997;29:418).

Si: Tenderness; edema; ecchymoses; angulation; crepitus; tendon or ligamentous instability about specific joint; perhaps auscultatory percussion in hip fractures (Clin Orthop 1977:9)—place stethescope over the pubic symphysis, percuss over the patella one at a time, and an ipsilateral fracture should have decreased sound conduction.

Crs: Extremely variable depending on what type of fracture, the cause, and patient's overall health. Osteoporotic fractures may not be amenable to reduction or repair, and therapy should be tailored toward osteoporosis treatment [including exercise (Brit J Sports Med 1999;33:378)].

Cmplc: Non-union; open fracture (skin not intact); vascular or neurologic compromise.

Diff Dx: Rupture of ligaments with or without avulsion injury; stretching of ligaments, aka sprain [ankle review (Am Fam Phys 2001;63:93)]; tendon rupture [elbow—(Orthop Clin N Am 1999;30:95)]; tendonitis (acute inflammation) or tendinopathy (overuse syndrome) (BMJ 2002;324:626).

Lab: Potential need for CBC with diff, type and screen, and EKG, if pt needs operative repair and has age-related anesthesia concerns.

Increase plasma homocysteine level associated with increased risk of hip fracture—numbers here are based on age-related levels and can either be viewed as number of standard deviations away from the norm versus quartile type distribution—the risk based on this level independent of other risks such as bone mineral density (Nejm 2004;350:2033)

X-ray: Plain radiographs [facial only need single 30° occipitomental for screening with CT for further delineation—this does not include mandible (J Trauma 2002;52:688)], and children may need comparison views from the contralateral side, although utility of comparison views controversial (Ann EM 1992;21:895); with CT or MRI, if unable to adequately assess if true fracture [such as femoral head cortical fracture (Am J Roentgenol 1990;155:93)] and would be operative repair (as seen in some hip fractures), or if vertebral body fracture and assessing for retropulsion or posterior element involvement. Simple mandibular views as good as pantomographic for mandibular fractures (Acad Emerg Med 2000;7:141). Special rib films are not clinically indicated, but chest films are helpful to look for associated injuries with complaint of traumatic rib pain (Am J Roentgenol 1982;138:91). Algorithms for CT dependent on area in question, eg, Le Fort facial fractures use coronal CT, whereas zygoma with axial (Am J Neuroradiol 1991;12:861)—give the radiologist clinical info.

Bone scan becoming of limited use in this arena (specifically because it does not give other information about the anatomy in question).

Emergency Management:

- Splint, ice, elevate, and npo pending evaluation.
- Immediate pain control, consider iv access or appropriate block—do block only after distal neurovascular exam is completed.
- Traction splint (Hare, Sager) for femur fractures.
- If possible, reduce to anatomic alignment fractures causing vascular compromise, and get post-reduction films.
- Any fracture with neurologic or vascular compromise needs immediate ortho referral.
- Open fractures need iv antibiotics (consider cefazolin 1-2 gm iv), update Td if needed, and emergent ortho consult.
- Fractures that involve articular surfaces need urgent (< 24 hr) ortho follow-up.
- If no fracture, treatment of contusion/sprain/strain based on clinical grounds with splint, immobilization, ice, elevation, NSAIDs, and/or po narcotics. 2-4 wk follow-up.

Specific Considerations:

Fractures of weight bearing joints/bones need to be assessed carefully and approach these with the consideration that ortho should be immediately involved in all of these:

- *Toe digits*—Reduce if angulated, ortho referral if joint space involved or unable to reduce; treat with buddy tape and/or cast boot.
- *Foot* (Semin Roentgenol 1994;29:152; Radiol Clin N Am 1997;35:655; Am Fam Phys 2002;66:785)—Look carefully for tarsal-metatarsal dislocations [Lisfranc's (Clin Orthop 1963;30:116; Radiology 1976;120:79)]; a transverse fracture of the fifth metatarsal [Jones Fracture (J Bone Joint Surg [Am] 1978;60:776)] and for calcaneal fractures—these necessitate

immediate ortho referral. Other fractures will be referred based on extent of injury and may need further studies or perhaps second radiographic opinion to decide on extent of injury, such as fifth metatarsal avulsion fractures. If no immediate referral, splint/cast boot and 1-2 wk follow-up.

- *Ankle* (Curr Opin Peds 2000;12:52)—Ankle fractures are classified on which malleoli (lateral—fibula, medial—tibia, posterior—tibia) are involved and whether or not the Mortisse is intact. Most significant is the lateral malleolus; a lone lateral malleolus fracture may have an abnormal Mortisse view with ankle instability because the deltoid (tibial-calcaneal) ligament is ruptured on the medial side—although isolated anterior talofibular sprain with inversion ankle injury is very common (Foot Ankle Int 2000;21:138). All unstable ankle fractures need ortho referral, whereas chip fractures are managed as moderate to severe sprains as long as no clinical or radiographic instability exists. Ankle taping helps with propioception (Med Sci Sports Exerc 2000;32:10).
- *Tibia*—Tibia fractures need to be non-weight bearing for treatment, and proximal tibia metaphysis fractures may have an arterial injury as well, especially with valgus angulation. Tibial shaft fractures associated with ligamentous injury to the ipsilateral knee (J Bone Joint Surg [Am] 1989;71:1392). Ortho referral/outpatient follow-up based on degree of injury/patient discomfort.
- *Fibula*—If it does not involve the ankle joint, usually does very well. Individual preference as far as splinting, and outpatient follow-up.
- *Knee* (Emerg Med Clin N Am 2000;18:67)—Look carefully for tibial plateau fractures and intercondylar eminence fractures (Tibia), the latter being the attachment of the anterior cruciate ligament. Patellar fractures and tibial tubercle fractures can sometimes be difficult to judge, as normal variants may show separate osseous bodies in these locations. The knee can

suffer significant ligamentous and internal derangement without bony fracture, and those with traumatic hemarthroses or ligamentous instability should have ortho referral (Injury 1984;16:96). As stated above, these aforementioned considerations limit the applicability of the Ottawa Knee Rules. Remember to assess for vascular compromise if displaced fracture or dislocation of the knee. The aforementioned fractures and all epiphyseal fractures also need ortho referral.

- *Femur*—The femoral shaft fracture may lead to local hemorrhage with a hematoma collection of approximately 1 L not being unusual—use a traction splint (Injury 1973;5:35)(eg, Hare, Sager) to stabilize femur. No true findings of hemodynamic instability in those with closed femur fractures.

  Hip fractures (J Trauma 1970;10:51; Am J Orthop 1999;28:497) include femoral head, femoral neck, intertrochanteric fractures, and subtrochanteric fractures— these are sometimes difficult to diagnose. Look carefully at the trabeculation pattern, as it should be uninterrupted. Also look carefully for wedge shaped defects in the head of the femur and consider AVN. In adolescents, consider Slipped Capital Femoral Epiphysis (SCFE), that has increased incidence noted in those that are obese (Clin Orthop 1996:8). Ortho referral for all of these, and those with femoral neck fractures do better if operation within 12 hr (Injury 1992;23:83). Prevent hip fractures with fall prevention, treatment of bony disease, and hip protectors (Am J Orthop 1998;27:407). Consider femoral nerve block for analgesia (20 cc of 0.5% bupivicaine 1 cm lateral to the femoral pulse fanned out in a 90° arc) (Ann EM 2003;41:227)

- *Pelvis* (Emerg Med Clin N Am 2000;18:1)—The ring usually breaks in two spots, search for the second when seeing the first—diastasis of the pubic symphysis may be the second fracture location. Hemorrhage, bladder rupture, and urethral injury are potential major complications of pelvic fractures. Look for associated fractures in the hip; if blood is seen at the urethral opening, do a urethrogram to document an intact urethra before placing a urinary catheter. Ortho referral electively for individual ramus, coccyx, or pubic symphysis fractures with no other problems (all acetabular fractures need immediate referral). General Surgery or Interventional Radiology may need to be involved for unstable pts, as well (Am Surg 1998;64:862). Geriatric pts have problems with this fracture secondary to other co-morbid problems (Am J Emerg Med 1997;15:576). X-rays not necessary in neurologically and hemodynamically intact adults with blunt trauma, negative physical exam, and no anemia (J Trauma 1995;39:722); pts with GCS > 13 and with or without intoxication need no x-ray, if clinically no suspicion for pelvic fracture (sensitivity 93%) and missed fractures with this approach did not require surgical intervention (J Am Coll Surg 2002;194:121).

- *Vertebral Body*—Traumatic vertebral fractures, those with retropulsion of the body fragments (Neurosurgery 1979: 250), those with rotational fracture-dislocation (J Bone Joint Surg [Am];1970;52:1115) or posterior element involvement should have CT imaging (J Bone Joint Surg [Am] 1978; 60:1108) to look at the spinal canal, although those with single level and minimal anterior compression would probably do OK with just plain films—BAFL (Big Air, Fractured Lumbar) is a term coined with regard to those who snowboard and have minimal and single level anterior compression fracture. Transverse fracture through a vertebral body is a Chance fracture, and is associated with seatbelt use (Am J Roentgenol Radium Ther Nucl Med 1971;111:844). Cervical spine has special issues, (see p 480) and consider neurosurgical referral. Vetebral body fractures due to osteoporosis may benefit from calcitonin for both osteoporosis treatment and pain control.

- *Rib*—Rib fractures should be used as markers for associated injuries, such as:
  1) Look for associated pneumo/hemo-thorax on chest films;
  2) High rib fractures (1-3) may be associated with great vessel injury (J Trauma 1990;30:343) and look for widened mediastinum, pleural effusions or associated history and physical to decide on further testing—eg, CT, TEE, Aortogram (Ann Thorac Surg 1983;35:450);
  3) Low rib (9-12) fractures may have associated local organ injury, eg, diaphragm, kidneys, liver, spleen;
  4) Multiple rib fractures in a row have a higher likelihood of underlying lung injury (flail chest is 3 or more adjacent ribs fractured each in 2 or more locations and moving counter to the rest of the chest wall);
  5) Three or more rib fractures in general associated with a higher likelihood of other significant injuries (J Trauma 1990;30:689). If secondary injuries, appropriate referral. Rib belts do convey some comfort (Am J Emerg Med 1990;8:277). For those with severe pain, an intercostal, interpleural (J Emerg Med 1994;12:441) or epidural block may be used.
- *Clavicle*—"A clavicle fracture will heal as long as both ends are in the same room"— Anonymous. If no complications from the fracture [underlying vessel injury rare (J Trauma 2000;48: 316)], then outpatient follow-up with figure of 8 immobilization or sling and swathe—fractures of the medial ⅓ of the clavicle should invoke the same thought process for vessel injury as high rib fractures.
- *Scapula*—Most significant as marker of significant trauma, look for associated injuries. Glenoid, coracoid, and acromion fractures with ortho referral, others may sling if no other associated problems and outpatient ortho follow-up.
- *Shoulder*—This implies the humeral head (anatomic neck) and be sure to exclude co-incident dislocation (J Trauma 1999;46:

318). Most of these fractures are treated with shoulder immobilization (via spica splint or pre-packaged tool), but those with rotation of the humeral head may necessitate immediate surgical intervention. Both anatomic neck and surgical neck fractures are at risk for AVN to the head of the humerus, especially if rotation of the humeral head has occurred—those with rotation or displacement need immediate ortho referral, otherwise 2-5 d follow-up OK.

- *Humerus*—Humeral shaft fractures are usually managed non-operatively despite how significant the x-rays may look. Radial nerve palsy may occur in 10-20% of people, and most of those resolve without operative intervention. Due to the fact that a radial nerve injury may occur with manipulation/splinting, consider ortho consult for splint application.
- *Elbow* (Emerg Med Clin N Am 1999;17:843)—We usually speak of intercondylar fractures in adults and supracondylar fractures in children as being significant here. Radial head fractures may occur, and are usually treated with a posterior splint plus a sling and 1 wk ortho follow-up. In an adult, a simple non-displaced condylar fracture can be posterior splinted with 1 wk follow-up, but any displacement or rotation of the condyles necessitates immediate ortho referral. In children, a supracondylar fracture may go onto a myriad of problems [neurologic (Orthop Clin N Am 1999;30:91), vascular (Int Angiol 1995;14:307), non-union, etc], so get ortho involved early for even non-displaced fractures. If a posterior fat pad or billowing anterior fat pad is seen (Injury 1978;9:297), treat as an occult elbow fracture if none is obvious.
- *Radius/Ulna*, a partnership (Emerg Med Clin N Am 1992; 10:133)—If you see an isolated fracture of either bone, look carefully at the complete length of its partner. Look carefully at the radial styloid and radial-ulnar joint on the radiographs to be sure fractures or disruptions have not occurred here—minimal

injuries here can have significant consequences and necessitate urgent ortho referral. Any radius/ulna fracture with more than approximately 10° of angulation or greater than 25% displacement needs ortho consult. Specifics: Monteggia fracture is an isolated proximal ulna fracture with a radial head dislocation; a Galeazzi fracture is a distal radius fracture with a distal radial-ulna joint dislocation; a Colles fracture is a distal radial metaphysis fracture/ulna styloid fracture with dorsal angulation of the fractured segment; a Smith fracture is a distal radial metaphysis fracture with volar angulation. A risk factor for distal radius/ulna fracture is being left-handed, or being naturally left-handed but forced to be right-handed (Am J Epidem 1994; 140:361).

- *Carpal bones* (Emerg Med Clin N Am 1993:703)—Proximal row radius to ulna is Scaphoid, Lunate, Triquetrum, and Pisiform over Triquetrum, with the second row radius to ulna as Trapezium, Trapezoid, Capitate, and Hamate. All fractures here may be difficult to diagnose on plain radiographs, and the most important fractures are to the lunate and scaphoid. The scaphoid crosses both rows, which makes it more susceptible to injury. To the radial side of the scaphoid is a triangular soft tissue density that is disrupted if the scaphoid is fractured (variable reliability). Both of these fractures can go onto AVN (AVN of lunate is Kienbock disease), so Thumb spica splint if clinically suspected with ortho follow-up in 3-7 d. Some advocate slight extension when splinting for scaphoid fractures (J Bone Joint Surg [Br] 1999;81:91). Fractures of the pisiform and hook of the hamate may sometimes be diagnosed with a reverse oblique x-ray, where the wrist is angled toward supination (J Emerg Med 1998;16:445). Wrist guards do help prevent these and distal forearm fractures (Ann EM 1997;29:766).
- *Metacarpals* (Occup Med 1998;13:549)—Most important to assess the cascade (rotational alignment) if fracture noted in

the shaft or neck; thus, have the patient bring the fingers to the palm with the nail beds showing. Trade names: fifth metacarpal neck fracture known as Boxer's fracture and thumb metacarpal fracture involving the metacarpal-carpal joint is a Bennett fracture—a Bennett fracture needs immediate ortho referral. Most metacarpal fractures can be treated in a radial or ulnar gutter splint with 1-2 wk follow-up. Immediate ortho referral for fractures that are cleanly transverse (these have a predisposition to rotate), if the shafts are rotated, more than 15° of angulation of second or third metacarpals, or more than 30° of angulation of fourth or fifth metacarpals.

- *Hand digits*—Articular surface fractures should be reduced and referred urgently to ortho; shaft fractures that are transverse or comminuted require a radial or ulnar gutter splint. Trade names: Chip fracture of distal phalanx at the extensor tendon insertion is a Mallet finger—splint this joint (DIP) in extension for 2-3 mon and refer for ortho follow-up.

- *Mandibular*—Mandibular fractures are common, and the decision for admission vs outpatient follow-up (next day) has to do with whether the pt can protect the airway and the amount of displacement. To clinically diagnose, look for facial asymmetry, malocclusion, and have pt bite on a tongue depressor placed over the molars (one side at a time) (Am J Emerg Med 1998;16:304); if pt can oppose you twisting the tongue depressor so that it breaks, then most likely not a fracture; if cannot oppose, a fracture more likely. More than 25% displacement, or if the airway appears to be at risk (inability to swallow or control the tongue), then the pt should be admitted. Remove loose teeth from fracture site unless essential for splinting, clear liquids only, and next day follow-up if discharged from ER. Place on prophylactic antibiotics such as PCN VK 500 mg tid due to high likelihood of gum, dental, or wound site infection.

- *Facial bones* (Plast Reconstr Surg 1979;63:26)—These are fractures of the zygoma, orbital floor, maxilla, mandible, and nasal bones [in descending order (J Trauma 1989;29:388)]; and others (cribiform plate, pterygoids, etc.). Look for cranial nerve deficits and facial asymmetry for keys to correct diagnoses. Maxilla fractures carry the Le Fort classification (Plast Reconstr Surg 1980;66:54), and other midface variations also occur (Int J Oral Surg 1980;9:92); maxillofacial surgeons should be consulted when suspected—the upper dental plate will move independent of the rest of the head. Orbital floor fractures may show entrapment of an intraocular muscle clinically, and look for secondary globe trauma—ophthalmology consult, but they usually advocate delayed repair for isolated orbital floor fractures. The zygoma may show a fracture line, but always compare the contralateral side and look for cheek flattening of affected side. Nasal fractures if isolated and closed do not need x-rays, but the diagnosis of open fracture can be made by having the pt gently blow out the nose while occluding both nares—if air escapes through an open wound, this is an open fracture and will necessitate antibiotics such as cephazolin 1-2 gm iv as well as deep and superficial wound closure. Epistaxis is seen in zygoma fractures, nasal bone fractures, and cribiform plate fractures—put bloody nasal discharge on gauze and see if halo of clear fluid encompasses the spot of blood; if so, this is a CSF leak, give antibiotic, such as cephazolin 1-2 gm iv, and consult neurosurgery. No correlation of facial fractures with closed head injury (if closed head injury not clinically suspected) except for those in car accidents—they have a 1.5 increased risk for closed head injury (Ann EM 1988;17:6). Conversely, facial fractures do not help prevent injuries to the brain (Arch Surg 1999;134:14).

16.4 Gout/Pseudogout

Curr Opin Rheumatol 1999;11:1; Am J Med 1967;43:322; Radiology 1977;122:1; Nejm 2003;349:1647

Cause: *Gout* is due to hyperuricemia due to 2 possible reasons—either increased production due to a transferase deficiency (possibly genetic with sporadic penetrance) or increased tissue breakdown (Arthritis Rheum 1965;8:765), or decreased renal tubular excretion of urate. White blood cells may ingest the crystals, but the main problem is then deposition of uric acid in joints and other tissues.

Pseudogout is calcium pyrophosphate crystal deposition.

Epidem: *Gout* due to a transferase deficiency is seen 20:1 male:female, with males affected in fourth decade of life, females postmenopausal. The secondary type seen in those with leukemia (especially if treated), polycythemia, hemolytic anemia, starvation, diuretic therapy, lead ingestion (Nejm 1981;304:520), and alcoholics due to increased urate production and perhaps decreased excretion. Increased risk of gout with diet that has a high percentage of meat and seafood (which were used as surrogate markers of purine), and no increased risk with a diet where purine is a moderate component, and decreased risk of gout with a diet that has a high percentage of dairy products (Nejm 2004;350:1093).

Pseudogout has an increased incidence in neuropathic joints, hemochromatosis, hypothyroidism, hypomagnesemia, hyperparathyroidism, gout, RA, osteoarthritis.

Pathophys: *Gout* depends on uric acid physiology. Uric acid is normally 100% filtered, 100% resorbed, and 100% excreted in distal tubule. This may be competitively inhibited by lactate, ethanol, and ketone bodies. Perhaps increase in uric acid production correlating with hypertriglyceridemia (Metabolism 1989;38:698). Podagra comes from traumatically increased synovial fluid from which water is resorbed at night faster than urate, leading to a gouty attack.

Pseudogout occurs with poly ingestion of crystals resulting in enzyme release in the joint and subsequent inflammation.

Sx:

- *Gout*—Family hx (50%); podagra (84%)—inflammation of first mcp joint of big toe; low dose ASA (< 4 gm) precipitates or worsens.
- *Gout or pseudogout*—other painful arthritides.

Si:

- *Gout*—podagra; tophi of ear > elbow > finger > foot.
- *Pseudogout*—arthritis of knee > mcp > wrist > shoulder.

Crs: Acute *gouty* attacks last 1-14 d, symptom free between attacks but with increasing frequency over the years, without treatment permanent damage ensues.

Cmplc: *Gout*—osteoarthritis; no increase in pseudogout; renal stones, but the nephropathy is only associated with lead-related gout.

Diff Dx: *Gout*—Sarcoid arthritis which also improves with colchicine; Reiter syndrome; septic arthritis; RA; pseudogout: osteoarthritis; Lesch-Nyhan syndrome—choreoathetosis, dystonic spasticity, self-mutilation.

Pseudogout—Calcium oxalate deposition in renal failure, septic arthritis (Jama 1979;242:1768).

Lab: *Gout*—hyperuricemia non-specific and is seen in idiopathic without gout, hemolysis, leukemia, diuretics, psoriasis, Fanconi syndrome, chronic beryllium disease, Down syndrome (and never get gout), starvation, lead poisoning, and alcoholism. False hypouricemia seen with ASA, allopurinol, and x-ray dyes; false hyperuricemia with methyldopa and L-dopa. Perhaps serum creatinine to assess renal function before initiating colchicines (J Rheumatol 1991;18:264) and hypophosphatemia secondary to impaired renal tubular phosphate transport (Nephron 1992; 62:142).

- *Joint fluid* with long thin urate crystals, some inside WBCs, negatively birefringent.
- *X-ray* with soft tissue swelling, possible erosions.
- *24-hr urine* for uric acid $\geq$ 1 gm.

    Pseudogout with joint fluid showing rhomboid and positively birefringent crystals; may be small enough to require oil immersion lens.
- *X-ray* with semilunar calcifications of joint cartilages.

Emergency Management:

Gout:

- Colchicine 0.6 mg po q 1 hr up to 7 mg, or iv dosing of 1 mg q 12 hr (J Clin Pharmacol J New Drugs 1969;9:410; Jama 1987;257:1920)
- ACTH 80 IU im/iv then 40 IU 12 hr later, especially if symptoms >1 wk.

Gout and Pseudogout:

- Indomethacin 50 mg po tid or qid, then rapid 1 wk taper.
- Intra-articular or systemic steroids.

Gout prevention:

- Colchicine 1-2 mg po qd (Arthritis Rheum 1974;17: 609)
- Probenecid 1-3 gm po qd in divided doses, start with 0.5 gm—prevents resorption and good if 24-hr urine with urate < 600 mg.
- Sulfinpyrazone 800 mg po qd in divided doses—same conditions for use as Probenecid.
- Allopurinol 200-400 mg po qd if 24-hr urine with urate > 600 mg or renal disease and if failure of probenecid (Am J Hosp Pharm 1989;46:1813)—decrease dose to 100 mg qd in

anuria to prevent rash, fever, or hepatitis syndrome, or tophi; can precipitate attack.

16.5 Septic Arthritis

J Am Ger Soc 1985;33:170; Rheum Dis Clin N Am 1997;23:239; J Rheumatol;1999;26:663

Cause: Immunosuppression, chronic joint disease, overlying skin disease or artificial joint as template for *Staphylococcus* or other Gram-pos bacteria to infect, although Gram-neg and anaerobes seen in those with joint replacements or if elderly.

Epidem: Approximatley 30% incidence in those > 60 yr of age; 1-2% risk in those with joint prosthesis; decreased *Haemophilus influenza* type B infection with vaccination (J Bone Joint Surg [Br] 1998;80:471).

Pathophys: Either direct introduction through skin or hematogenous spread of offending organisms to joint space.

Sx: Painful joint; fevers; chills.

Si: Red hot joint with palpable effusion.

Crs: Sepsis if unrecognized/untreated.

Cmplc: Septic shock; may occur in the setting of gout or pseudogout (J Rheumatol 1983;10:503)

Diff Dx: Hip and children: Transient synovitis (Ann EM 1992; 21:1418)—physical exam and laboratory evaluation rarely helpful and consider diagnostic aspiration by ortho consult. Rarely *Mycobacterium marinum* (J Cutan Med Surg 1999;3: 218). May see red hot joint in RA, osteoarthritis, gout, and fracture.

Lab: CBC with diff; ESR; blood cultures; tap bursa/joint for gram stain and culture [review of taps (Am Fam Phys 2002;66:283)].
  * *Joint fluid* with low viscosity, poor mucin clot, usually 80-200K WBCs/mm^3, but 95% with > 20K, >75% of WBCs are polys,

low glucose, pos Gram stain and culture—consider anaerobic cultures, especially if monoarticular or h/o puncture wound (Ann EM 1981;10:315).

- *X-ray* (Am J Roentgenol 1995;165:399): consider radiographs for osteomyelitis/erosion evaluation, perhaps US of hip in children if effusion is suspected; MRI (J Vasc Surg 1996;24:266), bone scan or CT if plain films equivocal—review article (Rheum Dis Clin N Am 2003;29:89).

Emergency Management:

Bursitis (J R Soc Med 1999;92:516):

- Needle tap for diagosis, and splint affected joint; consult ortho before opening bursa and placing drain as many differing opinions regarding this practice.
- Antibiotics such as cephalexin or dicloxacillin or erythromycin—iv antibiotics, such as cefazolin considered if lymphangitis; iv antibiotics advised if systemic response to infection.
- Pain control: Acetaminophen, NSAIDs, narcotics.
- Next day follow-up, ortho consult/admission if lymphangitis or worse clinical picture.

Arthritis:

- Aspirate joint—Ortho referral for aspiration if joint is prosthetic and the diagnosis of a prosthetic septic joint can be difficult (confusing) (Nejm 2004;351:1645).
- Irrigate joint if septic, consider ortho referral so that done in operating theater.
- Antibiotics: Cefazolin 1-2 gm iv, consider antipseudomonal coverage if diabetes mellitus or sickle cell history—such as ciprofloxacin 400 mg iv (J Infect Dis 1985;151:291).
- Perhaps NSAIDs of some benefit if due to *Staphylococcus aureus* (J Orthop Res 1997;15:919)
- Consult Ortho/Medicine for admission, early mobilization for hand joints (Ann Plast Surg 1999;42:623).

Chapter 17

Otolaryngology

17.1 Barotrauma

Am Fam Phys 1992;45:1777

Blast Injury

Nejm 2005;352:1335

Cause: Direct blows to the external ear with pressure wave damage to the tympanic membrane; closed space bomb explosion (Am J Otol 1993;14:92); rapid changes in atmospheric pressure as seen in non-pressurized aircraft, SCUBA diving (Ear Nose Throat J 1999;78:181,186) or hyperbaric (dive) chambers (Undersea Hyperb Med 1999;26:243).

Epidem: Common in SCUBA divers, with pulmonary barotrauma seen in those with lung cysts or end-expiratory flow limitation (Thorax 1998;53:S20).

Pathophys: Rapid changes in pressure can cause systemic effects from higher to lower pressure gas phase shifts. Association with closed space bomb explosion conveys significant injury possibilities for pt. Middle ear (TM) perforation benign in SCUBA diving, but inner ear perforation can lead to inner ear dysfunction problems such as hearing loss, dizziness, tinnitus, and vertigo.

Sx: Ear pain, sinus pain, chest pain, difficulty breathing, abdominal pain.

Si: TM perforation is both sensitive and specific for barotrauma—unless Valsalva or other pressure-equalizing phenomenon has occurred, including myringotomy tubes. Hypesthesia in the infraorbital area on ipsilateral maxillary barotraumas (Undersea Hyperb Med 1999;26:257). Also look for sc emphysema, subconjunctival hemorrhage, absence of breath sounds over usual lung fields, lack of bowel sounds with peritoneal signs—perforation.

Crs: Extremely variable, with full spectrum of simple TM perforation to multiple organ breaches—lung, bowel, skin.

Cmplc: Deafness, respiratory failure, peritonitis.

Diff Dx: Perforated TM from acute otitis media.

Lab: None for isolated ear trauma; CBC with diff, BMP and UA to guide fluid therapy in SCUBA accidents; multisystem trauma evaluation for bomb explosions.

Emergency Management:

Isolated TM rupture:
- Oral pain meds, NSAIDs and narcotics.
- Antibiotic ear drops, either corticosporin otic suspension (not solution) or gentamicin ophthalmologic drops, eg.
- Follow-up with primary physician in 2 wks, perforation needs to be followed until closed. Perhaps patching/hyaluronan by ENT (Acta Otolaryngol suppl 1987;442:88).
- No SCUBA diving, surface diving, or swimming deeper than 3 feet in water—use earplugs when swimming until healed.

SCUBA accident:
- O_2
- Iv fluid, resuscitation guided by hematocrit and urine specific gravity.
- Refer to hyperbaric chamber.

Bomb or other environmental explosion (Toxicology 1997;121:17):
- Trauma resuscitation, with trauma or general surgery consult.

17.2 Epiglottitis

Jama 1974;229:671; Ped Emerg Care 1989;5:16; Am J Emerg Med 1996;14:421)

Cause: *Haemophilus influenzae*, type B usually in adults, rarer now in the immunized child; *Staphylococcus, pneumococcal* disease, rarely other type strep. Rarely due to thermal injury (Peds 1988; 81:441).

Epidem: Now more common in adults with HIB vaccine in peds; mortality rate 1.2% (Laryngoscope 1998;108:64).

Pathophys: Obstruction of upper airway by edematous epiglottis.

Sx: Extremely sore throat (95%), more than the dysphagia (94%), plus respiratory distress over 6-24 hr—mainly in peds.

Si: Epiglottis or other supraglottic structures inflamed and edematous by direct or indirect laryngoscopy, need to sit erect (21%), muffled voice (54%), fever (50%), drooling (40%), stridor (15%) (Am J Dis Child 1988;142:679); pharynx is often normal (50%).

Crs: Lingual cellulitis; lingual abscess (Am J Emerg Med 1998; 16:414).

Cmplc: Sudden and unpredictable airway obstruction, 7% mortality without prophylactic airway (vs recognition of event); decreases to 1% with airway placed.

Lab: CBC with diff; blood culture.

X-ray: Soft tissue lateral neck looking for abnormal soft tissue swellings with or without air/fluid levels; look for swollen epiglottis (thumb sign) with loss of air in the vallecula (Ann EM 1997;30:1).

Emergency Management:
- Do not startle children, perhaps blowby O_2.

- Unknown value of racemic epi nebulizer (Anesth Analg 1975;54:622).
- Iv access in adults and cooperative children.
- Ceftriaxone 1-2 gm iv (J Paediatr Child Hlth 1992;28:220) (third generation cephalosporin).
- Equivocal, but advocate for use of iv steroids (methylprednisolone 125 mg or dexamethasone 15 mg) (J Ped Surg 1979;14:247).
- Early airway in operating theater is controversial, even in peds.

17.3 Epistaxis

Cause: Bleeding from nare(s) may be due to trauma externally such as nasal fracture, direct mucosal trauma, foreign body in nare, sinusitis, cocaine use, HT, thrombocytopenia, carotid artery aneurysm, or bleeding disorder.

Epidem: Common, most resolve with conservative treatment (Otolaryngol Head Neck Surg 1993;109:60); 5% are posterior bleeds, and these are associated with previous epistaxis and HT (Ann EM 1995;25:592). Medical issues/habits associated with persistent bleeds are HT, aspirin use, and alcohol abuse (Arch Otolaryngol Head Neck Surg 1988;14:862).

Pathophys: Exposed vessel bleeding are those that usually come to medical attention, or those with extensive mucosal involvement or hematologic/bleeding disorders.

Sx: Blood from nare.

Si: Look for blood running down pharynx with patient head neutral, with noted blood suggestive of posterior bleed—if head has been rested back, then blood in posterior pharynx will not help distinguish anterior from posterior bleeds; check the septum for perforation; multiple petechiae or ecchymoses to implicate systemic process; co-incident hemotympanum (J Emerg Med 1988;6:387).

Crs: ENT consult for repetitive, uncontrollable, or briskly flowing anterior bleeds, and all posterior bleeds.

Cmplc: Anemia, hypoxia, bleeds elsewhere, if systemic problem; sinusitis, if packing or other obstructive method used as treatment.

Lab: If elderly, with multiple medical problems, significant bleed, or anticipating admission, consider ordering—CBC with diff; PT/PTT; and/or Type and screen (J Laryngol Otol 1999;113: 1086; 2000;114:38)

Emergency Management:

All bleeds:
- Pinch nose below bridge; ice over nose.
- Head forward slightly (neck flexed).
- Trial of oxymetazoline HCl 0.05% (Afrin) nasal spray, most will resolve with this and pressure alone (Ann Otol Rhinol Laryngol 1995;104:704).
- Address HT if needed, with either acute treatment, or follow-up with primary physician for treatment; HT is a ubiquitous problem in those with spontaneous bleeds (Ann EM 2000;35:126).

If a brisk bleed:
- Soak cotton ball with cocaine 4% or oxymetazoline HCl 0.05% (Afrin) nasal spray, and place in nare that is bleeding—if bleeding stems, this is an anterior bleed. Then pinch nose for 10 min.
- If bleeding does not stem, follow posterior bleed instructions.

Anterior bleeds:
- Pack with Vaseline gauze, Merocel pack, Gelfoam, or Surgicell—packing goes smoother if viscous lidocaine, instead of surgilube, is used to facilitate insertion.
- Trial of cautery if able to get clear site, may use silver nitrate.

- Trial of microfibrillar collagen (J Otolaryngol 1980;9:468), if able to get clear site. Hold pressure for 3 min once collagen placed over site.
- Use nasal drops as needed to keep packing moist and to stem bleeds.
- Pack out in 1-2 d, 3 d at the most.
- Keep in cool environment. Avoid bending and straining. Hold nose if sneezing, and expel force through the mouth.

Posterior bleeds:
- Posterior pack, with viscous lidocaine for insertion. Single balloon packs with a procoagulant sleeve effective (Rapid Rhino).
- Dual balloon packs: Inflate distal balloon first, then proximal balloon—do only $\frac{1}{2}$ the amount of balloon capacity, and add more if needed (J Oral Maxillofac Surg 1982;140:317).
- Foley catheter may be used if posterior pack is not available (Surg Neurol 1979;11:115); perhaps umbilical cord clamp at external nares to secure position (J Otolaryngol 1996;25:46).
- O_2 if hypoxic; antibiotic prophylaxis for sinusitis, such as cefazolin 1 gm iv.
- ENT consult for admit if pt requires hemorrhage control, pain control or if hypoxic.

Thrombocytopenia:
- Transfuse platelets if < 50K and symptomatic (epistaxis counts).

17.4 Foreign Bodies (FB)—Nasal, Aural, Pharyngeal

Cause: Usually volitional, rare bug.

Epidem: Usually children 2-4 yr of age.

Sx: Pain, decreased hearing if aural; purulent nasal discharge if nasal.

Si: Noted FB, ubiquitous malodor with nasal FBs (Jama 1979;241:1496)

Crs: To operating theater with ENT, if unable to remove.

Cmplc: Pharyngeal FBs may be aspirated; aural FBs may cause a perforation; batteries cause tissue destruction (Jama 1986;255:1470).

Lab: Suspected pharyngeal FB should have radiographs if not visible on exam—soft tissue neck, CXR, if necessary, and AXR, if necessary.

Emergency Management:

Nasal (Am J Emerg Med 1997;15:54):

- Have pt occlude contralateral nare while closing mouth and forcing air out of occluded side.
- Variation: Have parent give puff of air in child's mouth while holding unaffected nare closed, or use Ambu-bag (Practitioner 1973;210:242; Am J Emerg Med 1996;14:57).
- Try to grasp with smooth forcep—4% cocaine pre-procedure may help.
- Crazy Glue on small stick (cotton swab) and touch object—wait a few minutes and then remove.
- Five or six French balloon catheter lubricated with 2 or 4% lidocaine, snaked past the FB, inflated, and withdrawn (Ann EM 1980;9:37).

Aural:

- Mineral oil or lidocaine instilled to "kill" potential bug is not advocated—may have unrecognized TM perforation, and sterile saline works just as well.
- Try smooth forcep delivery.
- Locate object with otoscope, sit right on top of it with ear speculum (disposable), open magnifying end and place wood stick (cotton swab) with crazy glue inside of speculum and "marry" object to stick and speculum, wait a min, and remove.
- Flushing may work—stop if any pain, and do not try if noted TM perforation.
- Dark room/light usually does not work for insects—cannot turn around.

Pharyngeal, visualized:
- If easy to reach and pt cooperative, remove object.
- If infant, turn infant head down, extend neck, and finger sweep to remove visualized object.

Pharyngeal, non-visualized (with x-ray):
- If object not found, may be radiolucent or abrasion in pharynx from FB—if symptoms still present next day, follow-up with ENT if no airway compromise.
- If FB in skeletal muscle (top ⅓) esophagus or higher, ENT consult to remove. If lower, see Esophageal FBs p100.

17.5 Otitis Externa

BMJ 1980;281:1616; Emerg Med Clin N Am 1995;13:445; Am Fam Phys 2001;63:927, 941

Cause: Allergic; seborrheic; infectious (J Otolaryngol 1984;13:289): bacterial (*Staphylococcus* spp., *Pseudomonas* spp.) most common, fungal—aka Otomycosis *(Aspergillus niger)*—if chronic, viral is rare *(H. simplex, H. zoster)*.

Epidem: Bacterial is most common. Bacterial/fungal—Swimmer's Ear. More common in those with allergies or prolonged water exposure, not with local trauma (J Laryngol Otol 1993;107:898).

Pathophys: Bacterial—local furunculosis that then becomes more diffuse.

Sx:

> *Allergic:* 1+ pain, 3+ itching.
> *Seborrheic:* 1+ pain, 1+ itching.
> *Bacterial:* 3+ pain, especially with movement of pinna.
> *Fungal:* 1+ pain, 3+ itching.
> *Viral:* 1+ pain with *H. simplex;* 3+ pain with *H. zoster.*

Si:

> *Allergic:* Acute with weeping small vesicles; chronic with fissures and scales.

Bacterial: Pain with pressure on tragus and pinna traction; erythema and edema (stenosis) of external ear canal.
Seborrheic: Greasy scales; dandruff.
Fungal: Looks like wet newspaper; black discharge is diagnostic.
Viral: Vessels in ear may rupture, or form hemorrhagic bullae.

Crs: Variable.

Cmplc: Bacterial may go onto malignant otitis externa, a severe form of perichondritis, now only a problem in pts with resistant organisms or diminished resistance, eg, in pts with diabetes, cancer, AIDS, etc.

Diff Dx: Mastoiditis.

Lab: Consider culture of drainage, especially if chronic.

Emergency Management:

All types:
- Avoid water in ear.
- Topical Auralgan for pain.

Allergic:
- Antihistamines; topical steroids.

Seborrheic:
- Keep hair away from ears; topical steroids.

Bacterial/fungal:
- Remove wax/debris usually by speculum/irrigation—relatively painless.
- Domeboro's solution, boric acid 4% (J Laryngol Otol 1987;101:533), or 9:1 alcohol:vinegar solution drops to acidify area, which prevents *Pseudomonas* spp. growth; use wick if stenosis (no stenosis and wick will fall right out) either from commercial source or roll a piece of tissue paper—helps delivery of therapy (Eye Ear Nose Throat Mon 1974;53:458).
- Topical antibiotics and steroids (Corticosporin or Cipro HCl) drops qid (Ear Nose Throat J 1978;57:198), or ofloxacin

(Floxin) drops bid; if TM perforation, use corticosporin otic suspension or antibiotic eye drops (Gentamicin ophthalmologic solution (Curr Med Res Opin 1993;13:182) to avoid damaging the ossicles.

- Glycerin with non-aqueous acetic acid to decrease swelling by hydroscopic action (Vosol) or with steroid (Vosol HC) are both effective (Curr Ther Res Clin Exp 1974;16:431).
- Systemic antibiotics, eg, dicloxacillin 500 mg qid; malignant external OM, treat with ceftazidime 1-2 gm iv (Ann Otol Rhinol Laryngol 1989;98:721; Rev Inf Dis 1990;12:173) or fluoroquinolones, such as ciprofloxacin 500 mg bid or levofloxacin 750 mg qd (Can Med Assoc J 1994;150:669; Am J Otolaryngol 1988;9:102)

Viral:
- Analgesia; occasionally local antibiotics and oral acyclovir although no supporting data.

17.6 Otitis Media

BMJ 1980;281:1616; Emerg Med Clin N Am 1995;13:445; Nejm 2002;347:1169)

Cause: Three types.
- *Acute (AOM):* 70% are bacterial—pneumococcus up to 50%, but this will change with heptavalent pneumococcal vaccine (Nejm 2001;344:403), *Moraxella (Branhamella) catarrhalis* up to 30%, *Haemophilus influenzae* up to 25%, but lower in immunized children, and other streptococci. Viral in approximately 30% pre-pneumococcal vaccine.
- *Chronic:* Above plus *Staphylococcus* spp., *Proteus, Pseudomonas*.
- *Serous:* Fluid secretion without organism, usually, although ⅓ may have organisms.

Epidem: Some viral infections predispose, eg, RSV, *influenza*, adenovirus. Childcare outside home and parental smoking also increased risk of acquiring, breast feeding is protective, and pacifier use appears equivocal (Clin Infect Dis 1996;22:1079). Serous OM often follows infectious resolution.

Pathophys: Rhinitis and sinusitis spread along eustachian tube. Pharyngeal closure of eustachian tube may cause ear pain with normal ear exam—Eustachian Tube Dysfunction. Infants and young children have flat (horizontal) and slightly curved Eustachian tubes that may have difficulty draining the middle ear.

Sx: Pain, decreased hearing, sense of fullness or water sloshing.

Si: No pain with manipulation of external ear; bulging or retracted tympanic membrane (TM) with loss of normal landmarks (light reflex), with erythema (erythema is the least helpful sign), and fluid visualized if able to see through the TM. Lack of TM movement with pneumatic otoscopy (Ped Infect Dis J 2000; 19:256).

Crs: AOM usually begins clearing in 48 hr, but fluid may persist for 2-3 wks. Serous OM lasts for months and may have associated hearing loss. Severity of episode related to previous attacks, and use of antibiotics both prophylactically and previously. Elective surgical intervention for recurrence with complications may be recommended such as ear tubes, adenoidectomy, or tonsillectomy.

Cmplc: All rare:
- Ossicle necrosis, especially of incus
- Chronic otitis with granulomas and polyps
- Mastoiditis
- Meningitis and encephalitis
- Lateral sinus thrombosis
- Facial nerve paralysis in chronic OM—treat with surgical decompression
- Labyrinthitis

- Chronic serous OM
- Hearing acuity decreases if chronic, but no diminished verbal/intellectual abilities with delayed tubes (Nejm 2001;344:1179)

Lab: None if > 28 d of life, and if not septic. Acute phase reactants (ESR, CRP) not helpful in differentiating AOM from other acute invasive bacterial processes (Am J Dis Child 1992;146:1037). Tympanometry or acoustic otoscopy helpful if diagnosis in question (Ann EM 1989;18:396).

Emergency Management:

AOM:

- Antibiotics by mouth (Ped Infect Dis J 1994;13:1054), although current pediatric prescription practice probably not justified (many reasons—diagnostic criteria, strength of study data, placebo controlled studies lacking) (Brit J Gen Pract 1998;48:1861): amoxicillin 40-80 mg/kg qd divided tid is first line (Jama 1991;266:2249); or TMP/SMX (4 TMP/20 SMX per kg per dose) bid to a max of 160 TMP/800 SMX; or amoxicillin clavulanate 90/6.4 mg/kg divided bid; or cefaclor 250 mg tid; or azithromycin 10 mg/kg on d 1 and 5 mg/kg, d 2-5. Treatment length has varied from 2-10 d for po medications (BMJ (Clin Res Ed) 1985;291:1243).
- If no po possible, ceftriaxone 50 mg/kg up to 1 gm im with lidocaine—single dose treatment (Peds 1993;91:23).
- Advocate ibuprofen 10 mg/kg each 6-8 hr for pain (Fundam Clin Pharmacol 1996;10:387), although no difference between acetaminophen 15 mg/kg each 4 hr.
- Topical Auralgan may be helpful (Arch Ped Adolesc Med 1997;151:675).
- Decongestants and antihistamines of no help (Ann EM 1983;12:13), and may actually worsen with analogous dry sinus syndrome—fluid not able to drain from ear.

- Have peds < 4 yr of age recheck with primary care in 4 wks.

Serous OM:
- Antibiotics may help (Arch Otolaryngol Head Neck Surg 1997;123:695), may try for 2-wk course, but many will clear spontaneously.
- Steroids times 7-14 d.
- Recheck with primary care in 4 wks.

Chronic OM:
- Pseudomonas coverage—fluoroquinolones if > 15 yr of age.
- ENT follow-up in 1 wk or less.

17.7 Parotitis/Parotid Duct Stone

Arch Otolaryngol Head Neck Surg 1992;118:469

Cause: Mechanical (stone), Stensen duct abnormalities, infectious (eg, mumps, TB), drugs (anticholinergics), irradiation.

Epidem: Bacterial parotitis is bilateral approximately 20% of the time and not uncommon postoperatively. *Streptococcal pneumoniae* and *Haemophilus influenzae* common in chronic cases (Ped Infect Dis J 1997;16:386).

Pathophys: Inability to effectively drain the gland allows bacteria to flourish if due to calculi or duct problem; the gland itself is primarily inflamed if due to systemic infectious or irradiation cause; drugs may cause parotitis secondary to causing ineffective drainage or cause direct inflammation of the salivary tissue. Chronic inflammation perhaps secondary to local release of kallikrein.

Sx: Painful neck/face.

Si: Tenderness, fluctuance, and erythema over parotid; oral inspection may show drainage from Stensen's duct.

Crs: Weeks to clear, longer in the elderly.

Cmplc: Abscess, osteomyelitis, facial nerve palsy (Arch Otolaryngol Head Neck Surg 1989;115:240), sepsis.

Diff Dx: Enlarged parotid may not be an acute infection, consider—
- Chronic Infection: Cat-scratch disease, atypical mycobacterial disease, actinomycoses, and TB.
- Enlargement without infection: alcoholism, malnutrition, celiac disease, DM, uremia, cirrhosis, cystic fibrosis, hypothyroidism, heavy metal poisoning, or drugs (eg, phenothiazines).

Lab: Gram stain and culture of drainage; consider CBC with diff and blood cultures, if febrile; other laboratories based on pt's hx and clinical exam.

Emergency Management:
- If parotid not draining, attempt to milk the gland—iv access with parenteral narcotics will probably be needed. Milk the gland by having one hand massaging the parotid, the other hand with one finger intra-oral below the duct and gently massaging it along its anterior/posterior course.
- Antibiotics to cover for penicillinase resistant *Staphylococcus* spp. until cultures are known, such as nafcillin 1-2 gm iv or ampicillin/sulbactam 1.5-3 gm iv; or dicloxacillin 500 mg qid or amoxicillin/clavulanate 875 mg bid po.
- Iv hydration and hold possibly offending medications if necessary; pain medicine.
- If unable to drain or to discharge to home, ENT consult for admission and further evaluation. Parotidectomy considered only if chronic and after failure of all conservative therapies (J Otolaryngol 1996;25:305).
- If OK for home, then use warm compresses, have patient suck on a lemon or lemon candy tid, and 1 wk follow-up with primary physician.
- Perhaps aprotinin (kallikrein inhibitor) for chronic cases (Arch Otorhinolaryngol 1985;242:321).

17.8 Peritonsillar Abscess (Quincy Abscess)

J Otolaryngol 1990;19:226; Arch Otolaryngol Head Neck Surg
    1993;119:521; Laryngoscope 1995;105:1

Cause: Group A, β-hemolytic *Streptococcus pyogenes* (J Otolaryngol
    1998;27:206); rarely group C or D that is an extension from
    pharyngitis; *Peptostreptococcus; Fusobacterium;* with anaerobes in
    75% of cases.

Epidem: Most common deep head and neck abscess.

Pathophys: This may set up a tonsillar vein phlebitis, rarely pro-
    gressing to PE.

Sx: Sore throat; difficulty swallowing; drooling.

Si: Asymmetric tonsillar pillars; dysphonia; dysphagia; trismus.

Crs: Most will drain spontaneously.

Cmplc: Recurrent infection and abscess formation.

Lab: Throat culture.
   • *X-ray:* Soft tissue lateral neck series if extending down into
     neck and looking for air/fluid level.

Diff Dx:
   • Peritonsillar cellulitis—may exactly mimic peritonsillar abscess
     (Arch EM 1990;7:212), except at 1-d follow-up after par-
     enteral antibiotics, trismus as measured from incisor to incisor
     is better in patients with cellulitis (Laryngoscope 1988;
     98:780); unfortunately, no threshold value exists.
   • Infectious mononucleosis—rare to have secondary abscess.

Emergency Management:

If airway appears at risk:
   • Iv for pain control (narcotics), antibiotics (ceftriaxone 2 gm,
     or clindamycin 900 mg), and steroids [dexamethasone 12 mg
     in adult or higher (Otolaryngol Head Neck Surg 1983;91:
     593)], and ENT consult with patient in ER.

If airway is patent:

- Treat as outpatient with PCN 500 mg tid, cephalexin 500 mg tid, second generation cephalosporin, such as cefuroxime 250-500 mg bid (Arch Otolaryngol 1982;108:655), or clindamycin 300 mg qid; or perhaps iv ceftriaxone 1-2 gm with next day follow-up.
- Steroid taper (prednisone 40-60 mg qd for one wk or dexamethasone 8-12 mg divided qd for 5 d—taper these doses if pt has received other exogenous steroids within the last mon).
- Oral narcotics; salt water gargle.
- ENT consult in ER for needle aspiration (Otolaryngol Head Neck Surg 1981;89:910), outpatient treatment still feasible.
- Call ENT to arrange 1-d follow-up; interval tonsillectomy in those with h/o tonsillitis (Ear Nose Throat J 2000;79:206).

17.9 Streptococcal Pharyngitis

Nejm 2001;344:205

Cause: Group A, β-hemolytic *Streptococcus pyogenes;* rarely group C or D.

Epidem: Respiratory droplets; foodborne; carrier state in 15% of the population.

Pathophys: Possibly due to some breach in the mucosa or increased bacterial load or relative immune state nadir—all theoretical. Treatment to prevent ARF (Peds 1995;96:758), and perhaps to shorten clinical course and infectious potential.

Sx: Sore throat; abdominal pain [although not predictive of *Streptococcus pharyngitis* (J Fam Pract 1998;46:159)]

Si: Fever; pharyngeal edema, erythema or exudates; soft-palate or widespread petechiae (Am J Dis Child 1969;117:156); anterior cervical adenopathy; normal abdominal exam.

Crs: 10 days without treatment.

Cmplc: Acute glomerulonephritis; acute rheumatic fever—currently < 1:10,000 without treatment, and < 1:100,000 with treatment in adults, not seen in peds < 3 yr of age; peritonsillar abscess— see p 357.

Diff Dx: Chlamydia—TWAR; viral—eg, EBV (mono), rhinovirus, adenovirus, parainfluenza virus, RSV, coxsackie; mycoplasma; non-Group A *Streptococcus*; periodic fever, such as familial mediterranean fever (FMF) or periodic fever, *aphthous stomatitis*, pharyngitis, and adenopathy (PFAPA) syndrome (J Peds 1999;135:98); *Legionella*; gonorrhea; diphtheria.

Table 17.1   Scoring System by Centor

Finding	Points
History of fever (> 38°C)	1
No cough	1
Tender anterior cervical lymphadenopathy	1
Tonsillar exudate (or edema)	1
[age modifications (Can Med Assoc J 2000;163:811-5)]	
3-14 years of age	1
15-44 years of age	0
≥ 45 years of age	−1

Centor, Witherspoon, Dalton, Brody and Link, The diagnosis of strep throat in adults in the emergency room, *Med Decis Making* 1981;1:239.

Scoring System:

The original scoring system of Centor gives a 56% probability for a positive throat culture if all 4 points acquired. The age modifications as validated by McIsaac give a sensitivity of 85% and specificity of 92% for accurate Group A *streptococcus* identification, if the modified score is 4 or higher.

Lab:

Controversial: Treatment is geared toward preventing acute rheumatic fever, and cultures and rapid *Streptococcus* tests are

90% sensitive at best. Treating everyone based on clinical grounds *may* miss some cases, but it would be highly unlikely that in the group of 10% that the culture misses would be the 1:10,000 person who goes on to acute rheumatic fever. Alternatively, culture those pts not believed to need treatment (they should at least have pharyngeal erythema) and empirically treat all others (J Fam Pract 1975;2:173) or treat if pt has a Centor score of 3 or 4 (Ann IM 2001;134:509), although this will result in overtreatment (Jama 2004;291:1587). Best practice is probably an empiric treatment for those with all pos risk values (Centor score of 4, or modified Centor score $\geq$ 4), and culture before treatment for everyone else (except for those with sore throat/pharyngitis with pos lab test in other family member).

Rapid Strep vs Culture: Most labs "back up" their rapid strep with cultures—this is because the latex agglutination tests have an approximately 87% pos predictive value and 96% neg predictive value (J Fam Pract 1986;22:245). Some believe that teleologically a 2-d wait period was helpful in bolstering the pt's immune response, and this still prevented ARF. Since it appears to make no difference, if necessary to order a test on every pt—order just one. The idea that the marginal cost incurred by ordering both tests is offset by preventing 17 cases of rheumatic fever (Peds 1990;85:246) is flawed, unless no pt follow-up is provided for cultures ordered.

Thoughtful ordering: Those who are immunosuppressed, septic, have an abscess, glomerulonephritis, recurrent strep throat, a large group outbreak or if considering parenteral antibiotics, then a quantitative culture (Lancet 1976;2:62) would be helpful. May also help to culture patient, if considering treating family.

Emergency Management:
- Antibiotics po: PCN VK 50 mg/kg divided bid to a max of 500 mg/dose for 7-10 d (Peds 1996;97:955); or Macrolide, such

as azithromycin 12 mg/kg per single qd dose to a max of 500 mg for 5 d (Am J Med 1991;91:23S); or first generation cephalosporin, such as cephalexin 50 mg/kg divided bid to a max of 500 mg/dose for 7-10 d; or clindamycin (warn patients about diarrheal side effect and predisposition to go onto *Clostridium difficile* colitis with clindamycin use) 20 mg/kg divided tid for 7-10 d.

- Antibiotics parenteral: PCN G benzathine—1.2 million U im in adults, 900,000 U im in peds > 60 lbs, and 300,000-600,000 U im in peds < 60 lbs; or PCN G benzathine 900,000 units and PCN G procaine 300,000 units combined as single im dose (Jama 1976;235:1112).
- Perhaps steroids, if severe or to shorten the time to pain control—may try single dose therapy of either oral dexamethasone 0.6 mg/kg (Ann EM 2003:601) or im dexamethasone 10 mg for ages 12-65 yr (Ann EM 1993;41:212); helps pain in 24 hr. Best to treat pain with pain medication (narcotic, eg, depending on symptoms or degree of cellulitis).
- Abbreviated or simple qd dosing for antibiotics that are usually tid or qid has not been shown to be effective (Antimicrob Agents Chemother 1996;40:1005).
- ENT referral outpatient if > 3 episodes per year over several years for consideration of tonsillectomy/adenoidectomy—this decreases recurrence.

17.10 Retropharyngeal Abscess

J Laryngol Otol 1997;11:546

Cause: Direct trauma [eg, candy cane (that was not well masticated before swallowing), fishbone (Ann Otol Rhinol Laryngol 1990;99:827)]; extension from pharyngitis or other head/neck infection.

Epidem: Usually Group A, β-hemolytic *Streptococcus* in peds; *Staphylococcus, Streptococcus, Klebsiella, Neisseria* and other Gram-negatives and anaerobes in adults.

Pathophys: Inoculation into fascial space that is contiguous with mediastinum.

Sx:

> *Peds:* Airway obstruction.
> *Adults:* Painful to swallow.

Si:

> *Peds:* Drooling, stridor, dysphonia, dysphagia, meningismus, cervical adenopathy.
> *Adults:* None, or as with peds (J Emerg Med 1996;14:147).

Crs: More serious in peds and older adults.

Cmplc: Mediastinitis, empyema (Thorax 1994;49:1179), airway obstruction, jugular vein thrombosis, sepsis.

Diff Dx: Retropharyngeal perforation—may be managed as outpatient in healthy adolescent or young adult with amoxicillin/clavulanate and steroids and next day follow-up; epiglottitis; pharyngeal foreign body; retropharyngeal hemorrhage (Jama 1973;226:427); meningitis in peds.

Lab: Blood tests if septic—CBC with diff; blood culture.
- *X-ray:* Soft tissue lateral neck, look for swelling in the prevertebral space, or air, or air/fluid level (J Otolaryngol 1999;28:134)—infants may have air here that disappears with inspiration and is thus a normal variant (Ped Radiol 1993;23:186); CXR, if respiratory symptoms or abnormal lung sounds; CT of neck, if simply prevertebral edema without air.

Emergency Management:
- Iv access.
- Antibiotics iv dosing: ampicillin/sulbactam 1.5-3 gm, clindamycin 600-900 mg and aminoglycoside, or ceftriaxone 1 gm with metronidazole 500 mg, eg.

- Consider methylprednisolone 125 mg iv or dexamethasone 15 mg iv, although lack of compelling data.
- ENT consult for admission.

17.11 Sinusitis

Emerg Med Clin N Am 1999;17:153; Nejm 2004;351:902

Cause: Viral, *Pneumococcus* spp., *Haemophilus influenzae*, *Streptococcus*, *Staphylococcus*, *Moraxella catarrhalis*, sometimes anaerobes, chronic may be fungal.

Epidem: Occurs at any age > 2 yr; anywhere from 0.5-5% of URIs complicated by acute sinusitis (Ped Infect Dis 1985;4:S51).

Pathophys: Edema around sinus ostia blocks drainage; all sinuses drain to medial meatus (Ostial Meatal Complex—OMC) except posterior ethmoidals to superior meatus, sphenoid to sphenoethmoid recess (posterior to the concha), and nasolacrimal duct to inferior meatus.

Sx: Fever; headache; maxillary toothache; purulent nasal discharge; outpatient trial of decongestant without relief.

Si: Rhinitis (90%); postnasal discharge; dental caries (10%); purulent material on middle turbinate; sinus tenderness with palpation or percussion; loss of sinus transillumination (for frontals—light below and pointing upwards from medial supraorbital rim; and for maxillaries—light at medial inferior orbital rim and pointing downwards while looking in mouth); Infraorbital nerve hypesthesia in maxillary sinusitis; noting sinus fluid is sensitive, but not specific for acute bacterial sinusitis.

Crs: May be chronic.

Cmplc: Meningitis/intracranial sepsis (J Laryngol Otol 1995;109:1061); lateral sinus thrombosis; osteomyelitis.

Lab: None unless septic—cultures and plain radiographs are nonspecific.

- *If septic,* CBC with diff, blood cultures, and other evaluation based on hx and physical exam.
- *X-ray:* Radiographic imaging may show fluid or not, with a lack of fluid not excluding bacterial sinusitis, and a fluid level possibly denoting viral, allergic or fungal sinusitis, or trauma. If diagnostic dilemma, CT is the better test (Acad Emerg Med 1994;1:235).

Emergency Management:

If septic (usually seen in frontal or ethmoidal sinusitis):

- O_2, iv access for fluid resuscitation and antibiotics.
- Antibiotics: ceftriaxone 2 gm iv; or ampicillin/sulbactam 3 gm iv; or cefuroxime 1.5 gm iv.
- ENT consult for admission.

If not septic:

- Local nasal decongestants like epinephrine drops 0.5-2% or phenylephrine 0.25% in saline qid for 4-5 d.
- Antibiotics for oral therapy: Amoxicillin (40-80 mg/kg/d divided tid to max 1500 mg/d) first line in peds and adults, except with ethmoidal and sphenoidal when need penicillinase-resistant penicillin like amoxicillin/clavulanate 875 mg bid (peds—90 mg/kg/d of amoxicillin component divided bid), TMP/SMX DS 1 pill bid (peds—4 TMP/20 SMX per kg per dose bid to a max of 160 TMP/800 SMX), cefpodoxime 200 mg bid (Pharmacoeconomics 1996;10:164), cefprozil 250 mg bid, cefuroxime 250-500 mg bid (Drugs 2001;61:1455) (peds—30 mg/kg/day divided bid)—short courses appropriate in healthy pts, eg, < 5-d courses of bacteriocidal antibiotics as effective as 10-14-d courses (Drugs 2003;63:2169) and first line antibiotics as efficacious as more expensive alternatives (Jama 2001;286:1849).

- Perhaps some benefit with intranasal steroids: fluticasone (Flonase) 2 sprays each nostril qd or triamcinolone— (J Allergy Clin Immunol 1998;102:403; Allergy 2000;55:19) vs (Laryngoscope 2002;112:320).
- Outpatient follow-up in 1-2 wks with primary care doctor if first evaluation and with ENT, if becoming a chronic problem.
- For URIs in general, vitamin E did not help cure nursing home participants, but may convey some protective effect (but this is not well-elucidated) (Jama 2004;292:828).

17.12 Vertigo

Ann Otol Rhinol Laryngol 1968;77:193; Emerg Med Clin N Am 1987;5:211)

Cause: Perhaps viral (labyrinthitis); positional vertigo (Ann EM 2001;37:392) (Brain 1972;95:369)—either positional nystagmus that persists or benign paroxysmal positional vertigo (BPPV); cerebellar insult (hemorrhage). See Acute Stroke Syndrome (p251); or other central causes.

Epidem: BPPV idiopathic in half its cases (inner ear stones postulated), but may have etiologies such as head trauma or viral labyrinthitis; female:male 2:1; most commonly posterior semicircular canal (Neurol 1987;37:371).

Pathophys (Arch Otorhinolaryngol 1984;241:23): Stability conferred via 3 mechanisms: vision, proprioception, and semicircular canals (for rotational stability). Need 2 out of 3 of these intact to avoid vertigo, unless inaccurate input from one site, such as lesion along the vestibular tract including the semicircular canals, the eighth cranial nerve, or eighth cranial nerve lesion. A lesion may be stones not settling correctly in the semicircular canals. As far as the specifics for the induction of vertigo, this is all conjecture.

Sx: Room spinning, nausea, dizziness—in general these symptoms are more pronounced in those with inner ear disease.

Si: Horizontal nystagmus with otherwise normal neurologic exam including hearing; BPPV may be elicited with Hall-Pike (head-hanging) maneuver—move patient from sitting to supine with one ear down and symptoms/nystagmus occur after approximately 15 sec and pass in 2 min, and then repeat with the other ear down.

Crs: Labyrinthitis and BPPV may have chronic course.

Cmplc: Based upon underlying etiology.

Diff Dx: TIA/CVA—vertebrobasilar insufficiency; metabolic abnormality, arrhythmia or pump failure; anemia; CNS or cranial nerve tumor; CNS or cranial nerve infection; vasculitis; medication reaction.

- Meniere's disease—with tinnitus and decreased hearing; use salt, caffeine, and ethanol restriction; may try antihistamines, antivertigo meds as listed below, diuretics such as thiazides and benzodiazepines for symptoms; refer to ENT as outpatient.
- Cerebellar-pontine angle tumor—diagnosed with auditory evoked potentials.
- Inner ear hemorrhage—acute with hearing loss.
- Temporal bone fracture—usually with trauma hx and severe hearing loss.
- Seizure.

Lab: None, but Head CT without contrast, if suspect cerebellar hemorrhage or skull fracture or other acute CNS event; head MRI, if suspect CNS neoplasm (Clin Imaging 1998;22:309).

Emergency Management:

Labyrinthitis and BPPV:

- Iv benzodiazepines (lorazepam, midazolam, or diazepam) of equivocal efficacy (J Otolaryngol 1980;9:472), but relaxes patient.
- Meclizine 25-50 mg po q 6 hr (Arch Neurol 1972;27:129).

- Dimenhydrinate (Dramamine) 50-100 mg po q 4-6 hr or scopolamine 0.4- 0.8 mg po q 8 hr or scopolamine (Transderm) patch 1.5 mg/72 hr.
- Outpatient primary care follow-up.

Labyrinthitis:
- Consider corticosteroid taper (begin with prednisone 40 mg po) if presenting within first 24 hr.

BPPV:
- Canalith Repositioning Procedure (Epley maneuvers) (Otolaryngol Head Neck Surg 1992;107:399; Am J Otol 2000;21:230).
- Homeopathy effective, specifically Vertigoheel (Heel, Inc.) (Arch Otolaryngol Head Neck Surg 1998;124:879).

Chapter 18

Pediatrics/Pediatric Surgery

18.1 Bronchiolitis/RSV

Peds 1999;104:1334; Nejm 2001;344:1917; Am Fam Phys 2004; 69:325

Cause: Respiratory Syncytial Virus (RSV).

Epidem: Peak incidence from November-April. Major issue in immunocompromised, premature infants, and cardiopulmonary disease in peds < 2 yr of age (Jama 1999;282:1440).

Pathophys: Bronchial infection/reactivity.

Sx: Respiratory distress.

Si: Tachypnea with wheezing.

Crs: Refractory course despite β-agonist treatment almost defines this disease process; fever associated with more severe clinical course (Arch Dis Child 1999;81:231). Lifelong increased chronic course of airway hyper-reactivity in children if bronchiolitis after 1 yr of age (Am J Respir Crit Care Med 2000;161:1501), but this is not found if disease affects one only as an infant (< 12 mon of age) (J Peds 1999;135:8).

Cmplc: Respiratory failure.

Diff Dx: Adenovirus; parainfluenza virus; foreign body; pneumonia; human metapneumovirus (Nejm 2004;350:443); cystic fibrosis, if recurrent; occult bacteremia in children 2-36 months of age is rare, and the approach of routine pan-culture is not supported by current literature (Arch Ped Adolesc Med 2004; 158:671).

Lab: Nasal wash RSV; capillary blood gas, pulse oximetry, and CXR, if significant distress.

Emergency Management:

- Isolation—prevent nosocomial spread.
- O_2; iv fluids, if in extremis.
- Nebulized racemic epinephrine (1 mg in 2 cc NS) in extremis (J Peds 1993;122:145) although routine use of 4 cc of 1% epinephrine nebulized with 3 treatments q 4 hr did not impact length of stay or ability of early for early discharge from hospital in those admitted (Nejm 2003;349:27).
- Albuterol neb 2.5 mg per treatment or 10 mg/hr continuous.
- Consider steroids (controversial)—parenteral, oral, or inhaled—parenteral study (Peds 2000;105:E44) vs budesonide inhaled study (Arch Dis Child 1999;80:343) and fluticasone inhaled study (Eur Respir J 2000;15:388).
- Heliox (70:30 Helium:O_2) may be of some benefit for both clinical severity score and need for ICU in those with moderate to severe symptoms—age group 1 mon to 2 yr (Peds 2002;109:68).
- Nitric oxide data are equivocal (Intensive Care Med 1999:81).
- Pediatrics consult for admit if not responding or stable, may need intubation +/− aerosolized ribavirin as inpatient—con (Am J Respir Crit Care Med 1999;160:829).
- Next day follow-up with peds if well enough to go home, consider home albuterol nebs (every 3-4 hr). Outpatient follow-up may include RSV immune globulin (each month in high-risk infants).

18.2 Cat-Scratch Disease (a Form of Cervical Adenitis)

Ped Infect Dis J 1997;16:163; 1985;4:S23

Cause: *Bartonella (Rochalimaea) henselae* and *quintana*, a small pleomorphic Gram negative, probably rickettsial organism. Sometimes *Afipia felis* (J Clin Microbiol 1998;36:2499).

Cervical adenitis itself is usually a self-limited viral (adenovirus, enterovirus, CMV, Epstein-Barr, *herpes simplex*) disease which resolves quickly, but can be caused by *Staphylococcus*, *Streptococcus*, and anaerobes (Clin Peds (Phila) 1980;19:693); less likely anaerobes, atypical organisms, cat-scratch disease, and toxoplasmosis.

Epidem: From young cats, infected for a few weeks; transmit via bites, scratches, and fleas, thus common name is a misnomer. 80% of cases in pts under age 21.

Pathophys: 7-14 d incubation. *Bartonella spp.* also found in bacillary angiomatosis and bartonellosis (Int J Dermatol 1997;36:405).

Sx: Bite or scratch from kitten (90% positive); papule at site of scratch.

Si: Fever; signs of scratch or bite with papule noted; adenopathy with 40% of nodes suppurative; potentially many ocular findings including Parinaud's oculoglandular syndrome (infection of eye surface and regional lymphadenopathy) (Curr Opin Ophthalmol 1999;10:209).

Crs: Usually self-limited, even with complications.

Cmplc: Encephalopathy (J Peds 1999;134:635); encephalitis (10%); osteolytic bone lesions; conjunctivitis; purpura; mesenteric adenitis.

- *Immunocompromised patients:* disseminated disease; bacillary angiomatosis—looks somewhat like Kaposi's sarcoma; peliosis hepatitis—sometimes seen in the immunocompetent.

Diff Dx (rare): TB and other mycobacterium (Clin Peds (Phila) 1997;36:403); *Haemophilus influenzae;* syphilis; fungal; *Yersinia pestis.*

Lab: CBC with diff showing mild eosinophilia; ESR; liver function tests, if systemically ill; obtain CSF, if neuro changes and look for increased protein; *Rochalimaea henselae* titer of > 1:64 is 84% sensitive and 96% specific. PCR may be needed (Hum Pathol 1997;28:820).

Emergency Management:

Mild disease (only papule at site):
- No rx, outpatient follow-up in 2-3 d with primary physician.

Moderate/severe disease:
- Ciprofloxacin 500 mg po bid; or azithromycin 500 mg d 1 followed by 250 mg d 2-5 (pediatrics—10 mg/kg d 1 followed by 5 mg/kg d 2-5) (Ped Infect Dis J 1998;17:447)
- Pediatrics—TMP/SMX (4 TMP/20 SMX per kg per dose) bid to a max of 160 TMP/800 SMX.
- Erythromycin 500 mg po qid for disseminated forms; second line is Doxycycline 100 mg po bid.
- May also consider gentamicin, ceftriaxone, cefotaxime, or amikacin.
- Primary care consult for admission, if moderate or severe disease.

18.3 Child Abuse

Hosp Community Psychiatry 1992;43:111; J Med Assoc Ga 2000;89:5

Cause: Potentially anyone—parents, caregivers, strangers.

Epidem: Linked to parental unemployment/poverty, especially fathers (Child Abuse Negl 1998;22:79). Adolescent mothers at higher risk than older counterparts, especially if they had been abused (Child Abuse Negl 2000;24:701). False allegations or misinterpretation uncommon (2.5%) (Child Abuse Negl 2000;24:149).

Pathophys: Abuse or neglect in the physical, sexual, or emotional (verbal) realm.

Sx: Sleep disorders; nightmares; inappropriate sexual play; school and developmental problems; phobias; depression.

Si: Delay in seeking rx. Recurrent injury; patterned bruises; fractures; head injuries; retinal hemorrhages; facial and oral injuries (Child Abuse Negl 2000;24:521). Injuries inappropriate for age, not consistent with hx, and to different body planes.

Crs: Potentially fatal; intervention requires a team approach with state agencies, police, social work, and other specialty organizations.

Cmplc: Failure to thrive; may impact all aspects of life, including long-term neurobehavioral problems (J Child Psychol Psychiatry 2000;41:97).

Lab: Consider radiographic bone survey if evidence of trauma (J Am Acad Orthop Surg 2000;8:10); forensic photos.

Emergency Management:
- Pediatrics consult for admission.
- Department of health/human services referral.

18.4 Croup

Nejm 2001;344:1917; Ped Pulmonol 1997;23:370; Ped Clin N Am 1999;46:1167

Cause: Parainfluenza virus, and others.

Epidem: 3:100 under age 6 yr; 1.3% must be hospitalized; adult croup does exist (Chest 1996;109:1659).

Pathophys: Two forms, and both occur mainly at night with child in recumbent position—whether this is due to fluid shifts with consequent edema or meridian causality is unknown.
Acute laryngotracheitis—follows 2-3 d of URI.

Spasmodic croup—no antecedent illness; acts like hypersensitivity syndrome.

Sx: Barky cough.

Si: Cough like a seal bark; tachypnea; hoarseness or other voice change; inspiratory stridor; accessory respiratory muscle use; cyanosis when severe.

Crs: Most self-limited, protracted course with *H. simplex* (Acta Paediatr 1996;85:118); Increased risk of asthma in school aged children with recurrent croup, with a higher risk if family h/o asthma (approximately 37%) (Acta Paediatr 1996;85:1295).

Cmplc: Hypoxia.

Diff Dx: Aspirated foreign body; epiglottitis; bacterial tracheitis—such as diphtheria; congenital anomaly—such as vascular ring.

Lab: None.

- *X-ray:* May be done to exclude other causes of airway obstruction, look for tracheal edema (steeple sign) (Radiol Clin N Am 1998;36:175).

Emergency Management:

- Most pts improved at ER secondary to cool night air and upright posture.
- Mist tent or humidified O_2.
- Racemic epinephrine 0.25-1 cc of 2.25% solution neb (Ped Emerg Care 1996;12:156), although L-epinephrine 5 cc of 1:1000 neb (cheaper and more available) perhaps as efficacious (Peds 1992;89:302). Observation time after epinephrine use is debatable (Ann EM 1995;25:331).
- Heliox 70/30 may be helpful in mild to moderately ill children (Acad Emerg Med 1998;5:1130).
- Steroids (BMJ 1999;319:595)—Dexamethasone 0.6 mg/kg po (Jama 1998;279:1629) or im (Acta Paediatr Scand 1988; 77:99); or prednisone 1-2 mg/kg po; or methylprednisolone 2 mg/kg iv; or nebulized dexamethasone (4 mg) or budesonide

(Pulmicort) 2 mg in 4 cc nebulized (Brit J Gen Pract 2000; 50:135; Drugs 2000;60:1141). Oral dexamethasone 0.6 mg/kg tastes better than other steroid elixirs, and will decrease the length of illness, the chance of a return for a recheck, and allow better sleep—thus, even mild cases would benefit from this single dose therapy (Nejm 2004;351:1306).

- Outpatient follow-up next day with primary physician if home, with trial of steam from shower or cool night air if recurrent. If severe, pediatrics/primary care consult for admission.

18.5 Hirschsprung Disease

Dig Dis 1994;12:106; Crit Rev Clin Lab Sci 1999;36:225

Cause: Unknown, probably many types of Hirschsprung disease with complicated genetic inheritance (Proc Natl Acad Sci USA 2000;97:268).

Epidem: Usually in infants with male:female 1:4.

Pathophys: Aganglionic segment of colon, variable in length from a few cm in rectum to all rectum and descending colon. No neurons in this segment resulting in constant contractions and no relaxation—eventually with intestinal obstruction; seen as acute in infants, chronic in children and teenagers.

Sx: Abdominal pain; chronic constipation.

Si: Distended and tender abdomen.

Crs: Variable.

Cmplc: Dehydration.

Diff Dx: Encopresis in 5-8 yr olds—they will have occasional "huge stool"; chronic idiopathic intestinal obstruction; other sphincter malfunctions where pts can be conditioned to control stools; intestinal neuronal malformations (Eur J Ped Surg 1999;9: 91); Chagas' disease; allergic colitis (eg, milk allergy) (Ped Radiol 1999;29:37).

Lab: Metabolic profile; CBC with diff.

- *X-ray:* 3-view abd series if obstructed or looking for megacolon.

Emergency Management:
- Iv fluid if dehydrated; pain control with iv meds.
- General surgery consult if obstructed.
- Pediatrics/primary care follow-up if constipation, with consideration of gi/general surgery follow-up for anorectal manometry (screening) (Eur J Ped Surg 1999;9:101) or rectal biopsy—definitive rx is to bypass aganglionic segments, with variable responses to surgery (J Ped Surg 1999;34:1152) vs (Am J Gastroenterol 2000;95:1226).

18.6 Hypercyanotic Episode of Tetralogy of Fallot

Cardiovasc Clin 1973;5:1; Ped Ann 1996;25:339

Cause: Congenital malformation.

Epidem: Approximately 8% of all CHD; approximately 60% of cyanotic CHD; 85% of adults cyanotics with CHD.

Pathophys: VSD and pulmonic stenosis of varying positions and severities; and dextroaorta with right-sided aortic arch (25%), and right ventricular hypertrophy.

Sx: Cyanosis onset after 3 mon of age, unless pulmonary atresia complete; dyspnea; squatting relieves symptoms.

Si: Cyanosis; clubbing (Semin Arth Rheum 1985;14:263); loud systolic murmur along left sternal border, which is absent in severe cases; P_2 decreased.

Crs: Variable with degree of impairment and depending on other congenital problems; potential pregnancy problems when of age (J Clin Anesth 1993;5:332).

Cmplc: Hypoxic spells with possible neurologic compromise; paradoxical emboli; brain abscess (Arch Neurol 1983;40:209); anemia;

SBE; pneumonia, hemoptysis; gout; pulmonary artery dissection; CHF.

Diff Dx: (lesions occurring 5% or greater of all CHD)—Pulmonary atresia with VSD, severe form of tetralogy of Fallot; pulmonary atresia with intact ventricular septum—right to left shunt through patent foramen ovale, possibly a severe form of pulmonary stenosis is approximately 5%; transposition of the great arteries—TGA is approximately 5%.

Lab: CBC with diff; metabolic profile; TSH; ABG; EKG—persistent right axis deviation and RVH with strain.
- *X-ray:* small heart, boot-shaped, look for right sided aortic arch (Radiol Clin N Am 1980;18:411).

Emergency Management:
- O_2; Pediatrics/cardiology consult.
- Post-operative complications may include heart block or pulmonary insufficiency.

18.7 Intussusception

J Accid Emerg Med 1995;12:182

Cause: Largely unknown, postulated post-viral infection, or other reasons to give leading edge such as Meckel diverticulum, intestinal duplication, intestinal polyp, foreign body, or neoplasm. Post-operative intussusception may occur (Arch Surg 1987;122:1190) and older children and adults may have atypical presentations (J Emerg Med 1991;9:347).

Epidem: Most common cause of intestinal obstruction from ages 3 mon to 3 yr; male:female 4:1; is associated with oral rotavirus vaccine and is after the first dose and usually within 2 wks (Nejm 2001;344:564).

Pathophys: Bowel tract pushes caudally and is sleeved by distal segment.

Sx: Abdominal pain; vomiting; "currant jelly stool" which is blood mixed with mucus.

Si: Distended and rigid abdomen; possibly palpable mass in right upper quadrant; look for rectal prolapse; guaiac-positive stools.

Crs: Variable, more emergent course of action needed the younger the child; look for the triad intermittent abdominal pain, vomiting, and palpable right upper quadrant mass, with gross or occult blood as also significant (J Peds 1998;132:836).

Cmplc: Dehydration; intestinal ischemia; peritonitis.

Diff Dx: Appendicitis; foreign body obstruction—ileocecal valve region; hernia; gastroenteritis; infectious colitis; Meckel diverticulum, although this is usually painless.

Lab: CBC with diff; metabolic profile; consider type and screen.
- *X-ray:* 3-view abdominal series should show intestinal dilatation with air/fluid levels (Ped Emerg Care 1992;8:325); barium enema is both diagnostic and many times curative, if no evidence of perforation; perhaps US for low risk pts (J Peds 1992;121:182).

Emergency Management:
- Iv access for fluids, pain and nausea control.
- Pediatrics/surgical consult, with expectation to do barium enema or air pressure enema reduction (J Ped Surg 1986;21:1201), if no signs of perforation or shock.

18.8 Kawasaki Disease

J Peds 1991;118:680; Arch Dis Child 1991;86:185

Cause: Unknown.

Epidem: Incidence of approximately 5:100,000/yr; commonly presents as fever of unknown origin.

Pathophys: A mucocutaneous lymph node disease, with the immune response precipitating a vasculitis (Immunodefic Rev 1989;1: 261).

Sx: Prolonged fever; variety of rashes.

Si: Fever in peds 1-8 yr of age; striking non-exudative conjunctivitis; non-pitting edema; cervical lymphadenopathy; desquamation of skin on palms, perineum, trunk and lips; "strawberry" tongue.

Crs: Difficult diagnosis in those < 6 mon of age, consider ECHO of heart looking for coronary aneurysms in those with prolonged fever (J Peds 1986;109:759).

Cmplc: 25% get coronary aneurysms later, which may cause an MI if thrombosed (Intern Med 1992;31:774); cardiac conduction system may become infiltrated/scarred (Am Hrt J 1978;96:744); polyserositis which includes cardiac tamponade.

Diff Dx: Infantile periarteritis nodosa; adenovirus; measles; scarlet fever; RMSF; leptospirosis; EBV; JRA.

Lab: CBC with diff (look for anemia); ESR; metabolic profile; blood cultures; CK-MB and Troponin I for myocarditis (Ped Cardiol 1999;20:184); rapid direct fluorescent antigen test for adenovirus (Arch Ped Adolesc Med 2000;154:453); EKG—none of these overwhelmingly specific.

- *X-ray:* CXR.

Emergency Management:
- Pediatrics/primary care consult for admission
- IgG 2 gm/kg iv over 10 hr to prevent complications (Nejm 1991;324:1633; Peds Int 1999;41:1)
- ASA 100 mg/kg, with more free salicylate available compared to normals (J Peds 1991;118:456).
- Iv streptokinase (3,500 IU/kg over 30 min, followed by 1,000 IU/kg/24 hr) for acute MI (Cathet Cardiovasc Diagn 1995;35:139).

- Consider methylprednisolone 30 mg/kg qd × 3 d, if impending cardiac tamponade (Intensive Care Med 1999; 25:1137).

18.9 Pyloric Stenosis

J Paediatr Child Hlth 1993;29:372

Cause: Possibly genetic/sex-linked.

Epidem: M > F; 50% of affected mothers' children will have, 10% of affected fathers' offspring will have; 1:100 − 1:600 births.

Pathophys: Concentric muscular hypertrophy of pyloric smooth muscle, in which nitric oxide synthetase deficiency precipitates the disease.

Sx: Well and gaining weight for first 3-5 wks of life, and then non-bilious projectile vomiting.

Si: Palpable "olive" in right upper quadrant 70% of the time; our clinical diagnosis skills are declining (BMJ 1993;306:553).

Crs: Benign with surgical repair.

Cmplc: Dehydration.

Diff Dx: All uncommon—annular pancreas; duodenal atresia; Addisonian crisis due to congenital adrenal hypoplasia; antral diaphragm; eosinophilic gastroenteritis (J Ped Gastroenterol Nutr 1987;6:543).

Lab: Metabolic profile shows a hypochloremic, hypokalemic metabolic alkalosis—this metabolic derangement is becoming more uncommon (J Ped Surg 1983;18:394; Am J Emerg Med 1999; 17:67).

- *X-ray:* Upper gi barium study vs abdominal US—increased use of radiologic diagnostic testing has not led to a significant change in management (BMJ 1993;306:553), although is the standard for current diagnosis and perhaps allows earlier diagnosis if pts present earlier (Peds 1997;100:E9).

Emergency Management:
- IVF rehydration if needed; surgery consult.

18.10 SIDS

Emerg Med Clin N Am 1983;1:27; Acad Emerg Med 1995;2: 926; 1995;2:996; 1995;2:1077)

Cause: Sudden infant death syndrome (SIDS) with unknown cause, but some cases due to unrecognized abuse.

Epidem: 1.4 deaths:1000 live births in U.S.; familial tendency; increased incidence by sleeping prone, use of deformable mattress, swaddling, warm room, URIs, and exposure to passive cigarette smoke; associated with primary *Pneumocystis carinii* infection (Clin Infect Dis 1999;29:1489); no association with DPT immunizations.

Pathophys: Hypothesized that several sleep apneas (> 15 sec) precede fatal event.

Sx/Si: Deceased.

Crs: Medical examiner case.

Diff Dx: Trauma; smothering asphyxia; other types of abuse.

Lab: None; near SIDS requires full physiologic evaluation including Hgb F level (look for elevation) (Nejm 1987;316:1122; Med Hypotheses 2000;54:987); and EKG showing no shortening of QT with rate increase.

Emergency Management:
- Resuscitative efforts while looking for other treatable causes.
- Counseling to parents and report to medical examiner.

- Prophylactic measures of supine or side position; firm bedding; and apnea monitor have been equivocal in efficacy.

18.11 Volvulus

Semin Ped Surg 2003;12:229; J Ped Surg 1981;16:614; Am J Surg 1984;148:252

Cause: Rotation of gut around a pedicle that occurred during embryonic formation—usually in the portion of the gut supplied by the superior mesenteric artery (SMA), which is the midgut.

Epidem: Usually within the first month of life, M > F.

Pathophys: Twisting of the gut causes obstruction to luminal flow and interruption of the blood flow to the affected portion.

Sx: Bilious vomiting, which is usually early and indicative of more severe presentation if precedes other abdominal complaints (J Postgrad Med 2004;50:27), pain, bloating; less common with diarrhea and fever.

Si: Tenderness, guarding, possibly palpable mass if distal obstruction.

Crs: If not recognized and ischemic bowel not released, then may become gangrenous.

Diff Dx: Pyloric stenosis, intussusception; rare causes include gastric volvulus [these pts may lack abdominal bloating, vomiting, and pain (Ped Emerg Care 2001;17:344)], transverse colon etiology of volvulus (Chilaiditi syndrome), sigmoid volvulus (J Am Coll Surg 2000;190:717), wandering spleen.

Lab: Plain radiographs—look for the duodenal triangle in the right upper quadrant (air-filled duodenum with air-fluid level overlapped by liver edge) on upright film as sign of duodenal obstruction (Clin Radiol 1985;36:47); Upper gi with small bowel followthrough; CT if not definitive (Radiology 1997;204:507); US may show "whirlpool sign," which may be sensitive in those with malrotation (J Ultrasound Med 2004;24:397).

Emergency Management:
- IVF; NGT decompression; surgical consult.
- Consider air contrast barium enema, if sigmoid volvulus to reduce.

Chapter 19

Plastic Surgery/ Wound Repair

19.1 Bites

Curr Clin Top Infect Dis 1999;19:99; Nejm 1999;340:138

Cause: Human, domestic or wild animal bite, or awakening in a room/tent with a bat as additional occupant (Wis Med J 1996;95:242).

Epidem: *Pastuerella multocida* is in > 50% of animal bite and cat scratch infections; polymicrobial infections in human and mammalian bite wounds (Nejm 1999;340:85); Higher risk in animal control officers (Am J Public Hlth 1984;74:255).

Pathophys: Inoculation of bacteria—cat bites frequently become infected because of deep inoculation; possible rabies virus in unvaccinated or wild animal saliva; envenomations (see p 87).

Sx: Obvious wound; may lack obvious wound for those with bat bites.

Si: Wound—note tenderness, erythema pattern, adenopathy, depth, and discharge; evaluate distal neurovascular status, check for tendon injury.

Crs: Varies with potential need for rabies prophylaxis.

Cmplc: Cellulitis, lymphangitis, tenosynovitis, or osteomyelitis (Arch EM 1992;9:299); rabies; sepsis—infections more common in those who are immunosuppressed such as those with DM.

Lab: Uncomplicated bites without specific lab evaluation; consider CBC with diff, ESR, wound gram stain, and culture for those with more significant infections.

For assailant in human bites, obtain HIV, Hep B, and Hep C, if possible.

- *X-ray:* Consider for osteomyelitis, look for periosteal reaction—not seen acutely.

Emergency Management:

- Clean wound, soap, and water as good as anything else.
- Update/initiate Tetanus if needed (see p218).
- Treat for rabies if mammalian bite from unvaccinated animal such as dog, cat, bat, fox, raccoon, or skunk, with no quarantine ability of attacking animal, or if awakened with bat in the same room (see p208). Not usually seen in mice, squirrels, or other rodents, nor rabbits.
- For envenomations, see p87.
- Do not close wounds if possible, although those on the head and neck may be closed if repaired within 12 hr (Ear Nose Throat J 1998;77:216). If closing on other areas of the body, consider placing a drain and do not use tissue adhesives for any bite wound closures. Debride all devitalized tissue, surgical consult if this extends beyond the myofascial plane or into tendons, ligaments, joint spaces, or bone.
- Splint and elevate the injured area.
- Consider oral prophylactic antibiotics for human bites (Plast Reconstr Surg 1975;56:538), especially to any part of the hand, and all animal bites (Arch EM 1989;6:251). Human and Animal bites—first choice is amoxicillin/clavulanate 875 mg bid for 3-5 d, or clindamycin 300 mg qid combined with ciprofloxacin 500 mg bid or TMP/SMX DS 1 pill bid; second choices include doxycycline 100 mg po bid or cefuroxime 500 mg bid.

- If antibiotics for rx of minor infection, such as cellulitis or minimal lymphangitis (no adenopathy) in an otherwise healthy person, first dose iv, such as ampicillin/sulbactam 1.5-3 gm, home with amoxicillin/clavulanate 875 mg po bid or one of the previous choices under prophylaxis, but treat for 10 d, and have next day follow-up—probably in the ER.
- For more serious infections, iv antibiotic as above, and ortho/plastics/general surgery consult (one of these) for admission.

19.2 Topical and Local Anesthesia

Selection and site of appropriate anesthesia is important for surgical procedures. All infiltration should be done through the cleanest field possible, and nerve blocks should have sterile prep performed.

Lidocaine: An aminoamide, maximum subcutaneous infusion is 2.5-3 mg/kg (Nejm 1979;301:418). Thus, goal of 1% solution (1 gm/100cc) is approximately 0.3 cc/kg, or 21 cc in the 70 kg person. Gives approximately 2 hr of local anesthesia. Iontophoresis effective (J Dermatol Surg Oncol 1994;20:579), yet not a common ER modality.

The Role of Epinephrine: Added to local anesthetic solutions, such as lidocaine, its vasoconstrictive properties are such that duration of anesthesia and control of hemostasis is enhanced (Anesthesiology 1989;71:757), and may use a larger volume and dose of anesthesia, since it is absorbed into circulation slower and over more time. Do not use epinephrine in nerve blocks or locally into digits, tip of the nose, onto the ear, or penis. Although critical data of distal tissue necrosis lacking if epinephrine injected into a digit (Plast Reconstr Surg 2001;108:114), may consider use of 1 mg of terbutaline diluted at least 1:1 (depends on the area infiltrated) and inject this sc into affected area (Am J Emerg Med 1999;17:91).

The Role of NaHCO₃: Along with warming injected solution (hand-rub filled syringe or 40°C heater) and injecting slowly, buffering is thought to decrease the pain of injecting (Ann R Coll Surg Engl 2004;86:213; J Dermatol Surg Oncol 1990;16:842). The solution of lidocaine:bicarb is 10:1. May keep up to 2 wks with refrigeration at 0-4°C (J Dermatol Surg Oncol 1991;17:411).

The Role of Benzyl Alcohol 0.9%: Allows to increase amount of fluid injected if epinephrine is not an option or if lidocaine allergy. Works better than diphenhydramine (Ann EM 1998;32:650).

The Role of Diphenhydramine 0.5% (Benadryl): Allows to increase amount of fluid injected for local anesthesia if epinephrine is not an option or in lieu of lidocaine, since diphenhydramine is a weak anesthetic (Ann EM 1994;23:1328). Combined with lidocaine, the solution is prepared 1:1.

Bupivicaine (Marcaine): Long-acting (8-12 hr) anesthetic available in 0.25 or 0.5% solution; has a lower safety profile than lidocaine; do not use with epinephrine or bicarbonate. No need to combine with lidocaine for faster onset of action (Ann EM 1996; 27:490).

TAC (Ann EM 1980;9:568): Solution of 0.5% tetracaine/ 0.5% adrenaline/11.8% cocaine applied topically to face or scalp for 20 min to facilitate anesthesia in children. Avoid to tip of nose, directly onto ear, or on mucous membranes. No advantage over LET (see next), and LET avoids any issues physicians may have with using cocaine. Evidence of effect is with observed blanching to surrounding tissues, may need to boost anesthesia in some with 1% lidocaine locally injected. Application of such type topical anesthetics to children at triage will reduce rx time in the ER (Ann EM 2003;42:34).

LET (Ann EM 1995;25:203): Solution of 4% lidocaine/0.1% epinephrine/0.5% tetracaine used in the same circumstances as with

TAC, same onset of action, same parameters. Application of such type topical anesthetics to children at triage will reduce rx time in the ER (Ann EM 2003;42:34).

4% viscous lidocaine: For use in injured skin where TAC or LET cannot be used, takes 30-60 min for onset of action, and most children will need additional 1% lidocaine supplementation, but allows infiltration with much less pain.

EMLA (J Dermatol Surg Oncol 1994;20:579): Solution of lidocaine and prilocaine for use over intact skin, such as prior to iv access. For elective situations since requires 60 min for onset, and use occlusive dressing, such as Opsite or Tagaderm, when applied to facilitate action.

Local infiltration: 25-30 G needle for injecting; do the proximal edge first, since this will facilitate pain control for the distal edge. Injecting through the wound is less painful than going through the skin, but beware of debris. Inject slowly. Lidocaine has onset in 5-10 min, and bupivicaine 10-15 min.

Nerve Blocks

Post Grad Med J 1999;106:69,77; Am Fam Phys 2004;69:585; 2004;69:896

Digital Block Fingers: Injections are just distal to the MCP. The neurovascular bundle runs on both the radial and ulnar sides of the phalanx, with some dorsal nerves also crossing the proximal phalanx. Begin on either the radial or ulnar side of the proximal phalanx, while blocking the web area—raise a wheal using a 25-27 G needle, and then go deeper toward the bone, inject here, and then aim to the volar aspect, and inject a little more (total 1-1.5 cc). Keep the needle in, but skew the aim (almost completely withdraw to re-aim), so that the needle is now across the extensor (dorsal) surface, and put 1 cc or less through here. Now block the web area on the other side of the finger, exactly the same way as the first side. Total infiltration solution volume should be 3-4 cc, and remember not to use any epinephrine.

Digital Block Toes: Same approach as with the digital finger block, but it is important to get the plantar aspect of the toes. Begin on either the medial or lateral side of the proximal phalanx, while blocking the web area—raise a wheal using a 25-27 G needle, and then go deeper toward the bone, inject here, and then aim to the plantar aspect, and inject a little more (total 1 cc). Now place the needle more toward the plantar aspect, but within the anesthetized area, and put 1 cc of fluid across the plantar aspect. Now block the web area on the other side of the toe, exactly as done on the first side. Total maximum solution volume should be 3 cc, and remember not to use epinephrine. The hallux may need 0.5-1 cc injected across its dorsal surface, so that a ring-like area of anesthesia has been performed. Total maximum solution volume for the hallux is 4 cc.

Metacarpal Block: This is performed dorsally and just proximal to the MCP joint, and can accommodate more fluid than a digital block—it is not to be used for the thumb. Anesthetize the skin using a 25-27 G needle. Introduce the needle just ulnar and radial to the metacarpal in question, and position it so that the tip is just deep (in a volar sense) to the metacarpal. Inject while withdrawing the needle, placing approximately 3 cc in this space. Inject both sides—this is not a palmar approach.

Radial Nerve Block: Block the superficial branch of the radial nerve when anesthetizing the thumb. The anesthetized area will resemble a half circle. Infiltrate the dorsum of the hand just below the skin beginning at the proximal "snuff box" area and end at the proximal second metacarpal using a 25-27 G needle. The convexity of the half circle should be away from the thumb.

Median Nerve Block: Useful when working on the palmar aspect of the index or middle finger, and when working on the thumb. Imagine a line that is an extension of the radial side of the middle finger and extends to the wrist. Two tendons are palpable at the wrist on either side of this line—the palmaris longus on the ulnar side and the flexor carpi radialis on the radial side. The median nerve is deep to the flexor retinaculum between these two tendons (approximately 2 cm deep), and can be anesthetized with a 25-27 G needle.

Ulnar Nerve Block: Useful when working on the little finger or the ulnar side of the hand. On the volar aspect of the wrist, the last large tendon toward the ulnar side is that of the flexor carpi ulnaris. At the distal end of this palpable tendon, off to its medial aspect, runs the ulnar nerve. It is just deep to the tendon, approximately 1 cm deep, and can be anesthetized with a 25-27 G needle.

Auricular Block: When working on the ear, it is preferable not to inject directly into the skin of the ear. Just before the skin reflects onto the ear, anesthetize this area both anteriorly and posteriorly using a 25-27 G needle. The external canal may also have some vagal branches that will require local anesthesia.

Dental Blocks (Gen Dent 1982;30:414): Most common is the inferior alveolar nerve block. This nerve enters the mandible on the medial aspect (at approximately its midpoint in the anterior/posterior axis) of the body of the mandible (just in front of the tonsillar pillars)—it is about a finger's breadth superior to the top of the lower teeth. If the needle is placed a finger's breadth above the lower row of teeth anteriorly at the body of the mandible, and then aim posteriorly while keeping parallel to the teeth, the depth can be gauged by keeping the non-injecting hand on the posterior and anterior aspects of the mandible. Inject about 1 cc.

19.3 Wound Management

This is a review of key points, and not a substitute for proper training and practice. Adjunctive materials are available (J Emerg Med 1998;16:651).

All Wounds: Examine for foreign body (X-ray, if necessary), and check for involvement of tendons, joint spaces, ligaments, or bone. Check distal neurovascular function: it is not uncommon to have a small area of skin anesthesia distal to a laceration. Remember tetanus prophylaxis. Hand wounds < 2 cm in length without any of the complications noted above will not need suturing (J Fam Pract 2003;52:23). The conventional wisdom is that all nail bed injuries need repair, but those with intact nails and nail margins (such as those with crush injuries) will do just as well with rx of the subungual hematoma and no nail bed exploration (J Hand Surg [Am] 1999;24:1166).

Puncture Wounds: Special wounds in the sense that an inoculum of bacteria may be deposited and then quickly sealed over. Although potentially more serious, overall incidence of secondary infection is only approximately 6% (J Accid Emerg Med 1996;13:274). All these wounds should be cleaned and left open, and perhaps soaking tid in warm water. If the wound is completely sealed, conservative rx with surface cleaning and non-weight bearing for 24 hr and 1-2 d follow-up is OK (J Emerg Med 1995;13:291); providing a crosshatch so that drainage can occur may be appropriate in those not deemed reliable. Foot wounds are high-risk for *Pseudomonas aeruginosa*, especially if nail through sole of shoe [antibiotic of choice is ciprofloxacin in those > 15 yr of age (Clin Infect Dis 1995;21:194)] (Jama 1968; 204:262). Dirty wounds or wounds in high-risk pts (CHD, DM, HIV, etc) should have prophylactic antibiotics (first generation cephalosporin, such as cephalexin), and perhaps consideration of having polymicrobial infections in those with DM (J Foot Ankle Surg 1994;33:91).

Irrigation: Irrigate with copious amounts of sterile saline; and wounds that are heavily contaminated or need significant debridement should be treated in the OR. If elect to use antibacterial skin prep agents, such as iodophor or chlorhexidine, avoid getting these into the open wound, as these will destroy the healthy tissue in the wound. Pts with simple lacerations (children in this study) did just as well with tap water irrigation as with sterile saline (Ann EM 2003;41:609).

Sterile Field/Gloves: Advocate a clean area that is then bordered by sterile towels/drape to decrease chance of introducing infection—no critical data. Sterile gloves are also advocated, although the use of clean gloves in simple traumatic lacerations in those who are immunocompetent is as effective in preventing secondary infection, as are sterile gloves (Ann EM 2004;43:362).

Repair: Debride all devitalized tissue. Make edges smooth leaving an elliptical opening if possible, and undermine tissue to reduce tension if necessary. Stitches do not need to be water tight and, if too tight, may lead to skin necrosis. If a myofascial layer has been violated, it is not necessary to repair this, and it actually may be necessary to extend the defect to avoid a compartment syndrome as in the anterior tibial region. Tendon and joint capsule repair should be done by an orthopedic surgeon (OK to repair extensor tendons if trained to do so). Deep or heavily contaminated wounds may need a drain for 2-3 d to prevent abscess formation. Remember to close deep layers so that a potential space is not left (> 3 cm depth is considered necessitating a deep closure). The palmar aspect of the hand has a high propensity for infection (Arch EM 1987;4:211), and the palm itself should not be explored in the ER. Most body areas need to be repaired within 12 hr of injury, but the face can be delayed for 24 hr—this can be modified with surgical debridement and if this needs to occur, should be done by a surgeon.

- Staples (Ann EM 1989;18:1122): The fastest way to close a wound, thus useful for hemostasis control. Helpful in large or if multiple lacerations from a trauma. Also used primarily in locations where scar formation is not an issue, such as the scalp.
- Sutures: The basics of absorbable stitches deep, and non-absorbable or absorbable at the skin are important to remember. Absorbable stitches have similar cosmetic outcomes and same rates of infection compared to non-absorbable stitches (Acad Emerg Med 2004;11:730). Do not make stitches tight, and it is OK to run the stitch in incision injuries rather than place repeated simple stitches (J Trauma 2000;48:495). Use mattress stitches to evert the edges of wound and to help evenly distribute wound tension. Facial injuries require 5-0 or 6-0 stitches, hands/digits 4-0 or 5-0, and 3-0 or 4-0 for the trunk and extremities. Be sure to repair the nail bed/matrix, and place nail back in place or surrogate (aluminum foil) to preserve nail fold—recent data do show this as equivocal (J Fam Pract 2003;52:23). Far-near-near-far: a type of stitch that helps close a wound under tension by itself absorbing the tension, even without the snug knot. Enter far from the wound on side A; come up close to the end edge on side B; go in close to the edge on side A; and come up far from the wound edge on Side B. The term far is usually about 2 cm and near is about 0.5 cm; the knot is tied on top, but not over wound opening. In general, sutures better if wound gaping or if continued bleeding.
- Wound closure tapes: A tape that can hold minimally tense wounds that have good hemostasis. Use tincture of Benzoin on either side of the wound to help secure this tape. Best are Steri-strip, Nichi-strip, and Curi-strip (J Emerg Med 1987;5:451).

- Tissue Adhesive: Advocate octyl-2-cyanoacrylate for wounds with no tension, controlled bleeding, not a bite, and not over an extensor surface (J Peds 1998;132:1067; Acad Emerg Med 1998;5:94).
- Watchful waiting: It is not necessary to manipulate all wounds; puncture wounds, bites, and heavily contaminated wounds would do better with cleaning, no closure, and 1-2 d follow-up. Small scalp wounds that are not bleeding can also just be observed. If the scalp injury is from a relatively clean source, manipulating the wound with cleaning or repair is often not necessary, and wound can be left to heal on its own. Infection of scalp wounds is rare, unless retained foreign body.

Chapter 20
Procedures

20.1 Airway Management

The first step in every assessment is to evaluate for a secure airway. The following information is intended as a refresher, and does not substitute for hands-on training with an appropriate instructor. Always first open an airway by placing the head and neck in neutral position and then use a chin lift or jaw thrust. Any techniques that violate the skin should have sterile prep and drape performed. The cricothyroid membrane is bound by the inferior border of the thyroid cartilage above and the cricoid below. Use of topical anesthetics for some of these procedures may improve pt comfort and success, but benzocaine may cause methemoglobinemia (Arch IM 2004;164: 1192).

N.B. Peds do well with bag-valve-mask (BVM) out of hospital compared with ET for medical or trauma in urban environment (Jama 2000;283:783).

Oral Pharyngeal Airway (OPA): This curved plastic airway may be the first step in oral airway adjunct. This is sized by having one end resting on the tip of the nose and the other end resting at the angle of the jaw. Insert with the concavity upwards, and then rotate 180° when it is halfway in. The final position is with the flange at the lips. This lifts the tongue from the back of the throat, and is not for use in a conscious person. Adult size is 5-6, with smaller numbers for smaller sizes.

Nasal Pharyngeal Airway/Nasal Trumpet (NPA): This is sized as with the OPA, and the lubricated tip goes through a nare, and the flange rests at the external nare when done. Many people have asymmetric nare passages—if it does not work on one side, try the other. Size 8-9 in adult (internal diameter in millimeters) may be used on the conscious pt, but should not be used in those with maxillofacial trauma.

Bipap/CPAP: May be useful for those in respiratory failure of medical cause (CHF, COPD, pneumonia) if pt can tolerate the device and intubation not clearly needed (Nejm 2001;344:481). Not for asthma.

Of note, non-invasive pos pressure ventilation for respiratory failure after extubation does not change the pt's immediate future need for re-intubation or the incidence of short-term mortality (Nejm 2004;350:2452).

Combitube: A variant on the esophageal obturator airway (EOA), but with the ability to have both the side vent and distal end vent accessed for ventilatory support. In other words, the provider has the ability to be ventilate a pt independent of where the tip ends up (esophagus vs trachea). Is heat dependent, in that it becomes very stiff in a cold environment and may cause lacerations. Advance so that the teeth are between the two black lines on the tube, and then fill the blue balloon and then the white balloon. Vent attempting the blue port first—if not venting then try the white port. Two sizes, but even the small size necessitates the pt be > 5 ft in height. Currently is not available in a latex-free option.

Laryngeal Mask Airway (LMA): An anesthesia device that is a "save" device in emergency medicine, whose use would be considered for those in C-spine immobilization (Anaesthesia 1999;54:793) or when an endotracheal tube cannot be introduced successfully. The distal tip of this device sits in the posterior pharynx, is then inflated to "occlude" the esophageal opening, and air vents just proximal to this area direct air toward the larynx. Not as secure as an endotracheal tube, and may intubate through this device with an endotracheal tube, sometimes using fiberoptic assistance (Ped Anaesth 2000;10:53)—the intubating laryngeal mask airway is of equivocal emergency usefulness (Anaesth Intensive Care 1998;26:387; Anaesthesia 1996;51:389).

Orotracheal Intubation: This tube is placed through the mouth and into the trachea. Peds tubes are uncuffed and can be sized using the pt's little finger, or consulting a Broselow-Hinkle tape. Adult tubes are typically in the 7-8 range (internal diameter in millimeters), have an inflatable cuff. "Cricoid" pressure from an assistant helps (BURP—manipulate the thyroid cartilage in a Back or posterior, Up, and Rightward Pressure), and this is commonly known as the Sellick maneuver (Anaesthesist 1998;47:45). Confirmation of placement with checking for breath sounds over anterior lung fields and lack of sounds over stomach, CXR is confirmatory. Not uncommon to have right mainstem intubation, and simply withdraw the tube 2-4 cm. Caution in the prehospital realm with unrecognized misplacement [as high as 12% (Acad Emerg Med 2003;10:961), so perhaps two confirmatory maneuvers.

Nasotracheal Intubation: This can be done in a conscious adult pt, and the same caveats with NPA in re: facial trauma. The pt must have spontaneous respirations because listening and feeling for breath sounds at the end of the tube is the mechanism for guiding the tube into the trachea (J Emerg Med 1999;17:791). Lubricate the tip of the tube, insert through largest nare passage, and follow the breath sounds, with gentle back and forth rotation of the tube to facilitate placement. Application of oxymetazoline HCl 0.05% (Afrin) nasal spray and/or nebulzing 5 cc of 2% lidocaine with epinephrine prior to procedure may decrease nasal bleeding and pain. Advancing during early inspiration is the timing most important to pass through the vocal cords. May be facilitated with digital intubation guidance (J Emerg Med 1989;7:275). Possibly the right procedure for angioedema not adequately managed with NPA.

Digital Intubation: A deeply comatose pt with obscure landmarks may be digitally intubated (J Emerg Med 1984;1:317). Place two fingers of non-dominant hand past the tongue and behind the epiglottis. Pass the tube down along the hand and use the two fingers at the epiglottis to guide the tube into the trachea. Not uncommon to have left mainstem intubation (Am J Emerg Med 1994;12:466). Beck airway air flow monitor (BAAM) may be helpful with these type of intubations, produces a whistle noise that intensifies with placement into trachea (Prehosp Disaster Med 1993;8:357).

Rapid Sequence Intubation (Ann EM 1993;22:1008): A protocol for allowing paralysis of a pt who is difficult to intubate, secondary to jaw clenching such as seen in those with head injury or seizures. Different protocols exist with all meds iv. Use of this sequence necessitates knowledge of these drugs, and learning about preanesthesia.

Pt assessment is key with a standardized approach for airway dynamics—eg, Mallapati or more complete LEMON approach (*L*ook, *E*valuate, *M*allapati, *O*bstruction, *N*eck mobility).

Typically, pain and amnestic modulation can occur with a narcotic and a sedative (including barbiturates and benzodiazepines).

Premedicate: Use lidocaine in those with head injuries or eye injuries, atropine in children or in those with bradycardia, a narcotic for pain control and to block the sympathetic response, and a barbiturate, sedative, or benzodiazepine for amnesia. Special case for ketamine in those with status asthmaticus, but avoid in those with head injury (increases ICP).

- Lidocaine 1.5-3 mg/kg to blunt reflex ICP/intraocular pressure increases from initiating gag reflex with laryngoscope blade. This is equivocal at best—(Brit J Ophthalm 1987;71:546) vs (Anesth Analg 1986;65:1037; J Clin Anesth 1990;2:81). This potentiation of the hemodynamic effects associated with laryngoscopy can be blunted with viscous or aerosolized lidocaine directly on posterior tongue, as well (Anesth Analg 1986; 65:389; 1977:618, Acta Anaesthesiol Scand 1982;26:599, 1977;56:618).
- Atropine 0.01 mg/kg (0.1 mg minimum) for all children to block the reflex bradycardia. Wait 3-5 min, and then give muscle relaxants.
- Barbiturate: thiopental 1-5 mg/kg.
- Benzodiazepine: midazolam 0.1-0.2 mg/kg or lorazepam 0.02-0.04 mg/kg or Diazepam 0.1-0.2 mg/kg.
- Narcotic: morphine 0.1-0.2 mg/kg or fentanyl 2-10 μg/kg or alfentanyl 10-20 μg/kg.
- Propofol: 2-3 mg/kg.
- Etomidate 0.2-0.3 mg/kg.
- Ketamine 2-4 mg/kg. Do not use in those with head injuries (increased intracranial pressure), HT, penetrating eye injuries, or glaucoma.

Paralytic:
- Succinylcholine (depolarizing agent): 1.5 mg/kg, and should be used with caution in those with massive muscle trauma or other reasons for hyperkalemia, those with increased intraocular pressure, and in those with brain tumors giving an increased ICP—may be used as sole paralytic agent (Ann EM 1992;21:929).
- Vecuronium: (non-depolarizing agent) 0.01 mg/kg priming dose followed by 0.1- 0.2 mg/kg paralyzing dose. No vagolytic effect or histamine release.

PROCEDURES

- Atracurium: (non-depolarizing agent) 0.3 mg/kg (5 mg in normal adults) for penetrating injury into cavity such as eye or peritoneum. Not for pt < 5 yr of age.
- Rocuronium: (non-depolarizing agent) 0.6-1 mg/kg.
- Pancuronium (non-depolarizing agent): 0.01 mg/kg priming dose, followed by 0.1- 0.2 mg/kg paralyzing dose.

Once the muscle relaxant has been given, the Sellick maneuver must be employed and held until the airway is controlled to avoid regurgitation (BURP—backward, upward, rightward pressure)—as well as the usual monitors for heart rate, blood pressure, and O_2 saturation; also consider end-tidal CO_2 monitor. Working with the hospital anesthesia department can help provide protocols for individual ERs. This is safe in those with unknown or undiagnosed cervical spine injury in trained and facile practitioners with no worse neurologic outcomes secondary to intubation found in this series (EMJ 2004;21:302).

Gum Elastic Bougie: A 2-3 ft length of Teflon that facilitates intubation in those with anatomy that makes it difficult to visualize the vocal cords (Anaesthesia 1992;47:878), or if pt with C-spine immobilization (Anaesthesia 1993;48:630). This performs better than using a stylet (Anaesthesia 1996;51:935). The end of this Teflon rod has a slight bend to it, and snaking this past the epiglottitis and toward the larynx should place this rod within the trachea—moving the rod back and forth and feeling slight bumps (tracheal rings) is a pos sign whereas complete smoothness probably denotes esophageal intubation. Leave the rod in place, and pass an endotracheal tube over this. Passage of the ET tube over the bougie is facilitated by leaving the laryngoscope in place and rotating the bougie so that the bevel is facing vertically once it is sitting in the trachea (Anaesthesia 1990;45:774). Also, if trouble threading ET tube over Bougie, then try a smaller tube (eg, 7-0 instead of 8-0).

Retrograde Intubation: A time-consuming technique (Crit Care Med 1986;14:589) (not for the apneic pt) that relies on identification of the cricothyroid membrane, passing a needle through this membrane followed by a J-wire through the needle and the J-wire passed into the oral cavity. Put the J-wire into the distal side port of the ET tube (the Murphy eye) and then out through the proximal opening (ie, opening of ET tube out of body) (Anesth Analg 1974;53:1013). Keep the J-wire taut at this point. Pass the tube until it can no longer go forward; cut the wire where it enters the neck; pull the wire; and pass the tube into its final position. This is not as necessary now with the advent of the bougie, tube changer, lighted stylet, and, of course, broncho-scopic intubation. Some pre-packaged kits are available that use a catheter over the wire, with the ET tube passed over the catheter.

Translaryngeal Insufflation: Demand valve or oxygen wall units that can deliver 50 psi of pressure may be used in this set-up. The cricothyroid membrane should be punctured with a 14-G needle, and the plastic catheter advanced toward the carina after removal of the needle. Insufflate for 1-2 sec, and allow chest relaxation for 4-5 sec. The plastic catheter commonly bends and occludes.

Cricothyrotomy: This is a rapid surgical airway that is indicated in those with significant facial/oral trauma where endotracheal intubation is not possible or in those with complete airway obstruction. After the cricothyroid membrane is identified, make a vertical 4 cm inci-sion centered on the membrane, and make a horizontal incision through the membrane itself. Pass a hemostat or dilator [such as the Trousseau (J Emerg Med 1999;17:433)] through the mem-brane, and then a #4 Shiley tracheostomy tube or a #5 ET tube. Be sure that the tube is not positioned in the anterior medi-astinum. Sew this in place. Placement with a guidewire following the Seldinger technique is also available with similar operator profiles (ie, similar time of and complications of procedure) (J Emerg Med 1999;17:957; Anesthesiology 2000;92:687).

Esophageal Detector Devices: A device used to ensure correct tube placement (non-esophageal). Two examples are the Esophageal Detector Device (Tube Check) or the "turkey baster," and the end-tidal CO_2 detector. The bulb is squeezed and then placed on the end of the ET tube—if it quickly inflates (< 5 sec), then it is a tracheal intubation. If it slowly re-inflates (> 5 sec), then it is a presumed esophageal intubation; this device is not reliable in cold environments (the plastic gets too stiff) and the reinflation may cause a distal mucus plug to lodge in the ET tube (Ann EM 2004;43:626). The CO_2 monitor is placed in-line with the BVM and is situated between the ET tube and the BVM. The litmus paper inside the plastic housing turns yellow with CO_2 and this is good; stays purple without CO_2 and this is bad. Has been validated in those > 20 kg (Ann EM 2003;41:623).

Fiberoptic Devices: Passage of an ET tube can be facilitated with a bronchoscope, or a fiberoptic laryngoscope if it is the only device available (Lab Anim 2000;34:199). Place the tube over the scope to begin with, advance the scope into the larynx/trachea, and then advance the tube. This may be particularly useful in burn pts with evidence of facial burns. Also may be preferable in those with C-spine immobilization (Anesthesiology 1999;91:1253). If abnormalities on facial, oral, or neck exam are noted, early elective intubation is usually advocated, and this can be quickly done if the tube is in position over the bronchoscope. A fiberoptic stylet is also available, which functions similar to a gum elastic bougie with an eyepiece (Anesth Analg 1999;89:526).

20.2 Procedural (Conscious) Sedation

Curr Opin Peds 1995;7:309; Nejm 2000;342:938

Many situations abound in medicine where pts feel uncomfortable or cannot tolerate procedures that need to be done. For example, suture repair in pediatrics, I + D of abscess (Arch

Otolaryngol Head Neck Surg 1999;125:1197), chest tube placement, central line placement, foreign body removal, lumbar puncture, or perhaps CT or MRI exam. Large doses of medications with a combination of analgesics and sedatives can be used to provide pain control, anxiolysis, and amnesia. When we impair a pt's reflexes and mentation has been impaired, then procedural sedation has been induced.

At least in pediatrics and young adults, lack of preprocedural fasting did not increase (was not associated) the risk of adverse events (Ann EM 2004;44:454; 2003;42:636).

A variety of medications are available to help in these situations, and learning to use them should be done with direct preceptorship. Intravenous dosing is more effective for titrating to effect.

When using these drugs as procedural sedation, one is doing more than simple pain control or anxiolysis. Continuous cardiac monitoring, O_2 saturations, and blood pressures should be employed (Ann EM 1992;21:551); end-tidal CO_2 monitoring via divided nasal cannula may herald respiratory depression earlier than other measures (Ped Emerg Care 1997;13:189).

As well, many of the following medications can be used for RSI and when dosing for RSI, we may speak of the induction dose.

Opiates: The opiates for pain control include Fentanyl at 0.5-1 μg/kg and MSO_4 at 0.05-0.1 mg/kg. These work best iv, morphine may be given im, and fentanyl has a lollipop (Ann EM 1994; 24:1059).

Benzodiazepines: The benzodiazepines include midazolam at 0.05-0.07 mg/kg im, which may be helpful with ketamine im (equivocal); midazolam 0.01-0.03 mg/kg iv (Ann EM 1993;22:201) or perhaps up to 0.1 mg/kg iv; and lorazepam at 0.01-0.02 mg/kg iv.

Barbiturates: The barbiturates include thiopental at 3-5 mg/kg iv and 25 mg/kg pr, and iv use is an effective induction agent for RSI. Methohexital at 25 mg/kg pr is also useful (Am J Roentgenol 1993;160:577).

Chloral Hydrate: Chloral hydrate is 25-50 mg/kg either po or pr, and has found a niche in radiology studies (Am J Roentgenol 1995; 165:905).

Ketamine (Ann EM 2004;44:460): Ketamine is 1-2 mg/kg iv and 3-5 mg/kg im (Acad Emerg Med 1999;6:21). Medication of choice for RSI in asthma, and may be of some use combining with midazolam 0.05-0.07 mg/kg im and atropine 0.02 mg/kg im to prevent emergence reactions and hypersalivation, respectively. Midazolam controversial (Ann EM 2000;35:229 vs. Ann EM 2000;36:579), and many do not use midazolam routinely. All three (ketamine, midazolam, atropine) can be combined in the same syringe for im use in peds, and no iv is necessary using this protocol (Ann EM 1998;31:688).

Nitrous oxide: Nitrous oxide is a 50% nitrous oxide/50% oxygen mixture that is a "self-use" system (Acad Emerg Med 1998; 5:112), and remember that nitrous oxide causes bowel edema. Efficacy is equivocal (Ped Dent 2000;22:125).

Etomidate: Etomidate is an imidazole that is useful for procedural sedation at 0.1 mg/kg (Ann EM 2002;39:592), and for induction at 0.3 mg/kg iv (J Emerg Med 2000;18:13; Ped Emerg Care 2000;16:18) with favorable results with the usual caveat of more attention to respiratory depression in the elderly.

Propofol: Propofol is 0.5-2 mg/kg iv bolus, followed by 25-125 μg/kg/min infusion. This may be useful for procedural sedation, RSI and then to ICU pts (Acad Emerg Med 1999;6:975) and is safe in children for procedural sedation—one option is to bolus 2.5 mg/kg with a 200 μg/kg/min maintenance (Crit Care Med 2002;30:1231).

Reversal of medications may "wake" patients faster, but does not shorten time to discharge post-procedure [eg, flumazenil for benzodiazepines (Acad Emerg Med 1997;4:944)]—advocate for letting patients "lighten" on their own.

20.3 Intraosseus Technique

J Crit Illn 1993;8:539

An effective access technique in all pts. In children < 5 years of age or in those with significant osteoporosis or non-use of lower extremity, the site of insertion is the flat anterior portion of the proximal tibia. Clean with iodine, local lidocaine anesthesia if available, and place needle by puncturing skin, and then screwing into place. Angle of insertion is perpendicular to the long axis of the tibia. When "pop" is felt, aspirate marrow to confirm placement, and secure in place by screwing plate to skin surface (IO needle) and/or taping into place. In an IO needle, the center tap is removed by unscrewing the top of the needle, and the iv line is placed into the exposed receptacle.

In older children or adults, use the same sterile technique but use a site specific device such as a sternal or tibial device that provides the energy for line placement.

20.4 Nasogastric Tube

Passage of a tube into the stomach via the nasal passage. In an intubated pt, may elect for an orogastic tube. Keys to success for passing a nasogastric tube are lubrication; neck flexed, if possible; and local anesthetic. In an awake pt, consider 5 cc of 2% lidocaine or 4 cc of 10% solution (Ann EM 2004;44:131) nebulized as a pretreatment to facilitate tube passage.

20.5 Pediatric Bladder Catheterization

Suprapubic tap is less efficient than urethral catheterization, with no benefit as far as risk (Ann EM 1994;23:225). Additionally, suprapubic tap less likely to succeed if bladder is not full. Thus, the suprapubic tap is not advocated.

20.6 Ventricular Shunt Management

Malfunction or secondary infection are possible with indwelling shunts, and ventriculoperitoneal shunts are the most common today.

Malfunction is most common with proximal occlusion, and secondarily distal occlusion. The bladder(s) of the shunt can be palpated subcutaneously over the skull. If one bladder system, inability to easily compress it is consistent with distal obstruction, and slow filling (>2 seconds) is consistent with proximal obstruction. If two bladders, compress the proximal one first, and inability to easily compress the second bladder is consistent with distal obstruction; after releasing the distal bladder, lack of quick filling of the proximal bladder is consistent with proximal obstruction. Head CT may show ventricular enlargement. A shunt series is a series of plain film x-rays showing the course of the shunt.

Infection can occur at any site along the catheter, and may present as an acute abdomen or meningitis/encephalitis. If considering either of these conditions, neurosurgical consult is mandatory.

Chapter 21

Psychiatric/Substance Abuse

21.1 Chemical and Physical Restraint

This section addresses the issue of how to best help a violent and aggressive pt. The procedures surrounding chemical and physical restraint should provide a safe environment for the pt and the staff (HEC Forum 1998;10:244).

Initial physical restraints may include wrist and ankle restraints to a stretcher/bed (J Nurs Adm 1998;28:19). If the pt does not respond to this immobilization, it may be necessary to secure the chest, pelvis, and be sure that the gurney is anchored to the floor. If the pt is spitting or biting, a mask may need to be positioned, and someone should be available at all times to remove the mask, if a patent airway becomes an issue.

Chemical restraints are medications used to modify and subdue a pt's behavior so that the pt is not a danger to him/herself or staff. This will also allow for a medical evaluation. Some options that are initially dosed via the im route are midazolam 5 mg—this is perhaps the best (Acad Emerg Med 2004;11:744), haloperidol 5 mg, droperidol 2.5-5 mg (Ann EM 1992;21:407), diphenhydramine 25-50 mg, lorazepam 2 mg, olanzapine 2.5-10 mg im (Can J Psychiatry 2003;48:716; Arch Gen Psychiatry 2002;59:441; J Clin Psychopharmacol 2001;21:389; Am J Psych 2001;158:1149), or perphenazine (Trilafon) (Curr Ther Res Clin Exp 1972;14:478). Use with caution in the elderly and may want to use lower doses—if using for delirium, these medications may change the exam.

Once chemical restraints begin to work, physical restraints can be modified and eventually eliminated. Frequent reassessment and rx of underlying medical issues may help release pts from physical restraints in a timely manner.

21.2 Delirium

Am J Psych 1999;156:1; Geriatrics 1999;54:28, 36, 39; Dement Geriatr Cogn Disord 1999;10:310

Cause: Drugs (Intoxication discussed in next section); intracranial lesion or process, such as encephalitis, meningitis, amyloid or primary neoplasm or metastatic disease; systemic diseases such as infections (syphilis) or autoimmune phenomenons; ethanol or sedative withdrawal; drug abuse—eg, ecstasy (J Psychoactive Drugs 1999;31:167); metabolic, such as hyperammonemia, sodium disorders, hypoglycemia, etc; seizures.

Epidem: High incidence in elderly, with 15% developing this after general surgery; higher rate noted in those with dementia.

Pathophys: Dependent on process, but overall leading to CNS dysfunction (Dement Geriatr Cogn Disord 1999;10:330). Increased serum anticholinergic activity in the elderly (J Gerontol A Biol Sci Med Sci 1999;54:M12) and elevated serotonergic activity in general (Dement Geriatr Cogn Disord 1999;10:339).

Sx: Hallucinations, often visual but also auditory.

Si: Acute onset and fluctuating course; transient global disorder of cognition and attention. Inattention, loss of attention span is most prominent deficit; test by serial 7's; serial digits up to 7, such as phone numbers; spell "world" backwards; disorganized thinking or altered level of consciousness; may also "sundown"—exacerbated at night (Dement Geriatr Cogn Disord 1999;10:353).

Crs: Variable depending on underlying illnesses and cause. Prognosis/course may be guided by the Delirium Rating Scale (Psychosomatics 1999;40:193), which is a tool applied over time (eg, 24 hr).

Cmplc: Inherent with cause.

Diff Dx: Psychoses are not global; consider total global amnesia in pt who recovers in 1 d.

Lab: Directed by exam and past medical history. Consider metabolic (p221), intoxication (p411, p449), infectious (p185) and CNS (Neurology p249) work-up.

Emergency Management:
- Consider 1:1 staffing to watch pt.
- Consider medication to help calm pt—Chemical Restraints p 409.
- Medical evaluation as above, with medicine consult for admission.

21.3 Intoxication, Abuse, and Withdrawal

Nejm 2003;348:1786

Cause: Ingestion, inhalation, injection or dermal absorption of substance that alters brain function (J Emerg Med 1999;17:679).

Epidem: Unknown, but drug intoxication linked to trauma (Jama 1997;277:1769).

Pathophys: Per substrate.

Sx: Hallucinations, often visual but also auditory (may be seen in withdrawal, too).

Si: Variable, from acute onset to fluctuating course; transient global disorder of cognition and attention. Inattention, loss of attention span is most prominent deficit; disorganized thinking or altered level of consciousness anywhere from agitation to coma.

Crs: Variable depending on underlying illnesses and cause.

Cmplc: Inherent with cause.

Diff Dx: If febrile, consider CNS infection (meningitis, encephalitis) or NMS; hypoglycemia; head trauma or other CNS pathology.

Lab: Rectal temperature with hypothermia thermometer if low; CBC with diff; glucoscan; metabolic profile with Ca and Mg levels; liver profile; acetaminophen level; salicylate level; ethanol level, especially in all trauma pts (J Trauma 1999;47:1131, 1139); measured vs calculated osmoles; methanol, ethylene glycol or isopropyl alcohol level, if suspicion by hx or if metabolic acidosis without other cause; serum levels of specific drugs based on hx, clinical exam, metabolic abnormalities, EKG, or positive indicator found on urine drug screen if necessary (Brit J Clin Pharmacol 1999;48:278).

UA; urine toxic drug screen—this is not infallible, such as quinolones converting the opiate test to a false pos (Jama 2001;286:3115); Wood's lamp evaluation of urine to assess for ethylene glycol; the use of marijuana is rising in young black men and women, young Hispanic men, and remains high in young white men and women (Jama 2004;291:2114).

- *X-ray:* Consider head CT without contrast to check for bleed.

Emergency Management:
- Airway; intubate, if necessary.
- Staffing with 1:1 watch, if needed.
- Iv access, with fluid resuscitation, if needed.
- Consider D50, naloxone; give thiamine 100 mg iv.
- Physical/chemical restraint, as needed.

Alcohol:
- Ethanol withdrawal may be treated with iv lorazepam 2 mg, or other benzodiazepine or chlordiazepoxide (Librium) orally, if able. Treat tremors, HT, and tachycardia to avoid delirium

tremens. Seizure rx, as on p284. No effect on clearance with iv NS (J Emerg Med 1999;17:1) or coffee.

- Methanol intoxication (Med Toxicol 1986;1:309) may lead to blindness (Arch Ophthalm 1999;117:286) and other complications with ingestions as low as 15 cc of a 40% solution. Rx is with iv $NaHCO_3$ to maintain normal pH and ethanol (Am J Kidney Dis 1987;9:441) to maintain level > 100 mg/dL. Institute rx if methanol suspected; do not wait for the serum level to return (intoxication usually with level > 20 mg/dL). Iv Ethanol is 10% Ethanol in D_5W—bolus 10 cc/kg, then 1.6 cc/kg per hr infusion. Also give folate 50 mg iv q 4 hr. Hemodialysis for those with CNS dysfunction, visual complaints or methanol level > 50 mg/dL. Do not withhold ethanol rx pending dialysis (Nejm 2001;344:424). 4-methylpyrazole (Fomepizole) may substitute for ethanol rx at 15 mg/kg load, then 10 mg/kg every 12 hr iv for a total of 4 doses. (J Toxicol Clin Toxicol 1999;37:777; Intensive Care Med 1999;25:528) and N-acetylcysteine (Drug Alcohol Depend 1999;57:61) may be of some use.
- Isopropranolol intoxication should be treated with supportive therapy; consider iv $NaHCO_3$ if acidosis with hypotension, and dialysis for pts who are hemodynamically unstable, have significant CNS or respiratory depression or if serum level is > 400 mg/dL.

Cocaine Intoxication:

- Use iv benzodiazepines to treat tremors, anxiety, and vasospasm. Vasospasm of coronary arteries and intracerebral arteries may cause acute coronary syndrome and acute stroke syndrome, respectively.
- Treat hyperthermia with cool mist and cooling blanket, usually no benefit with acetaminophen, avoid ASA.
- Seizure rx on p284, use phenobarbital before dilantin in these cases.

- Acute coronary syndrome rx should be ASA, TNG, benzodi-azepines, and narcotics. Avoid β-blockers (α activity would then be unopposed) and thrombolytics may be useful although probably vasospastic and possible secondary thrombotic etiology.
- HT crisis with iv benzodiazepines and nitroprusside—not labetalol.
- Mules (cocaine transporters who have swallowed packaged condoms) who have no signs of toxicity should be given oral charcoal and Golytely. If symptomatic, general surgery referral for package removal—not endoscopy.
- Chest pain—if an individual has chest pain and is placed at low to moderate risk for cardiac injury, perhaps a 9-12 hr observation, and then OK to discharge to home as long as no ischemic findings, such as neg markers, normal EKG (including no arrhythmias), and no further chest pain (Nejm 2003;348:510).

Narcotic Abuse:
- Reversible with naloxone 0.1 mg/kg, up to 2 mg iv. Use higher doses in those with propoxyphene (Darvon), pentazocine (Talwin), and methadone intoxication.
- Short half-life of naloxone may necessitate repeated dosing or drip—0.4 mg/hr titrated to effect.

21.4 Medical Screening Exam

Acad Emerg Med 1997;4:124; Nejm 2004;351:476

This is a term applied to those who come to the ER with psychiatric issues, but first need a medical evaluation. Even those pts with an emotional or stressful nidus accounting for increased psychiatric lability or somatization may have a significant medical condition that needs attention.

If a pt has had a medical evaluation previously, and no presenting symptoms have changed, further laboratory evaluation may not be necessary in the setting of a stable physical exam.

If a pt has not been previously evaluated or has an abnormal exam, then further medical evaluation may be necessary.

Intoxicants can also lead to coping or behavioral problems, and these may need to be screened, as well. Indiscriminate and universal toxicology screening is not supported by the literature (Am J Emerg Med 1984;2:331; J Emerg Med 2000;18:173). On the other hand, those with intentional overdose or any ingestion with suicidal overtones should be screened for both salicyclates and acetaminophen (Am J Emerg Med 1996;14:443) (see Delirium in previous section). Occult infections, metabolic abnormalities, or CNS lesions are more common in the elderly presenting for the first time for psychiatric evaluation. The value of random thyroid function testing (TSH) is equivocal in the young and more helpful in the elderly.

The most important part of the exam is the mental status and neurologic exam.

In psychiatric cases that are not clear cut, disposition can be difficult. No historical data (suicidality, homicidality, hallucinations) in a pt's evaluation or screening tool exists that helps us decide who needs emergent hospitalization, and who will benefit from other type of disposition. Many of the assessment issues must also balance social needs.

Chapter 22

Pulmonary

22.1 Aspirated Foreign Body

Ann Surg 1972;175:720

Cause: Usually accidental, may be anything that can be inhaled, such as small pieces of toys, coins, candy, and peanuts.

Epidem: Common in infants.

Pathophys: Inhalation of object in mouth or nose with lodging in larynx or bronchopulmonary tree.

Sx: Dyspnea; stridor; hemoptysis.

Si: Wheezing; tachypnea; decreased lung sounds in one lobe.

Crs: Benign if not obstructing entire airway/lung, and able to be retrieved with a bronchoscope.

Cmplc: Asphyxia; pneumothorax; pneumonia; pulmonary edema (Ped Emerg Care 1986;2:235).

Diff Dx: Asthma, croup, pneumonia.

Lab: X-Ray—CXR with expiratory film if radiolucent foreign body to look for area that does not symmetrically compress. If unable to locate foreign body, do lateral neck x-ray and abdominal x-ray to locate the foreign body (Radiol Clin N Am 1998;36: 175).

Emergency Management:
- O_2 if hypoxic, keep pt calm.
- Iv access.

- ENT or pulmonary consult immediately if in trachea, mainstem bronchus or beyond (Endoscopy 1977;9:216).
- If severe respiratory distress or impending respiratory failure, consider rapid sequence intubation. Look for FB in larynx, remove with Magill forceps, and intubate. If cannot locate the FB, intubate and try to push object down one mainstem to oxygenate and ventilate the contralateral lung.

22.2 Asthma

Ann IM 2000;132:219; Nejm 2001;344:350

Cause: Innumerable allergens, with genetic susceptibility— Chromosome 5—, and is also found more often in those with atopy susceptibility.

Epidem: Approximately 5% of U.S. population and increasing; seen more in low income groups; common in those with first and second hand smoke.

Pathophys: Airway inflammation with decreased airway lumen size, bronchial edema, and increased mucus production. Inflammatory airway secretions with eosinophils, but neutrophils predominate (Am J Respir Crit Care Med 2000;161:1185), and mast cell infiltration of airway smooth muscle (Nejm 2002;346:1699). Also, hypothesized that the effect of glucocorticoids mediated by a glucocorticoid receptor and the C/EBPα binding protein in bronchial smooth muscles—those with glucocorticoid resistant disease may lack C/EBPα (Nejm 2004;351:560). Multiple types including allergic; exercise-induced; infectious—approximately 25% of those with bronchiolitis go on to asthma, bronchiectasis, chronic bronchitis, and eventually some form of COPD; and emotional stress.

Morning wheezing due to circadian decrease in epinephrine and steroids. ASA sensitivity is a direct action on kinin receptors by acetyl groups, may be genetic as well. Food sulfites may precipitate an exacerbation, as may exposure to cigarette smoke.

Sx: Dyspnea; wheezing; exercise or cold induction of symptoms; opiate or ASA exacerbation induction.

Si: Wheezing, check with exertion or cough, if lung exam is normal at rest; dyspnea; nasal polyps correlates with atopic type; cyanosis, papilledema, pulsus paradoxus are three late signs.

Crs: Overall mortality has not increased.

Cmplc: Status asthmaticus—respiratory arrest with respiratory acidosis as most common mode of death (not arrhythmia); multifocal atrial tachycardia (Chest 1990;98:672) associated with hypoxia, theophylline, and catechol treatment; allergic asthma in mother associated with premature labor and respiratory distress syndrome of the newborn. Minor complication of mild hypokalemia in those with β-agonist therapy (Ped Pulmonol 1999;27:27).

Diff Dx: Aspirated FB in the young and elderly; croup; CHF in the elderly and peds with heart disease; vocal cord dysfunction; conversion reaction; pulmonary emboli, rarely.

Lab: If toxic or severe case—CBC with diff; ABG; blood cultures and sputum sample.

Peak flows poor predictor of severity in the ER (Am J Respir Crit Care Med 1996;154:889), length of speaking time just as useful (Am J Emerg Med 1998;16:572).

- *X-ray:* Chest film if severe, febrile, or not following classic asthma pathway.

Emergency Management:

Med Lett Drugs Ther 2000;42:19

- O_2, if hypoxic.
- Control airway, rapid sequence intubation if pt losing consciousness or in 1 word or less dyspnea and not responding—safer to do earlier rather than later, ie, do not wait for pt to have cardiopulmonary arrest (Crit Care Med 1993;21:1727).

When intubated, permissive hypercapnia (underventilating) is safe and appropriate (Chest 1994;105:891).

- β-agonists—nebulized albuterol at 0.1-0.15 mg/kg up to 5 mg/dose if > 40 lbs, may select as continuous at 10 mg/hr, all suspended in NS; terbutaline (Brethine) 1 cc in 2 cc of NS; or bitolterol (Tornalate)—all probably equally effective. Inhaler with spacer as effective as nebulizers, if able to use effectively (J Peds 2000;136:497) and 5 puffs every 20 min in adult (Chest 2002;121:1036)—10 puffs equivalent to unit dose of albuterol nebulizer.

- Ipratropium (Atrovent) is not approved for long-term maintenance (Nejm 1992;327:1413) but the literature supports acute use to decrease hospitalization in children with asthma (Nejm 1998;339:1030); consider dosing with albuterol at 0.5 cc in nebulized solution (Duoneb) for those with severe exacerbations or not responding to β-agonists, definitely not a chronic rx choice (Plotnick, L. H. and F. M. Ducharme (2000). "Combined inhaled anticholinergic agents and beta-2-agonists for initial treatment of acute asthma in children." Cochrane Database Syst Rev 2).

- Steroids—Hydrocortisone (100-300 mg every 6 hr), dexamethasone (4-8 mg every 8 hr), methylprednisolone (1-1.5 mg/kg iv every 12 hr) and prednisone (1-2 mg/kg qd) all equal at appropriate doses and give in ER; route of administration does not matter as far as onset of action or efficacy (6-8 hr or longer for onset of action). Outpatient rx should include a short course of steroids which may be extended depending on patient history (Rowe, B. H., C. H. Spooner, et al. (2000). "Corticosteroids for preventing relapse following acute exacerbations of asthma." Cochrane Database Syst Rev 2). Consider inhaled steroids such as triamcinolone or budesonide, and perhaps some benefit in combining oral and inhaled steroids (Jama 1999;281:2119).

- MgSO$_4$ 2 gm iv or nebulized (2.5-3 cc isotonic) (Am J Med 2000;108:193) may help in severe cases (Rowe, B. H., J. A. Bretzlaff, et al. (2000). "Magnesium sulfate for treating exacerbations of acute asthma in the emergency department." Cochrane Database Syst Rev 2), but not suggested for routine use in any pts, especially peds (Ann EM 2000;36:572).
- Aminophylline may be considered in severe cases, load at 5.6 mg/kg over 20-30 min, then 0.5 mg/kg/hr; decrease dose in those with CHF, liver disease, pneumonia, or h/o cardiac dysrhythmia.
- Consider Heliox (60-80% helium), probably better in sick pts (Chest 1999;116:296) vs (Am J Emerg Med 2000;18:495). Albuterol nebulized with Heliox 80:20 had better spirometry after 3 treatments when compared with albuterol nebulized with air (Am J Respir Crit Care Med 2002;165:1317).
- IVF important in severe cases, will need NaCl and KCl to reverse chloride depletion, be wary of pulmonary edema—ie, avoid fluid overload!
- Antibiotics if bacterial focus or severe: Consider TMP/SMX DS 1 pill bid or see options under CAP (p425)—caution with those on theophylline.
- May consider NaHCO$_3$ for severe acidosis if intubated, but do not overcorrect.
- Internal medicine/primary care ER consult for those needing admission, outpatient follow-up with steroid taper for those with good response to rx—peak flows ideally > 80% predicted. As well, intervention in pediatric pts with home intervention on allergens and tobacco smoke will decrease morbidity (Nejm 2004;351:1068).
- Salmeterol (Serevent), montelukast (Singulair), zafirlukast (Accolate), zileuton (Zyflo), cromolyn (Intal), nedocromil (Tilade) and the decision for outpatient theophylline (Slo-bid,

Theodur) should be part of the outpatient physician's realm or perhaps to help get pt off of ventilator.

- Heparin is anti-inflammatory, its exact role in asthma has not been elucidated (Ann Pharmacother 2001;35:1161).
- The role of 40 mg of nebulized furosemide to be determined, and one study claims a modest success (J Asthma 1998;35:89).

22.3 Community-Acquired Pneumonia (CAP)

Nejm 2002;346:429; Ped Infect Dis J 2000;19:251; Allergy Asthma Proc 2000;21:33; J Am Ger Soc 2000;48:82

Cause: (By age)

Ped Infect Dis J 2000;19:293

0-28 d: *E. coli,* group B streptococcus; less commonly *Staphylococcus aureus,* RSV, *Enterobacter* spp.

28 d to 5 yr: RSV, rhinovirus, *Streptococcal Pneumoniae,* parainfluenza virus, adenovirus; less commonly *Chlamydia.*

5 to 15 yr: *Streptococcal pneumoniae,* Influenza A, adenovirus; less commonly *Mycoplasma.*

Adults: *Streptococcal pneumoniae, Haemophilus influenzae* (more common in smokers), Atypicals (more common in young adults), including Mycoplasma and *Chlamydia;* less commonly aspiration (unless good history for such), *S. aureus,* Gram negatives, and *Legionella.*

Epidem: Much more common in immunosuppressed individuals who constitute 60% of hospital admissions for pneumonia; worse prognosis in the elderly if elevated BUN, hypotensive or respiratory rate > 30 breaths per min; incidence of 1.62:1000 population with males > females (Eur Respir J 2000;15:757). *Acinetobacter* in foundry workers (Ann IM 1981;95:688). Increased risk of acquiring CAP for those on gastric acid suppressing medications, and this is a dose-dependent phenomenon for those on PPI's (but not H_2-blockers) (Jama 2004;292:1955).

Pathophys: Most likely either inoculation from airborne respiratory droplets, or part of systemic problem with hematogenous spread, or aspiration (look to the hx).

Sx: Cough, fever, dyspnea, sputum production, pleurisy, altered mental status in the elderly.

Si: Fever > 101°F, rales (80%), consolidation changes (30%), dullness, increased tactile fremitus, whispered pectoriloquoy, "E" to "A" changes (egophony), vesicles on tympanic membrane (bullous myringitis).

Crs: Poor prognostic factors (see Table 22.1) include age > 65 yr, T < 37°C, mental confusion, tachypnea, elevated BUN, hyponatremia, pleural effusion (Thorax 2000;55:219); or if nursing home-acquired (Chest 2000;117:1378).

Table 22.1   Patient Outcomes Research Team Score

The patient's age (subtract 10 if female)	
Nursing home resident	_____ (+10)
Coexisting	_____
Neoplastic Disease	(+30)
Liver Disease	_____ (+20)
CHF	_____ (+10)
CVA	_____ (+10)
Renal Disease	_____ (+10)
Physical exam findings	_____
Altered mental status	(+20)
Resp rate > 30 breaths/min	_____ (+20)
Systolic BP < 90 mm Hg	_____ (+20)
T < 35 or ≥ 40°C	_____ (+15)
Pulse ≥ 125 bpm	_____ (+10)
	_____

Table 22.1   continued

Laboratory
    Arterial pH < 7.35   _____ (+30)
    BUN > 30   _____ (+20)
    Na < 130   _____ (+20)
    Blood glucose > 250   _____ (+10)
    Hct < 30%   (+10)
    PaO_2 < 60 mm Hg   _____ (+10)
    Pleural effusion   _____ (+10)
Total (calculate the sum and find the appropriate class):   _____
Class I: Mortality < 0.1%
    Age < 50 years; No significant co-morbid disease; Vital signs normal or nearly
    normal; Normal mental status
Class II: Mortality approximately 0.6%
    PORT Score of 70 points or less
Class III: Mortality approximately 2.8%
    PORT Score of 71–90 points
Class IV: Mortality approximately 8.2%
    PORT Score of 91–130 points
Class V: Mortality approximately 29.2%
    PORT Score of > 130 points

(Nejm 1997; 336:243)

Cmplc: Lung abscess; sepsis; atypical types may go onto hemolytic anemia with cold agglutinins, myocarditis, or Guillain-Barré syndrome.

Diff Dx: Bronchitis—sputum does not differentiate bronchitis and pneumonia or automatically necessitate antibiotic use in the healthy population (J Gen Intern Med 1999;14:151; Lancet 2002;359:1648); sinusitis; influenza—prophylaxis best, rapid testing will not exclude diagnosis (Med Lett Drugs Ther 1999;41:121), and antibiotic drug therapy not useful in most.

Persistent coughs may be seen in those with TB, pertussis, aspirated FB, undiagnosed chronic lung disease, pulmonary neoplasm, PE, and postnasal drip.

Pleural effusion may be seen in CHF, cancer or other infections (TB); right-sided effusions may be sympathetic and due to gallbladder or liver disease (eg, sub-phrenic abscess, cholecystitis, amebiasis).

Lab: *If older child, adolescent, or young adult that is healthy, may consider CXR or treat empirically if not severely ill, for all others consider the following:*

CBC with diff; blood culture(s)—limited usefulness in those mild or moderately ill who are immunocompetent even if they are hospitalized (EMJ 2004;21:446; Respir Med 1999;93:208); also limited usefulness if lacking other co-morbid risk factors (HIV, malignancy, exogenous steroids, SCD, institutionalization, recent hospital stay) (Chest 1995;108:932); and rebuttal of the naysayers (Chest 1995;108:891); Serology if considering specific atypical; sputum gram stain and culture, usefulness is equivocal (Chest 2002;121:1486)—induced as good as spontaneous (Respiration 2000;67:173); UA and urine c + s for the very young and elderly, if septic; procalcitonin level elevation (> 0.1 $\mu g/L$) associated with more severe disease, and > 0.5 $\mu g/L$ associated with atypical organisms (Infection 2000;28:68); ABG if SaO_2 is low, eg, $< 92\%$.

- *X-ray:* CXR for infiltrate or other pulmonary lesion, look for pleural effusion, and do both right and left lateral decubitus films to ascertain amount/loculation—thoracentesis if moderate sized fluid pocket (parapneumonic effusion) for dx and rx.

Emergency Management:

Chemotherapy 2000;46:24

- O_2, if necessary.
- Iv access if moderately or severely ill, although ceftriaxone 1 gm iv may help all recover quicker as induction therapy. IVF

rehydration does not "bring out" infiltrates, and infiltrates will probably persist past clinical need for antibiotics.

- Inpatient: Iv 3rd generation cephalosporin (eg, ceftriaxone 1 gm iv, cefotaxime 1-2 gm iv every 8 hr) + macrolide [azithromycin 500 mg iv (Arch IM 2000;160:1294)]; consider vancomycin, if not responding to β-lactam; consider a fluoroquinolone [levofloxacin 750 mg iv, moxifloxacin 400 mg iv (Respir Med 2000;94:97), sparfloxacin (Pharmacotherapy 2000;20:461)] for β-lactam substitution and atypical coverage in adults.
- Outpatient (except for azithromycin, typical course may vary from 10-21 d): Macrolide as first choice such as azithromycin 500 mg d 1 then 250 mg qd for 4 more d, clarithromycin 500 mg bid or clarithromycin ER 1 gm po qd; doxycycline as second line treatment at 100 mg po bid. 3 to 4-wk follow-up with primary physician. Other options include the following: fluoroquinolones, such as levofloxacin 750 mg/d for 5 d (Clin Infect Dis 2003;37:752), or 500 mg/d for 10 d (check renal function if any concerns and decrease dose as appropriate); or gatifloxacin (Tequin) 400 mg once a day, moxifloxacin (Med Lett Drugs Ther 2000;42:15) (Avelox) 400 mg qd or gemifloxacin (Factive) 320 mg qd × 7 d (Med Lett Drugs Ther 2004;46:78) in the elderly, if many co-morbid problems and considering outpatient trial of rx. Critical pathway examples (Chest 2000;117:1368; Jama 2000;283:749).
- May consider telithromycin (Ketek), which is ketolide antibiotic (Med Lett Drugs Ther 2004;46:66)—derived form erythromycin. May be useful in macrolide resistant pneumococcal strains as option to fluoroquinolones, which would be dosed at 800 mg qd. It is costly and 1% of pts have blurred vision, diplopia, or difficulty focusing, which can be poorly tolerated (as well as usual antibiotic side effects).

22.4 Chronic Obstructive Pulmonary Disease

Nejm 2002;346:988

Cause: COPD is associated with bronchitis/hyperactive airways from smoking, recurrent infections; cystic fibrosis; α_1-antitrypsin deficiency (α_1-ATD), which is autosomal recessive and usually combined with smoking.

Epidem: Smoker type, onset usually 50 yr of age; M > F; increased incidence in cold, damp climates, or conversely with high levels of air pollution (Am J Epidem 1993;137:701). Seen from second-hand smoke. α_1-ATD has an approximately 5% incidence in U.S. and onset by age 45.

Pathophys: Proteases balanced by α_1-antitrypsin, with functional deficiency causing of α_1-antitrypsin causing loss of lung elasticity (too much elastase); smoke inactivates it and increases polys (which bring proteases) in lung capillaries.

Sx: Dyspnea on exertion of arms more than legs; chronic productive cough with bronchitis but not emphysema; wheezing.

Si: Barrel chest; diminished breath sounds; wheezing; PMI moves medially; forced expiratory time over trachea > 6 sec—75% sensitive and specific. The "Blue Bloater" is the pt with CHF, hypoxia, and hypercarbia. The "Pink Puffer" is the pt with weight loss, low pCO_2, moderate decrease in O_2 at rest, and possible left-sided CHF.

Crs: Pink puffer has better prognosis than Blue bloater because pulmonary HT is less. Stages of COPD per American Thoracic Society: Stage I is FEV_1 > 50% predicted, Stage II is FEV_1 36-50% predicted, and Stage III is FEV_1 < 35% predicted. This may be inferior to the BODE score, which is a composite from the body-mass index (B), obstruction of airway (O), dyspnea (D), and exercise capacity (E) in predicting death—the obstruction of airway is the FEV_1, the dyspnea is the score on the Modified Medical Research Council (MMRC) dyspnea scale, and the exercise capacity is the best of two 6-min walk tests (Nejm 2004; 350:1005).

Cmplc: Polycythemia; pulmonary HT; peptic ulcer disease; acute respiratory failure; lithium worsens disease; treat hypophosphatemia—impairs diaphragmatic contractility. ARDS outcomes (Nejm 2003;348:683).

Lab: If severe distress or toxic—CBC with diff; metabolic profile including phosphate and Mg; ABG.
- *X-ray:* CXR—air trapping, large lung fields, and narrow mediastinum are common.

Emergency Management:
- O_2; keep SaO_2 at 90-92%, if unsure about CO_2 retention.
- Consider Bi-Pap with levels 10/4 if attempting to avoid intubation, but patient still willing for intubation if this fails—this is not as effective as for those with CHF (Am J Respir Med 2003;2:343; Eur Respir J 1996;9:1240; Chest 1992;101: 385).
- β-agonists—nebulized albuterol at 0.1-0.15 mg/kg up to 5 mg/dose if > 40 lbs., may select as continuous at 10 mg/hr, all suspended in NS; terbutaline (Brethine) 1 cc in 2 cc of NS; or bitolterol (Tornalate)—all probably equally effective (Am J Med 1983;75:697). Inhaler with spacer as effective as nebulizers, if able to use effectively.
- Ipratropium (Atrovent) 0.5 cc in first neb and then every 6 hr (Respiration 1998:354).
- Steroids—Hydrocortisone (100-300 mg q 6 hr), dexamethasone (4-12 mg q 8 hr), methylprednisolone (1-1.5 mg/kg iv q 12 hr), and prednisone (1-2 mg/kg qd) all equal at appropriate doses, route of administration does not matter as far as onset of action or efficacy (Eur Respir J 2002;19:928). Not all COPD pts have equivalent response to steroid pulse, and this makes a

small difference to discharged pts from the ER (Nejm 2003;348:2618).

- Consider antibiotics: TMP/SMX DS 1 pill bid or see antibiotics for CAP p 426—will most likely help clear exacerbation sooner (Respir Med 1998;92:442).
- Aminophylline may be considered in severe cases, load at 5.6 mg/kg over 20-30 min, then 0.5 mg/kg/hr, less in those with CHF, liver disease, pneumonia, or h/o cardiac dysrhythmia.
- Blood gas and minute ventilation improvement with 2-wk treatment of medroxyprogesterone acetate 30 mg bid po and acetazolamide 250 mg bid po (Eur Respir J 2002;20:1130).
- Consider $MgSO_4$ 2 gm iv in severe cases, poor data.
- Internal medicine/primary care consult if requires hospitalization.
- Outpatient: If able to clear quickly, home with appropriate inhalers with scheduled times, prednisone taper, antibiotics, and 1-2 d follow-up with primary physician.

22.5 Massive Hemoptysis

Clin Chest Med 1994;15:147

Cause: Pulmonary vascular change (telangiectasia), TB (Radiology 1996;200:691), cancer, cystic fibrosis, trauma, massive PE, coagulation abnormalities.

Epidem: < 5% of those with hemoptysis with massive hemoptysis, but mortality in this small group ranges from 7-32%.

Pathophys: Erosion into bronchopulmonary tree; self-limited cases usually from irritation.

Sx: Coughing up blood.

Si: Look in nares, oral cavity for other source; examine skin for petechiae or ecchymoses to consider systemic coagulopathy.

Crs: Dependent on degree of bleeding; difficult to control true exsanguination.

Cmplc: Asphyxia.

Diff Dx: (minimal or limited usually)—Bronchitis; TB; mitral stenosis; nasopharyngeal, oral or gastrointestinal source; bronchiectasis.

Lab: Consider CBC with diff and PT/PTT if potential coagulopathy; get type and screen if pt exsanguinating.

- *X-ray:* CXR.

Emergency Management:
- O_2 if hypoxic, iv access, bed rest, and mild sedation for conservative rx (Arch IM 1983;143:287).
- Place in lateral decubitus position with affected side down.
- Selective mainstem intubation of unaffected side if possible, especially in trauma (J Trauma 1987;27:1123); will probably need Anesthesia consult.
- Correct coagulopathy and replace blood, if necessary.
- Pulmonary consult for emergent bronchoscopy (Chest 1989;96:473) or perhaps embolization (Arch Surg 1998; 133:862).

22.6 Pneumothorax

Cause: Trauma—either out of hospital (MVA, iv drug use) (Ann EM 1983;12:167) or iatrogenic (central lines, mechanical ventilation, emergency surgical airway) (Am J Emerg Med 1991;9:176; 1995;13:532; J Laryngol Otol 1994;108:69), bullous disease, postbiopsy via transthoracic or bronchoscopic approach (Thorax 1986;41:647).

Epidem: Spontaneous Pneumothorax (SP) incidence changing from primarily a bleb nidus to those with AIDS and non-AIDS/ non-bleb disease, which includes a host of diffuse interstitial lung diseases (Am J Surg 1992;164:528). No increase in risk of pneumothorax in those undergoing percutaneous pulmonary biopsies with h/o COPD (Chest 1994;105:1705), but is related to depth and size (small) of lesion (Radiology 1996;198:371).

Pathophys: Violation of pleural space with air trapping and expansion.

Sx: Dsypnea, chest pain.

Si: Decreased breath sounds over lung field, with perhaps "crackling" or "bubbling" heard that is louder than rales (Hamman's sign)—associated with both pneumothorax and pneumomediastinum (Chest 1992;102:1281); look for associated signs of sc emphysema in trauma; look for tracheal shift or hypotension to diagnose tension pneumothorax.

Crs: Those with spontaneous etiology or bullous disease may need thoracic surgery.

Cmplc: Tension pneumothorax—pt develops shock from pneumothorax with mediastinal shift to contralateral side as a feature.

SP recurrence higher in those that are tall, with less recurrence with smoking cessation (Thorax 1997;52:805).

Diff Dx: Catamenial pneumothorax occurs in females, it is recurrent SP that occurs with menses (Ped Emerg Care 1997:390).

Pneumothorax may be mistaken as Boerhaave's syndrome (J Accid Emerg Med 1999;16:235) or diaphragmatic hernia—congenital (Ann EM 1993;22:1221) or post-surgical.

Lab: None for Tension Pneumothorax (decompress first), otherwise CXR. Inspiration and expiration films increase yield of finding pneumothorax (Arch EM 1993;10:343). CT of chest in Multisystem trauma will show occult pneumothoraces that may need rx if pt going onto ventilator or to operating theater (Am J Roentgenol 1984;143:987).

EKG changes may be noted that mimic acute MI (Ann EM 1985;14:164).

Emergency Management:

Tension Pneumothorax:
- With sterile procedure, tap affected side going over the second rib in the midclavicular line, with over-the-needle catheter (14G) be careful of withdrawing the needle completely

because sometimes the catheter collapses, or use a 16G Verres needle, which automatically protrudes inner blunt tube when pleural cavity is entered (Crit Care Med 1978;6:378), or 16F McSwain Dart, which has its plastic tip formed into a flange post-insertion to maintain patency (Ann Surg 1980;191:760).

- Iv and O_2, conscious sedation if necessary.
- Chest tube.

Pneumothorax without tension physiology:

- O_2 and iv access.
- Procedural sedation with midazolam and narcotic of choice, eg fentanyl.
- After local sterile prep and anesthesia, chest tube, 32F for traumatic or those with fluid (hemothorax) component. May try simple aspiration (J Emerg Med 1986;4:437) although age > 50 yr, chronic lung disease or > 2.5 L of aspirated air associated with failure of this therapy (J Accid Emerg Med 1998; 15:317). Small tube with Heimlich valve an option in spontaneous or pneumothoraces.
- Post-needle biopsy of lung, having pt on affected side down or on the contralateral side has no influence on development of pneumothorax (Radiology 1999;10:59).

22.7 Pulmonary Embolus

Nejm 2003;349:1247; Chest 1998;113:499

Cause: Embolic clots to pulmonary arteries from systemic veins.

Epidem: Associated with h/o thromboembolic disease (Chest 1992;102:677); pregnancy, estrogen-containing birth control pills (Jama 1992;268:1689; Lancet 1996;348:983); hypercoagulable states from factor disorders or anti-phospholipid syndromes; prolonged rest state such as air travel > 3100 miles (Nejm 2001;345:779). Equivocal association with occult malignancy (Arch IM 1987;147:1907).

Pathophys: Thrombophlebitis causes thrombus, which breaks free and migrates to the lungs; it is possible to have small emboli chronically rather than one large one (one etiology for pulmonary HT). Calves and upper extremities are rarely the source; no signs or symptoms of DVT in 50% of pts.

Sx: Dyspnea—sudden or chronic; pleuritic chest pain; hemoptysis; fever; syncope—seen in massive PE.

Si: JVD; rales; wheezing; $P_2 > A_2$; BP cuff test for calf pain; cyanosis.

Crs: Resolves over 10-30 d; 80% overall survival; 75% of deaths within the first 2 hr; DVT clinically resolves in $^1\!/_3$ after 3 d of heparin.

Cmplc: ARDS; chronic pulmonary HT.

Diff Dx: Fat emboli—from bony fractures, 24-48 hr latency period, trial of methylprednisolone 1-1.5 mg/kg every 6 hr and other supportive care; Amniotic fluid emboli in pregnancy.

Scoring System: To delineate pt with low, medium or high risk, see Table 22.2 and Table 22.3.

Table 22.2   Canadian Scoring System

Criteria	Points
Suspected DVT	3.0
An alternative diagnosis less likely than PE	3.0
Heart rate > 100 bpm	1.5
Immobilization or surgery within previous 4 weeks	1.5
Previous DVT/PE	1.5
Hemoptysis	1.0
Malignancy (active treatment or within the last 6 months or palliative treatment)	1.0

• Score Interpretation

Score Range	Mean Probability of PE (%)	Risk
0-2 points	3.6	Low
3-6 points	20.5	Moderate
> 6 points	66.7	High

(Thromb Haemost 2000;83:416)

Table 22.3 Geneva Scoring System

Criteria	Points
Age 60-79 yr	1
Age > 79 yr	2
Prior DVT/PE	2
Recent Surgery	3
Heart rate > 100 bpm	1
$PaCO_2$ < 36 mm Hg	2
$PaCO_2$ 36-39 mm Hg	1
PaO_2 < 49 mm Hg	4
PaO_2 49-60 mm Hg	3
PaO_2 61-71 mm Hg	2
PaO_2 72-82 mm Hg	1
CXR with plate-like atelectasis	1
Elevation of hemidiaphragm	1
• Score Interpretation	

Score Range	Mean Probability of PE (%)	Risk
0-4 points	10	Low
5-8 points	38	Moderate
9-1 nts	81	High

(Arch IM 2001;161:92)

- Pulmonary Embolism Rule Out Protocol (Ann EM 2004; 44:490):

    Step 1: Must have pretest probability < 40% chance of having a PE to use this protocol. An algorithm for screening should determine if:

    a. High-risk on either the Canadian Scoring System or the Geneva Scoring System—if no, then go to "b" and if "yes," then pt is unsafe for this protocol.

    b. Pt is 50 yr of age or older; or any pulse rate (bpm) is greater than the systolic blood pressure—if "no," then go to Step 2 and if "yes," then go to "c."

c. Unexplained hypoxemia ($SaO_2 < 95\%$ breathing room air)—if "no," then go to "d" and if "yes," then pt is unsafe for this protocol.

d. Unilateral leg swelling—if "no," then go to "e" and if "yes," then pt is unsafe for this protocol.

e. Recent surgery requiring general anesthesia within the past 4 wks—if "no," then go to "f" and if "yes," then pt is unsafe for this protocol.

f. Hemoptysis—if "no" then go to Step 2 and if "yes," then the pt is unsafe for this protocol.

Step 2: Measure d-dimer and alveolar dead space (again, afore-mentioned high-risk pts and those screened out as noted above should not participate in this protocol). If neg d-dimer (normal d-dimer) and normal alveolar dead space ($< 20\%$), then no further work-up required. This will miss less than 1% of those with a PE at 90-d follow-up. If either d-dimer or alveolar dead space measurement is elevated, then further evaluation per your facility standards is required (such as CT angiogram, V/Q scan, leg duplex US, pulmonary angiogram).

Pts who are high-risk and not appropriate for this rule out protocol should undergo evaluation for PE, which may include imaging evaluation for PE or imaging evaluation for venous thrombosis.

Lab:

- *Alveolar Dead Space Measurement* (Anaesth Intensive Care 1999;27:452): Measure end-tidal CO_2 and the arterial PCO_2 in a pt breathing ambient air for two min. Measure 3 deeply exhaled CO_2 measurements before and after arterial puncture (each $PETCO_2$ measurement should be separated by 30 sec). Calculate alveolar dead space from the following equation:

$$\% \text{ alveolar dead space} = 100 \times (PaCO_2 - PETCO_2)/PaCO_2$$

- *Lab:* CBC with diff and PT/PTT if considering rx with antico-agulants or thrombolytics; ABG may be of real value in calcu-lating alveolar dead space, but cannot base further testing on pO_2 alone—$pO_2 < 80$ mm Hg with 10% false neg, $pO_2 < 90$ mm Hg with 0% false neg; d-dimer equivocal with latex agglu-tination tests including SimplyRed—(J Nucl Med 1993; 34:896) vs (Ann EM 2000;35:121); the ELISA d-dimer may be useful in excluding those with low to moderate risk (94% sen-sitive and 45% specific), but this was found on data dredging (subgroup analysis) (Ann EM 2002;40:133). It appears it is best to combine the results of d-dimer and alveolar dead space measurements, as noted in Scoring Systems (p 433).
- *Non-invasive tests:* Duplex US if unsure if pt is high or low risk to help interpret the utility of pulmonary test (V/Q scan, helical CT) (Am J Emerg Med 1999;17:271) (see Venous Thrombosis p179).
- *X-ray:* CXR to ascertain other reasons for hypoxia, look for pulmonary infarcts or newly elevated diaphragm—or perhaps future rule in lieu of ventilation phase of V/Q scan (Thromb Haemost 2000;83:412). V/Q scan [91% sensitive, 96% spe-cific (Clin Physiol Funct Imaging 2002;22:392)] to look for multiple mismatched defects, helpful if normal or low proba-bility with low index of suspicion, or high probability with high or moderate index of suspicion—otherwise not helpful (Jama 1990;263:2753). Helical CT to look for intraluminal clot in medium to large pulmonary arteries (Radiology 1997;205:447). Pulmonary angiography is the gold standard [not CT (Radiology 1997;205:453; Clin Radiol 2001;56: 838)], and should be used in cases where studies are persis-tently equivocal.
- *EKG:* Of no help in differentiating those with PE from those without PE—normal sinus rhythm is the most common under-

lying rhythm with PE, and most common abnormality is sinus tachycardia (J Emerg Med 2004;27:121).

Emergency Management:

- O$_2$ if hypoxic or dyspneic; iv access if unstable or if using unfractionated heparin.
- Heparin 5,000-10,000 U iv bolus, large dose for larger thrombus/emboli if considering clot consumption of heparin as an issue, then weight-based dosing/hr—OK in pregnancy (Chest 2004;126:401S).
- Studies of the following LMWH have been found to be effective: fragmin (Thromb Haemost 1995;74:1432), tinzaparin (Nejm 1997;337:663) and qd fondaparinux sc (5 mg if pt < 50 kg, 7.5 mg if pt 50 to 100 kg, and 10 mg if pt > 100 kg) can be effective in nonmonitored pts who are hemodynamically stable (Nejm 2003;349:1695); all low molecular weight heparins are not equivalent in action and efficacy.
- Ximelagatran at a dose of 36 mg bid for rx of VTE with or without pulmonary embolism is as effective as initial rx with enoxaparin followed by warfarin but may increase LFTs (approximately 9.6% of the time) (Jama 2005;293:681).
- Thrombolytics have some role but need further study—lower composite endpoint of death/recurrence but needs to be considered in the setting of increased bleeding episodes that have been fatal (Arch IM 2002;162:2537).
- Consider streptokinase to speed clearing with better PFTs and vein function; consider TPA if right heart failure with acute embolus (Lancet 1993;341:507).
- Alteplase with heparin in those with acute submassive pulmonary embolus with pulmonary HT or right ventricular dysfunction but without arterial hypotension or shock gives improved morbidity and mortality (Nejm 2002;347:1143).
- Medical consult for admission, with consideration of IVC umbrella, invasive radiology thrombolysis (rare) (Clin Cardiol 1999;22:661) or surgical embolectomy (rare).

Chapter 23

Rheumatology

23.1 Acute Rheumatic Fever (ARF)

Paediatrician 1981;10:158

Cause: Group A hemolytic (rarely non-hemolytic) *Streptococcus*, with presence of m-protein; post-*streptococcal*, upper respiratory infection × 2-3 wks, but bacteria must still be present.

Epidem: Children peak incidence between 5-15 yr of age (J Infect 1998;36:249); female:male 3:1; incidence of approximately 0.3:100,000 (Acta Med Scand 1988;224:587); see Pharyngitis p358.

Pathophys: Autoimmune theories with cross reacting antibodies between Group A strep and human tissues [such as T-cells (Clin Exp Immunol 1999;116:100)], but does not explain why only strep pharyngitis may go onto ARF.
- *Jones criteria* (Ped Ann 1999;28:9): for diagnosis need 2 major criteria or 1 major plus 2 minor criteria, and then also a pos ASO titer or culture or h/o scarlet fever.
- *Major criteria:* carditis; polyarthritis; erythema marginatum; sc nodules; chorea.
- *Minor criteria:* fever; arthralgias; distant h/o ARF; elevated WBC, ESR or CRP; long PR interval or other EKG abnormalities. Members of the same family tend to have same major sx.

Sx: Sore throat; fever; arthralgias—although transitory (Indian J Peds 1988;55:9).

439

Si: Erythema marginatum—associated with carditis; murmurs (valvular or non-valvular) which are associated with pericarditis; sc nodules at bony prominences that are associated with carditis; pneumonitis; serositis; polyarthritis of large joints; Sydenham's chorea may follow other signs (or symptoms) by weeks or months.

Crs: Less than 12 wks in approximately 90%; approximately 95% of those with murmurs appear by 2 wks of symptom onset.

Cmplc: Chronic cardiac valve disease; mitral regurgitation with Jaccoud's arthritis (ulnar deviation that can voluntarily correct); transient glomerulonephritis.

Diff Dx: Post-streptococcal reactive arthritis (J Intern Med 1999; 245:261); Familial Mediterranean fever (Clin Rheumatol 1999;18:446); septic arthritis; infective endocarditis; cat scratch disease; RA; immune complex disease; Still's disease; pustular psoriasis; dermatomyositis; inflammatory bowel disease; sarcoidosis; systemic lupus erythematosus (SLE).

Lab: CBC with diff; ESR; metabolic profile; UA; throat culture, if still inflamed; ASO titer or streptozyme test; consider anti-DNAase or anti-streptodornase titer; EKG.
  - *X-ray:* Look for interstitial pneumonitis.

Emergency Management:
  - PCN G 25-50 mg/kg qd divided bid po for peds, 500 mg po bid for adults; PCN G benzathine and procaine (bicillin C-R, or bicillin C-R 900/300) im single dose—this will be extended for years of prophylaxis in those with carditis.
  - ASA for all.
  - Corticosteroids: for all with severe carditis or pneumonia; optional if sick without murmur; not needed for murmur alone.
  - Medicine consult for admit if ill, otherwise 1-2 d f/u.

23.2 Behcet's Syndrome

Curr Opin Rheumatol 1999;11:53; JR Coll Physicians Lond 2000;34:169

Cause: Genetic and viral hypotheses.

Epidem: 27% of those affected with HLA B5 and B27; M:F 1.7:1 in Eastern Mediterranean type.

Pathophys: A vasculitis, onset in third decade of life. It is a multi-system disorder, and different classifications helpful for research, not as much in dx (Ann Med Interne (Paris) 1999;150:477).

Sx: Oral ulcers; genital ulcers; eye pain.

Si: Recurrent problems with the following—oral aphthous ulcers; genital ulcers with no preferred site, often painless in women; uveitis.

Crs: Each attack lasts 1-4 wks; unique pulmonary vasculitis is possible (Chest 1989;95:585); CNS disease has bad prognosis (Brain 1999;122:2183)

Cmplc: Blindness; cardiac problems; inflammatory arthritis; aseptic meningitis; thrombophlebitis; colitis; skin pustules.

Lab: CBC with diff; ESR; viral and bacterial cultures of ulcers.
  • *Diagnostic:* Saline shot challenge—delayed hypersensitivity reaction is diagnostic.

Emergency Management:

Ann Med Interne (Paris) 1999;150:576; Cochrane Database Syst Rv 2000;2
  • 1st line—ASA or indomethacin.
  • 2nd line—steroids: type, dose and route depend on manifestations.
  • 3rd line—azathioprine, cyclophosphamide or chlorambucil.
  • Poor data—colchicine (Clin Exp Dermatol 1989;14:298).

- Oral ulcers—try mixture of 1:1:1:1 mylanta:benadryl:tetracycline:prednisolone elixir, 5 cc, swish and spit qid for 1 wk. Thalidomide may be helpful.
- Medicine consult for admit if CNS manifestations or same day ophthalmology consult for uveitis, otherwise outpatient medicine f/u.

23.3 Temporal Arteritis

Semin Ophthalm 1999;14:109; Brit J Rheum 1996;35:1161; Jama 2002;287:2996

Cause: Autoimmune; aka Giant Cell Arteritis.

Epidem: 133:100,000; F:M ratio is approximately 2:1; usually in pts > 60 yr of age; occasionally associated with HLA DR4; associated with polymyalgia rheumatica (PMR) (Recenti Prog Med 1990;81:176; J Am Ger Soc 1992;40:515)

Pathophys: Arteritis of medium- and large-sized vessels. Sometimes with mild anemia and liver function abnormalities. Should spare the kidneys; equivocal association with thyroid disease (Rev Rhum Ed Fr 1993;60:493).

Sx (Lancet 1967;2:638): Fever; headache; visual changes—eg, diplopia or amaurosis fugax; scalp pain; sore throat; cough; claudication symptoms of leg, tongue and jaw; weakness; joint stiffness; malaise; weight loss.

Si: Fever; thickened temporal artery; retinal changes with ischemia or cherry red macular spot of retinal artery occlusion; synovitis; muscle tenderness.

Crs: Most resolve with rx over 1-2 yr, some refractory cases. Arthritis of temporal arteritis not associated with progression to RA (unlike PMR) (Rheumatology (Oxford) 2000;39:283).

Cmplc: Blindness; cranial nerve deficits; MI; CVA; thoracic aortic aneurysms and dissections 17 × more common in this population (Ann IM 1982;97:672); psychosis; hypothyroidism.

Diff Dx: Polymyalgia rheumatica—appears to be closely related to Temporal arteritis; Takayasu's arteritis—arteritis of large vessels.

Lab: CBC with diff, thrombocytosis with more significant disease (J Neuroophthalmol 2000;20:67); PT/PTT; ESR > 80 mm/hr, but significant cases will still be missed, and changing this to > 30 mm/hr appears to be appropriately more sensitive (Clin Rheumatol 2000;19:73), degree of elevation inversely correlated with degree of anemia (Arch Ophthalm 1987;105:965); metabolic profile with LFTs; total CPK, consider aldolase—if myalgias; UA; consider rheumatoid profile. Temporal artery biopsy is diagnostic.
- *X-ray:* Head CT or MRI to look for anatomic lesion of other cause if headache, visual disturbance or cranial nerve deficits. CXR for thoracic aortic aneurysm, with CT if wide mediastinum noted.

Emergency Management:
- If visual loss, give methylprednisolone 250 mg iv (Ophthalm 1992;68; J Rheumatol 2000:1484) and Medical consult for admission.
- If no visual changes, begin Prednisone 40-60 mg po qd × 12 wks.
- Arrange adult medicine follow-up, with temporal artery biopsy arranged through surgery—either directly arrange to have medicine assume this, or set up to have done within 1 wk.

Chapter 24

Tools

24.1 ACLS Guidelines

Circ 1998;97:1654; 2000;102:I129; Peds 1998;101:E13

These guidelines are opinions based on imperfect information. Best example, perhaps, is the study that shows that pts who receive ACLS medications do worse than those who do not (Ann EM 1998;32:544). This is because all people do better if their "code" is related to an arrhythmia treatable with electricity (Jama 1999; 281:1175). Even success at early resuscitation still carries a poor ultimate prognosis (Resuscitation 1998;36:95). This is constantly updated, and please refer to the American Heart Association literature for the latest algorithms.

24.2 APGAR Scores

Developed by Patricia Apgar (Ped Dev Pathol 1999;2:292) to quickly stratify neonates and give a prognosis for the first minutes of life (Arch IM 1999;159:125). Traditionally done at one and five min of life (see Table 24.1), has been extended to ten min and other longer time intervals in an attempt to give further prognostic information. A persistently low score (3 or less) from 5 to 20 min of life is an indicator of increased neonatal morbidity/mortality (Arch Ped Adolesc Med 2000;154:294; Nejm 2001;344:467); with a finding of 3 or less at 5 min associated with cerebral palsy (Jama 1984;251: 1843).

TOOLS

Table 24.1 APGAR Score

Indicator	Score		
	0	1	2
A: appearance	Blue/cyanosis	Pink body/blue extremities (acrocyanosis)	Pink body
P: pulse	None	< 100 bpm	> 100 bpm
G: grimace (stroke sole)	None	Weak	Cry
A: activity	None	Weak flexor tone	Strong tone
R: respirations	None	Weak	Strong; crying

24.3 Glasgow Coma Scale

Lancet 1976;1:1031; Acta Neurochir 1976;34:45

The Glasgow Coma Scale was intended as a research tool with measurements originally 24 hr after injury to predict mortality and morbidity (see Table 24.2). Its primary usefulness has been its ease of use (Clin Neurol Neurosurg 1977;80:100), helping different practitioners communicate, and showing improvement or deterioration of a pt with repeat evaluations. Acute changes in this scale are now used to triage patients (J Emerg Med 1984;2:1)—the motor component with systolic blood pressure is the strongest predictor of severe injury (Ann EM 2001;38:541). Its predictive value has not had rigorous evaluation (J Clin Epidem 1996;49:755), especially with regard to functional outcome (Am J Phys Med Rehabil 1996;75:364). Other tools exist (the APACHE scores (Intensive Care Med 1997;23:77), Acute Physiology Score, Reaction Level Scale, Simplified Acute Physiology Score, Therapeutic Intervention Scoring System, individual trauma scores, such as the Maine Trauma Score), which may be better indicators and pt stratifiers in those with sepsis or trauma, but getting prognostic data on those with head injuries is still incomplete

(J Trauma 1989;29:299). The APACHE II was found to be as predictive as the Glasgow Coma Scale in those with stroke (Stroke 1990;21:1280). The Baux Score, Edlich Burn Score, and Zawacki Score appear to be more prognostic in those with burns, and focus on size of burn and age of pt as bearing more weight prognostically (J Burn Care Rehabil 1991;12:560). As far as children, the Glasgow Coma Scale is not as predictive in those with severe traumatic injury (J Peds 1992;120:195), and mild abnormalities may be predictive of intracranial pathology (Neurosurgery 2000;46:1093). Other scales also exist for research methods, such as the Comprehensive Level of Consciousness Scale (J Neurosurg 1984;60:955). Add the best response from each category of eyes, verbal, and motor. This does not supplant a careful neurologic exam, and scores range from 3 (worst) to 15 (best).

Table 24.2   Glasgow Coma Scale

Indicator	Response	Score
Eyes	Open spontaneously	4
	Open to verbal stimuli	3
	Open to painful stimuli	2
	No movement	1
Verbal	Normally conversant/oriented	5
	Conversant/disoriented	4
	Inappropriate words	3
	Incomprehensible words (sounds)	2
	No response	1
Motor	Follows voice commands	6
	Correctly localizes painful stimuli	5
	Flexion-withdrawal to pain	4
	Decorticate posturing (flexion)	3
	Decerebrate posturing (extension)	2
	No response	1

TOOLS

Chapter 25

Toxicology

Med Lett Drugs Ther 2002;44:21; Crit Care Med 2003;31:2794

25.1 Activated Charcoal

Ann EM 2002;39:273; Vet Hum Toxicol 2002;44:182; J Toxicol Clin Toxicol 2004;42:101

The use of activated charcoal has become ubiquitous in overdose rx. Knowing the complications and significance of such is of paramount importance. One study found that multidose activated charcoal can lead to the following complications (Ann EM 2003;41:370):

- Aspiration (0.5% incidence with no deaths) vs 1.6% incidence with 8.5% mortality rate (control group with 0.4% mortality) in competing study (Crit Care Med 2004;32:88)
- Hypernatremia (6% incidence)
- Hypermagnesemia (3.1% incidence)
- Corneal abrasion (0.1% incidence)

Of note, gi obstruction was not seen in this series. Yet, a study of healthy volunteers finds that many minor effects can have an effect on ability to successfully complete an rx with activated charcoal, and the following effects were found when compared to controls (only those with differences shown here) (Hawaii Med J 2002;61:251):

- Constipation or abdominal fullness (50% incidence)
- Nausea (20% incidence)

- Vomiting (8% incidence), may be as high as 26% incidence (J Toxicol Clin Toxicol 2002;40:775)
- Diarrhea (8% incidence)

Finally, whether single-dose oral activated charcoal makes a difference in the rx of relatively low-risk, self-poisoned pts is controversial and looking at clinical deterioration, length of stay in the ER or hospital, and complication rates show no difference in one study (Am J Ther 2002;9:301). Important to note that significantly acute ingestions with potentially serious sequela (hydrocarbons including acetaminophen > 140 mg/kg, crack cocaine, mushrooms, caustic agents, heavy metals, lithium or iron) were all excluded from this study.

25.2 Acetaminophen

Acad Emerg Med 1999;6:1115; Ann IM 1999;130:52

Cause: Ingestion.

Epidem: Most common reason for call to Poison Control; increased risk of toxicity in those with chronic disease, malnourishment, or liver disease (interestingly, chronic alcoholism can lead to these risk factors).

Pathophys: Causes liver failure secondary to metabolite which depletes reduced glutathione and perhaps secondary release of mitochondrial Ca. Stages will be covered below, and Stage I is within 24 hr Stage II is 24-48 hr, Stage III is 72-96 hr, and Stage IV is 96 hr-2 wks.

Sx: H/o ingestion > 10 gm in adult in < 24 hr, peds > 140 mg/kg single dose.
Stage I: Nausea, vomiting.
Stage II: Abdominal pain, not urinating.
Stage III: Laboratory abnormalities.
Stage IV: Declaration of liver injury—either improving or failing.

Si: None specific

> *Stage I:* Clammy and pale skin.
> *Stage II:* RUQ abdominal pain.
> *Stage III:* Laboratory abnormalities.
> *Stage IV:* Declaration of liver injury—either improving or failing.

Crs.: Most LFT abnormalities are transient, yet may be the harbinger of a fatal reaction.

Cmplc: Co-ingestions (ethanol, anticonvulsants) can amplify toxic effects, or cause delayed symptoms and peak levels; nomogram not accurate in circumstances where co-ingested materials (cold remedies) alter uptake (Brit J Clin Pharmacol 1999;48:278).

Lab: Acetaminophen level at 4, 8, and 12 hr (see Figure 25.1) gives prognostic data (Am J Hlth Syst Pharm 1999;56:1081), and upon arrival to ER (Scand J Gastroenterol 1999;34:723); liver profile; salicylate level; ethanol level; CBC with diff; PT/PTT; urine toxic drug screen; EKG. Possible use of urine acetaminophen to r/o ingestion (J Toxicol Clin Toxicol 1999;37:769).

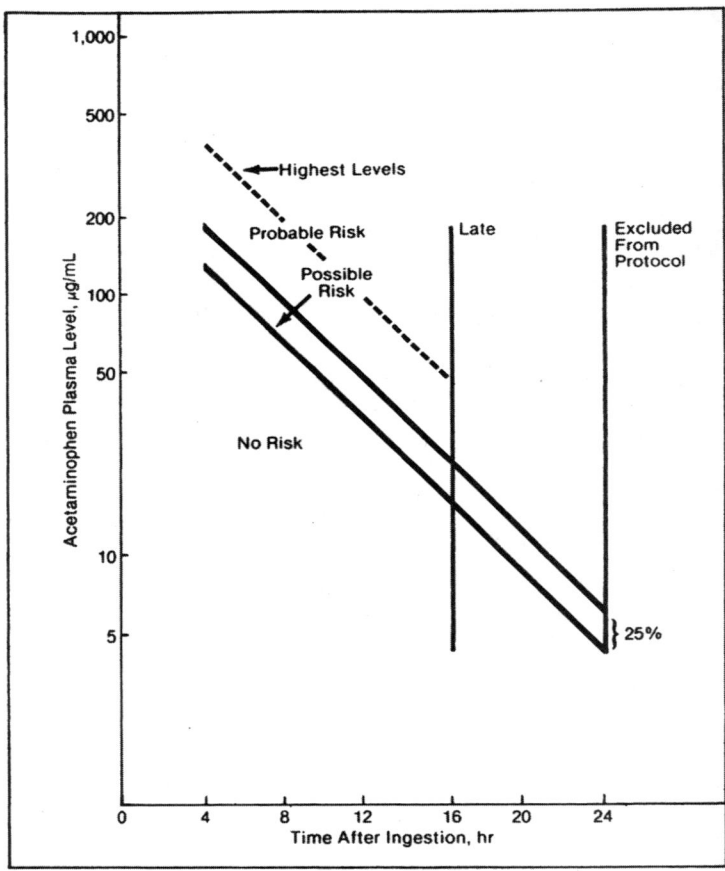

Figure 25.1 Study design nomogram. Possible risk is 25% below nomogram for multiclinic open-study purpose only. Reproduced with permission from Rumack BH, et al., Acetaminophen overdose. Arch IM 1981;141:380.

Emergency Management:

- Acetylcysteine po 140 mg/kg load then 70 mg/kg every 4 hr for a total of 18 doses (Arch IM 1981;141:380). Iv as efficacious (J Toxicol Clin Toxicol 1999;37:759) and use of the ingestion form for iv administration is safe (Ann EM 2003;42:9); doses are the same of 3% solution infused over 1 hr (Crit Care Med 1998;26:40).

- Activated charcoal 1 gm/kg (J Toxicol Clin Toxicol 1999;37:753) if given within an hr of ingestion; do not use Sorbitol as cathartic in these cases, but sodium sulfate instead, if cathartic needed. No data that charcoal impedes absorption of acetylcysteine, but some advocate giving extra acetylcysteine in loading dose such as 150 mg/kg. The usefulness of activated charcoal in acetaminophen overdose cases is being more scrutinized.

- Studies have shown that hypothyroidism and cimetidine-induced delayed gastric emptying may have had a small beneficial effect in certain populations, but PTU and cimetidine are not advocated as emergency medicine treatment.

25.3 Antidepressants

Jama 1987;257:521; Ped Emerg Care 1998;14:293)

Cause: Tricyclic antidepressants (TCAs) are discussed here, with MAO inhibitors and SSRIs (discussion in Acute Serotonin Syndrome on p249). St. John's Wort is a weak MAO inhibitor. Cyclobenzaprine (Flexeril) is similar to TCAs.

Epidem: Most common intentional OD which causes death, since narrow therapeutic window.

Pathophys: The mortal effect of TCAs has to do with Na-channel blockade in the myocardium. Na-channel blockade causes decreased ionotropic action, conduction defects (heart block, widening QRS, ectopic beats), and resulting hypotension (Am J Emerg Med 1988;6:439). The anticholinergic effects and α-blocking effects may cause symptoms, but these are usually secondary and not fatal.

Sx: Anticholinergic symptoms—dry mouth, dry skin, confusion, palpitations.

Si: Tachycardia, altered mental status, hypotension, seizures, coma.

Crs: When these problems occur, they do so rapidly—altered mental status (J Toxicol Clin Toxicol 1992;30:161), cardiac conduction defects, arrhythmias, and seizures are poor prognostic indicators (Am J Emerg Med 1986;4:496). Hypotension due to cardiogenic shock has high mortality.

Cmplc: ARDS (Chest 1989;96:852; Ann Pharmacother 1993;27:572), pancreatitis (J Toxicol Clin Toxicol 1994;32:425).

Diff Dx: Consider other similar toxic overdoses (wide QRS with seizures), such as cocaine, lithium, phenothiazines, antihistamines, carbamazepine, quinidine, quinine, propoxyphene, propranolol, phenothiazines, bupivicaine, and lidocaine.

Lab: EKG looking for right axis deviation (Ann EM 1989;18:348), wide QRS, or prolonged QT (Am J Cardiol 1986;57:1154); glucoscan; CBC with diff; metabolic profile; ABG; ethanol level; acetaminophen level; salicylate level; urine toxic drug screen.

Emergency Management:

- Airway, O_2
- Iv access, consider naloxone and thiamine 100 mg iv as overdose/coma protocol.
- Gastric lavage if within 1 hr of presentation, followed by activated charcoal 1 gm/kg—activated charcoal is the most important tool (J Emerg Med 1995;13:203); Be prepared to protect the airway if necessary, since sudden deterioration is a possibility.
- $NaHCO_3$ 1-2 mg/kg iv bolus, followed by 2 cc/kg/hr drip of 1 L of D_5W with 2-3 amps of $NaHCO_3$ added. Use $NaHCO_3$ if wide QRS (> 0.1 sec), refractory hypotension or cardiac

arrhythmias noted. Goal of rx is pH 7.50-7.55 (J Toxicol Clin Toxicol 2004;42:1).

- Lidocaine is second line drug for arrhythmias, and would avoid use of disopyramide, imipramine, procainamide, quinidine, flecainide, propafenone, β-blockers, and Ca channel blockers.
- Role of phenytoin to be elucidated for cardiac arrhythmias (Ann EM 1981;10:270).
- Benzodiazepines for seizures, followed by phenobarbital.
- Hypotension refractory to fluids and $NaHCO_3$ should be treated with norepinephrine 2-20 µg/min, avoid dopamine (Am J Emerg Med 1988;6:566).
- Refractory arrhythmia/complex widening, despite sodium bicarbonate and an alkalemic blood gas, and refractory hypotension, despite iv fluids and norepinephrine, may prompt use of hypertonic NaCl (7.5% solution) as a 200 cc bolus (Ann EM 2003;42:20).
- Perhaps Fab or single chain Fv fragment (sFv) fragments for desipramine overdose (Toxicol Lett 1995;82-83:801).
- Consider extracorporeal circulation, if not responding to usual methods (Am J Emerg Med 1994;12:456).
- Admission for continuous cardiac monitoring for 24 hr if not toxic (Jama 1985;254:1772).

25.4 Arsenic (Acute and Chronic Types)

Ann EM 2003;41:378

Cause: Insecticides and herbicides, especially crab grass killers.

Epidem: Arsenic associated water poisoning puts millions of people at risk in many parts of the world (Int J Hyg Environ Hlth 2003; 206:323; Bull World Hlth Organ 2000;78:1093; J Water Hlth 2003;1:73).

Pathophys: Blocks Krebs cycle.

Sx:

>*Acute:* Nausea, vomiting and diarrhea with esophageal and epigastric pain; immediate "rice water" then bloody stool; CHF (myocardiopathy), with risk of increased QT and torsades de pointes or ventricular tachycardia, treat with pacer or $MgSO_4$.

>*Chronic:* Vague malaise.

Si:

>*Acute:* Dyspnea, guaiac-positive stools.

>*Chronic:* Mees' lines in nails after 4-6 weeks of chronic exposure (r/o INH, thallium); hematuria especially in children; increased skin pigmentation with spared spots = "rain drops on a dusty table"; keratosis.

Crs: After several days mucous membrane inflammation, rashes, hematologic, ATN, encephalopathy, painful peripheral, sensory, and motor neuropathy after 7-14 d.

Cmplc: Lung cancer incidence increased (Jama 2004;292:2984); r/o similar toxicity from arsine gas from industrial exposure in semiconductor industry.

Lab:

- *Chemistries:* in *acute,* spot urine level; in *chronic,* arsenic tissue levels in bone, nails, hair (pubic best, since fast-growing and sweat adds Hg); normal levels = 3-13 μgm/100 gm; 24-h urine arsenic level, fewer false positives than blood levels, but will be back to normal when presents with neuropathy, but can bring it out with dimercaprol.
- *X-ray:* KUB shows radiodense cast of stomach or gi tract acutely.

Emergency Management:

- Dimercaprol (BAL, British anti-Lewisite) 3-5 mg/kg im q 4 hr over several d; within first 24-36 hr to chelate arsenic and reverse symptoms (Am J Emerg Med 1988;6:602). Few complications at these doses in adults or children (Am J Emerg Med 1995;13:432).

- Succimer, aka DMSA (2,3-dimercaptosuccinic acid) treatment (Am J Emerg Med 1995;13:432) (see Emergency Management in Lead p466 for dosing)
- D-penicillamine 125 mg or 250 mg po qd as alternative therapy (Vet Hum Toxicol 1981;23:164).

25.5 Benzodiazepine

Curr Opin Peds 1996;8:243; Drug Saf 1997;17:181

Cause: Ingestion or parenteral use of benzodiazepines; mixed overdoses common (J Forensic Sci 1997:155).

Epidem: Common intentional overdose, occasionally miscalculated medicine dosing.

Pathophys: CNS receptors activated, inducing anxiolysis and sedation.

Sx/Si: Nonspecific; sleepiness.

Crs: Most recover from pure ingestions; the elderly may present as being delirious.

Cmplc: Co-ingestions usually cause most problems with coma, respiratory depression, or hypotension; withdrawal from benzodiazepines may precipitate seizures—avoid this if at all possible.

Lab: Search for co-ingestions with ethanol level; acetaminophen level; salicylate level; CBC with diff; metabolic profile; urine toxic drug screen; EKG.

Emergency Management:

- Airway support; iv access and fluid bolus if hypotensive; consider activated charcoal 1 gm/kg po if < 1-2 hr since ingestion and competent airway.
- Do not reverse with flumazenil (Romazicon) (Crit Care Med 1992;20:1733; Am J Emerg Med 1992;10:184) unless adverse

side effect of parenteral sedation in ER or hospital inpatient who is not ethanol or benzodiazepine dependent. Otherwise, may precipitate seizure. Dose of flumazenil is 1 mg over 3 min every 1 hr prn.

25.6 Carbon Monoxide

Ann EM 1994;24:242

Cause: Carbon monoxide (CO) inhalation, from combustible sources.

Epidem: Common sources are car exhaust, cigarette or any fire smoke, gas appliances with closed space inhalation.

Pathophys: CO has a 200X affinity for Hgb than O_2, with a slow dissociation rate (Circ 1981;63:253A): It shifts the Hgb dissociation curve to the left, which means that it also decreases O_2 dissociation.

Sx: Cherry red skin; headache; dizziness; altered mental status (Arch Surg 1973;107:851)—30-40 mg% CO; coma— > 40 mg% CO.

Si: Cherry red skin; retinal hemorrhages.

Crs: Recovery may take months.

Cmplc: Ischemic heart and CNS disease.

Lab: Serum CO level (look for level > 10 mg%); ABG; CBC with diff for significant exposures to assess for anemia; screen for co-ingestions (see Benzodiazepines p 457) if possible suicide attempt.

Emergency Management:
- High flow O_2, with non-rebreather mask and 15 lpm flow rate; treat longer if pregnant (Science 1977;197:680)
- Use of hyperbaric O_2 is controversial [study showing efficaciousness with control group having 15 pts with cerebellar dysfunction prior to rx, vs 4 in hyperbaric group; mean time of CO exposure was 22 hr control vs 13 hr in treatment group—thus not truly identical comparison (Nejm 2002;347:1057)],

but would use if available (J Emerg Med 1985;3:443; Undersea Hyperb Med 1996;23:215); more efficacious if metabolic acidosis (J Accid Emerg Med 1999;16:96), pregnant, focal neurologic symptoms or if coincident cyanide exposure and inducing methemoglobinemia. Rarely helpful in cardiac arrest, even post resuscitation (Ann EM 2001;38:36).

- Exchange transfusion is controversial.

25.7 Cyanide

J Emerg Med 2000;18:441; Occup Med (Lond) 1998;48:427

Cause: Ingestion, inhalation, or transdermal absorption of cyanide (CN); past use of Laetrile (Ann EM 1983;12:449).

Epidem: Common inhalation toxin from house fires, yet overall serious toxicity from all sources is uncommon.

Pathophys: Cytochrome oxidase poisoning, which renders cells unable to use O_2 (J Toxicol Clin Toxicol 1987;25:121).

Sx: Non-specific, but may include headache and dyspnea; rarely history of "almond smell."

Si: Cyanosis if respiratory arrest; mental status change with coma possible.

Crs: Inhalation exposures usually recover rapidly with removal of pt from toxic environment.

Cmplc: Arrhythmias; metabolic acidosis; diabetes insipidus; seizures; respiratory arrest.

Diff Dx: Cocaine, ethylene glycol, isoniazid, methanol, salicylates, iron poisoning.

Lab: Serum CN level (look for level > 40µM/L); CO level; ABG—look for lactic acidosis (BMJ 1996;312:26)—plasma lactate level > 10 mmol/L sensitive for CN poisoning in smoke inhalation victims who do not have severe burns (Nejm 1991;325:1761); ethanol level; methanol level; ethylene glycol level; salicylate level; acetaminophen level; metabolic profile; CBC with diff; urine toxic drug screen; EKG.

Emergency Management: Consider calling for Lilly CN antidote kit, which contains amyl nitrite, sodium thiosulfate, and sodium nitrite (Am J Emerg Med 1995;13:524).

- O_2.
- Iv access.
- Amyl nitrite for inhalation or sodium nitrite ($NaNO_2$) 0.2 cc/kg of 3% solution or 300 mg bolus (maximum of 10 cc) iv—this leads to the formation of methemoglobin, which CN will bind to, but the nitrites may have other actions that are not fully elucidated; potentially dangerous in the setting of co-toxicity with CO.
- Sodium thiosulfate ($Na_2S_2O_3$) to form SCN, which can then be excreted, better than amyl nitrite; 12.5 gm iv in adult.
- Perhaps hydroxocobalamin (vit B12) to complex CN for acute treatment or preventative role in those receiving nitroprusside (Crit Care Med 1993;21:465).
- Dicobalt edetate (Kelocyanor) and 4-dimethylaminophenol (DMAP) used in Europe, no proven efficacy over the Lilly kit. Previous cobalt experiments without benefit (Proc Soc Exp Biol Med 1965;120:780).
- Research active using stroma-free methemoglobin solution (SFMS) (Am J Emerg Med 1985;3:519).
- If resuscitating pts with a cyanide overdose, it is possible to have significant exposure (J Forensic Sci 1989;34:1280), especially if ingestion (combination with HCl in the stomach can form hydrogen cyanide, which is expressed with burping).

25.8 Digitalis

Prog Cardiovasc Dis 1984;27:21; J Card Surg 1987;2:453

Cause: Ingestion or parenteral use of digitalis (digoxin, digitoxin), foxglove *(Digitalis purpurea)* or yellow oleander *(Thevetia peruviana)*.

Epidem: Common accidental overdose.

Pathophys: The primary clinical action of digitalis as a Na/K pump inhibitor is the same action that causes its lethality, with consequent heart blocks and arrhythmias. More common in people with renal disease since digoxin has renal elimination (Ger Med Mon 1966;11:316).

Sx/Si: Weakness, fatigue, yellow halos, other nonspecific findings.

Crs: Variable, with acute toxicity more likely to have gi symptoms and hyperkalemia, and chronic toxicity with more nonspecific findings.

Cmplc: Co-ingestion with β-blockers, calcium-channel blockers, and quinidine may increase toxicity.

Diff Dx: Rarely seen from toad venom bite in U.S.

Lab: Serum digoxin level; metabolic profile including calcium and magnesium (hypomagnesemia) (Am Hrt J 1970;79:57); EKG, with a myriad of arrhythmias, PVCs most common (Geriatrics 1965;20:1006); cardiac markers if EKG changes.

Emergency Management:
- Iv access and cardiac monitor.
- Activated charcoal 1 gm/kg po for acute poisoning.
- Digoxin antibody or Fab fragments (Digibind) (Conn Med 1986;50:835) for ventricular arrhythmias or bradyarrhythmias not responding to standard therapy (see next bullet). May also be used for hyperkalemia (Am J Emerg Med 1986;4:364). Dose is 40 mg of Fab (1 vial)/0.6 mg of digoxin (actual) (Clin

Pharmacokinet 1995;28:483), and number of vials = serum digoxin level × weight (kg)/100 (good estimate).

- Bradyarrhythmias—Atropine 0.5-1 mg iv, consider $MgSO_4$ 2 gm iv and cardiac pacing. Co-ingestion of β-blockers and Ca-channel blockers may make it difficult to use standard therapy. Perhaps try glucagon 1 mg iv, if β-blockers co-ingestion. **N.B.** *Do not use* $CaCl_2$ or other calcium compounds in digitalis overdose—may worsen cardiac effects of digitalis.
- Hyperkalemia—May use $NaHCO_3$, glucose, insulin, and kayexalate, but avoid $CaCl_2$ since may worsen cardiac effects of digitalis.
- Ventricular arrhythmias—consider lidocaine or phenytoin (Dis Chest 1968;53:263) or fosphenytoin; phenytoin/fosphenytoin bolus is the same as for seizures at 15 mg/kg. If no effect, consider $MgSO_4$ 2 gm iv. Quinidine, procainamide, and amiodarone should not be used since they depress AV node conduction.

25.9 Ethylene Glycol

Med Toxicol 1986;1:309; J Toxicol Clin Toxicol 1999;37:537; Crit Rev Toxicol 1999;29:331; Am Fam Phys 2002;66:807)

Cause: Usually inadvertent ingestion of antifreeze.

Epidem: Unsure, since not every intoxicated pt is screened for ethylene glycol ingestion, and pt likely has no clinical problems if the ingestion of ethylene glycol is minimal and pt is intoxicated with ethanol.

Pathophys: Alcohol dehydrogenase (ADH) converts ethylene glycol to glycolic acid, which is metabolized to oxalate; this process gives a metabolic acidosis with a high osmolar gap (Vet Hum Toxicol 1980;22:255). Glycolic acid is a physiologic marker that correlates with severity of disease (Toxicol Sci 1999;50:117).

Other metabolites include lactate and glycolate (Am J Clin Path 1966;45:46).

Sx/Si: Intoxication, with CNS effects of seizures and coma in severe cases.

Crs: Variable degrees of end-organ damage to the heart, lungs, and kidneys may occur if this overdose goes unchecked.

Cmplc: Respiratory, cardiac, and kidney failure may be the result of this end-organ damage.

Diff Dx: Ethanol, cocaine, salicylates, methanol, iron, isoniazid, and cyanide poisoning.

Lab: Ethanol level; ethylene glycol (look for level > 20 mg/dL), methanol, and isopropyl alcohol levels; ABG—metabolic acidosis may be lacking if coincident ingestion, such as lithium (Am J Kidney Dis 1994;23:313); metabolic profile including Ca and Mg; salicylate level; acetaminophen level; CBC with diff; EKG; UA; urine toxic drug screen; bedside black light (Wood's lamp) evaluation looking for urine fluorescence is a weak and variable outcome test (Ann EM 2001;38:49).

Emergency Management:

- Iv access.
- Thiamine 100 mg iv and pyridoxine 100 mg iv (J Nutr 1977;107:458).
- Correct calcium and magnesium deficiencies, if necessary.
- 4-methylpyrazole (Fomepizole) as first-line treatment (J Toxicol Clin Toxicol 1986;24:463; Toxicol Lett 1987; 35:307)—15 mg/kg load, then 10 mg/kg q 12 hr iv for a total of 4 doses.
- Iv ethanol is 10% ethanol in D_5W—bolus 10 cc/kg, then 1.6 cc/kg/hr infusion. An oral loading dose of 20-50% ethanol solution with maintenance of 20% solution po provides just as good, if not better results (Nejm 1981;304:21).

- Hemodialysis for those with CNS dysfunction, visual complaints, or methanol level > 50 mg/dL (Acta Med Scand 1984;216:409). Do not withhold ethanol rx pending dialysis.

25.10 Iron

Cause: Ingestion of either form—ferric or ferrous—in dose > 20 mg/kg.

Epidem: Common, and many prove to be accidental.

Pathophys: Direct corrosive effect on gi mucosa; iron salts are hepatotoxic; subsequent release of iron and ferritin leads to vasodilatory effect and shock (Adv Exp Med Biol 1994;356:239).

Sx: Nausea, abdominal pain, seizures; then 2-3 hr respite, then protracted/fatal seizures.

Si: Hematemesis; melena/hematochezia.

Crs: Systemic toxicity occurs in 4-40 hr post ingestion.

Cmplc: Possible late complications include gi strictures, obstruction, and perforation.

Diff Dx: Cocaine, ethylene glycol, isoniazid, methanol, salicylates, cyanide poisoning.

Lab: Serum iron level (look for level > 300 μgm%)—deferoxamine can interfere with this measurement and radioimmunoassays are unreliable here; TIBC (Ann EM 1999;33:73), and transferrin and ferritin (Ann EM 1991;20:532) are unreliable predictors; salicylate level; acetaminophen level; CBC with diff; metabolic profile including Ca and Mg; UA; urine toxic drug screen; urine for deferoxamine challenge test, with rose-colored change, if serum-free iron is present, is not a reliable indicator. Leukocytosis and hyperglycemia not indicative of severity in adults (Am J Emerg Med 1996;14:454).

- *X-ray:* Single view flat plate abdomen to look for iron tablets, low sensitivity and specificity.

Emergency Management:
- Iv access.
- Gastric lavage if < 2 hr, otherwise just activated charcoal 1 gm/kg po.
- Chelate with L1 (Brit J Haematol 1994;86:851), which also complexes aluminum; or
- Deferoxamine 1 gm iv bolus, then 15 mg/kg/hr continuous infusion—this is safe in pregnancy (Am J Hematol 1999; 60:24); start this immediately if pt is symptomatic.
- Perhaps magnesium hydroxide 4.5 gm po per gm elemental iron if < 1 hr post ingestion (Acad Emerg Med 1998;5:961)
- Consider L1,1,2-dimethyl-3-hydroxypyris-4-one (Deferiprone) (Toxicol Lett 1995;80:1)
- Hemodialysis, if renal failure.

25.11 Isoniazid

Cause: Ingestion of isoniazid (INH); from a toxicologic basis, this is similar to hydrazine.

Epidem: Uncommon.

Pathophys: INH inhibits glutamic acid decarboxylase, which leads to decreased GABA levels. This decarboxylase enzyme is pyridoxine-dependent.

Sx: Gi symptoms.

Si: Change in mental status including seizures or coma.

Crs: Seizures predispose to a metabolic acidosis.

Cmplc: Protracted seizures (South Med J 1976;69:294).

Diff Dx: Related to hydrazine. Consider cocaine, ethylene glycol, methanol, salicylates, iron, and cyanide poisoning.

Lab: Serum INH level (look for > 2 mg/L); ABG—profound acidosis (Am J Emerg Med 1987;5:165); CBC with diff; metabolic profile with calcium and magnesium; urine toxic drug screen; EKG.

Emergency Management:

- Iv access.
- Activated charcoal 1 gm/kg, but less helpful if > 1 hr post ingestion (Hum Toxicol 1986;5:285).
- Pyridoxine gm/gm of INH ingested; give 5 gm iv if unknown (Ann EM 1983;12:303). This is first-line treatment for seizures in these cases, as well (Jama 1981;246:1102).
- Benzodiazepines for protracted seizures such as lorazepam (see Grand Mal Seizures p 286).
- Hemodialysis rarely needed.

25.12 Lead

Nejm 1973;289:1289; 1973;289:1229

Cause: An acquired porphyria from lead (Pb) ingestion; found in paint, battery fumes, pottery glazes, smeltering, indoor firing ranges, radiator repair shops, moonshine; Tetraethyl lead from gas only results in encephalopathy, not porphyria or blood changes.

Epidem: Unknown incidence in adults and usually via work exposure, common in children (pica).

Pathophys: Pb chelates sulfhydryl groups of ALA dehydrogenase, ferrochelatase, and ALA synthetase. Induces gout and gouty nephropathy in adults—gouty nephropathy commonly associated with Pb intoxication.

Sx: Abdominal pain, better with palpation; associated family pet illness.

Si: Gingival margin lead line (Am J Hematol 1981;11:99), peripheral motor neuropathy (eg, wrist drop), neuroses, psychoses (Am J Psych 1984;141:1423).

Crs: Chelation helps avoid seizures, not other neurologic complications.

Cmplc: Hypothyroidism; gout; gouty nephropathy (Nejm 1981; 304:520); encephalopathy (50% mortality without rx, 3% with); mental and neurologic disabilities; HT (Environ Hlth Perspect 1988;78:57); look for creatinine > 1.5 mg %.

Diff Dx: Other causes of encephalopathy (CNS lesion, drugs, metabolic, infectious, CO) or psychiatric disorders.

Lab: CBC with diff, look for RBC stippling; serum Pb level (Arch IM 1987;147:697), all other tests for Pb not as accurate; metabolic profile and UA, if suspect renal involvement; consider TSH.
- *X-ray:* Acute ingestions may show lead pills in bowel; children with Pb lines at metaphyseal calcification areas.

Emergency Management:

All patients:
- Iv; O_2 if encephalopathy.
- For seizures, see Grand Mal Seizures p 284.
- If Pb pills noted in bowel, polyethylene glycol solution (Golytely) 1-2L po.

Level of 10-25 μg %:
- Find source, oral Fe to decrease Pb absorption, mandatory follow-up.

Level of 25-45 μg %:
- Find source, oral Fe, consider chelation.

Level of 45 μg % or higher:
- Chelation

Chelation Rx (J Peds 1968;73:1):
- EDTA (ethylenediaminetetraacetic acid) 1500 mg/m² iv for 24 hr 4 hr after BAL, 1000 mg/m² in children who are not encephalopathic (J Pharm Exp Ther 1987;243:804).

- BAL im (2,3-dimercaptopropanol) 75 mg/m^2 in adults, 50 mg/m^2 in children who are not encephalopathic.
- Succimer, aka DMSA (2,3-dimercaptosuccinic acid) (Clin Pharmacol Ther 1985;37:431), 10 mg/kg po every 8 hr × 5 d, then q 12 hr × 14 d.
- CDTA (cyclohexanediaminetetraacetic acid) (Arch Environ Contam Toxicol 1990;19:185).
- Perhaps zinc supplementation (Toxicology 1990;64:129).

25.13 Mercury

Nejm 2003;349:1731

Cause: Inhalation of inorganic Hg or vaporized Hg; ingestion of Hg, inorganic mercuric (mercurous) ions or salts or organic mercurials (eg, methyl, alkyl).

Epidem:

Inorganic: In miners, hatters, mirror makers, mercury factory or lab workers; accidental release (Environ Hlth Perspect 2002;110:129); mercury batteries (Peds 1992;89:747; Arch EM 1990;7:100).

Organic: Fish are major converters to methyl Hg when exposed to inorganic Hg, eg, in Minamata Bay; mercurial fungicides; low levels found in all fish may not impair childhood development (Jama 1998;280:701). Organic Hg preservatives in interior latex paint, now removed (Nejm 1990;223:1096).

Pathophys: Brain is primary target, exact action unknown (*in vitro* differs from *in vivo*).

Sx:

Vapor inhalation: Acutely chemical pneumonitis, gingivostomatitis, noncardiac pulmonary edema; chronically neuropsych symptoms, tremor, acrodynia.

Inorganic salt ingestion: Gradual onset (months to years) abdominal pain, gi bleeding, nausea, vomiting, diarrhea, shock, renal failure, CNS toxicity including erythism (shyness, decreased attention, decreased memory, decreased intellect).

Organic [see case report of fatal minor spill exposure of Dartmouth chemistry professor (Nejm 1998;338:1672)]: Rapid onset (days to months), dysarthria, ataxia, leg cramps, restricted visual fields, muscle weakness, personality changes, desquamative rash, occasional gastroenteritis.

Si: *Inorganic:* Fine tremor of face and tongue, may progress to coarse.

Crs: Variable, but also suggestion of cardiac risk.

Cmplc: *Inorganic:* Nephrotic syndrome; perhaps ALS syndrome.
Organic: Nephrotic syndrome (Ann IM 1977;86:731).

Lab:

- *Chemistries:* for *elemental* and *inorganic* exposures: whole blood urine levels followed by 24 hr urine collection for Hg ($> 100\text{-}200$ µg/L significant) and creatinine.

  Organic: blood Hg; urine (as above); and hair analysis, but commercial lab heavy metal results unreliable (Jama 2001; 285:67).

- *X-ray:* Head CT may show brain atrophy in chronic exposure.

Emergency Management:

- *Elemental:* succimer*, aka DMSA (2,3-dimercaptosuccinic acid) may help.
- *Inorganic:* bowel irrigation with polyethylene glycol solution and chelate with BAL* until enteritis resolves, followed by succimer* (Ann EM 2002;39:312); or consider 2,3-dimercaptopropane-1-sulphonate (DMPS), which is a chelating agent [which was studied with use of continuous veno-venous hemodiafiltration (Crit Care 2003;7:R1)]; may consider d-penicillamine at 125 mg or 250 mg qd (J Anal Toxicol 1982;6:120).
- *Organic:* succimer*, possibly vit E as an anti-oxidant.
  *see Emergency Management in Lead p467 re: dosing.

25.14 Salicylate (ASA)

Drug Saf 1992;7:292

Cause: Ingestion of > 10 gm of ASA in adult; topical treatment absorption (Cutis 1992;50:307).

Epidem: Common in all ages, and many times unintentional.

Pathophys: Oxidative metabolism uncoupling, with early stimulation of respiratory centers as well; CNS stimulant; gastric irritant.

Sx: Nonspecific; dizziness, abdominal pain, nausea.

Si: Fever and hypermetabolic state; confusion; seizures; hematemesis or melena.

Crs: Variable with mild cases requiring iv fluid for dehydration and alkalosis, severe cases (see "Cmplc").

Cmplc: CNS ischemia secondary to decrease in CNS ATP and cerebral edema; pulmonary edema; altered glycemic control, with hypoglycemia common in peds; cardiac arrhythmias; and rarely renal failure.

Nomogram not accurate in enteric coated formulations, or for dosages spread out over time, such as acute ingestion on top of chronic therapy (Ann EM 1989;18:1186); some salicylate assays cross react with diflunisal (J Emerg Med 1987;5:499).

Diff Dx: Sepsis, cocaine, ethylene glycol, isoniazid, methanol, iron, and cyanide.

NSAIDs (Drug Saf 1990;5:252) usually not as severe as salicylates, with major problem if coingested with anticoagulants—the antiplatelet effect increases risk of bleeding. Gi (ulcers) and renal (interstitial nephritis, metabolic acidosis, failure) side effects are most common with overdose, with less likely pulmonary (bronchospasm), hepatic (hepatitis), anaphylaxis, and CNS (aseptic meningitis). Rx is supportive.

Lab: Salicylate level at admission and 6 hr post ingestion (see Figure 25.2); ABG (respiratory alkalosis followed by metabolic alkalosis); acetaminophen level; ethanol level; CBC with diff; PT/PTT; metabolic profile; UA; urine toxic drug screen; EKG.
- *X-ray:* Abdominal flat plate to look for salicylates in gi tract.

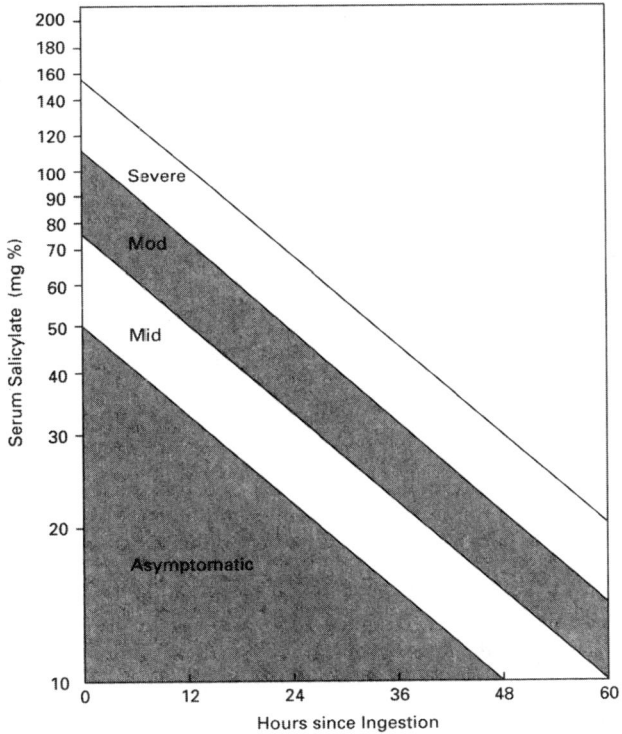

Figure 25.2 Nomogram relating serum salicylate concentration and expected severity of intoxication at varying intervals following the ingestion of a single dose of salicylate. Reproduced with permission from Done AK, Salicylate intoxication: Significance of measurements of salicylate in blood in cases of acute ingestion. Peds 1960;26:800.

Emergency Management:

- Iv access.
- Activated charcoal 1 gm/kg po, most effective when repeated every 4 hr × 3 (Ann EM 1988;17:34); with cathartic, such as sorbitol (Ann EM 1990;19:654) or $MgSO_4$ (Arch IM 1984;144:48).
- Vit K for prolonged protime (controversial if no clinical effects of prolonged PT).
- Intravenous glucose, for ASA-induced hypoglycemia.
- Metabolic acidosis treated with iv $NaHCO_3$, 2-3 amps in L of D_5W at 100 cc/hr, and follow serum pH and urine pH > 7.5 (J Toxicol Clin Toxicol 2004;42:1). Consider dialysis if severe, correct lytes—still treat with alkalinization if going to dialysis (Clin Nephrol 1998;50:178).
- Consider hemodialysis for initial level > 120 mg% or 6-hr level > 100 mg%; or if renal failure, pulmonary edema, or persistent CNS problems, consider exchange transfusion if pt too small for hemodialysis (Vet Hum Toxicol 2002;44:224).

25.15 Theophylline

J Emerg Med 1993;11:415

Cause: Usually iatrogenic (Ann IM 1991;114:748), with aminophylline or oral theophylline used for chronic lung disease; this chemical has a narrow therapeutic window and has many interactions with other medications, and is influenced by thyroid function (Clin Pharm 1988;7:620).

Epidem: Becoming more uncommon as use of theophylline is waning; increased risk if > 60 yr of age, increased levels secondary to drug interactions (eg, some antibiotics, estrogens, allopurinol, cimetidine) and lower levels cause more toxicity in chronic users (Ann IM 1993;119:1161).

Pathophys: Unknown, but many hypotheses with theophylline interaction with phosphodiesterase-2 (PDE-2), cAMP, prostaglandins, release/synergism with catecholamines and adenosine antagonism. These interactions may occur at some level, but not known which are predominant at the levels that are regularly used (usually < 20 μg/ml). Reaction to theophylline also appears to be idiosyncratic and avoiding toxicity is only reliably done via serum levels (Jama 1976;235:1983).

Sx: Headache, irritability, gi upset, agitation (as with other methylxanthines such as caffeine); seizures.

Si: Tachycardia, hypotension, seizures, coma.

Crs: Variable—dependent on level and chronicity.

Cmplc: Status epilepticus, ventricular arrhythmias (rare), rhabdomyolysis (rare).

Lab: CBC with diff looking for leukocytosis; metabolic profile, looking for metabolic acidosis, hypokalemia, hypophosphatemia, and hypomagnesemia; theophylline level; EKG, looking for ectopic beats, sustained arrhythmias rare (Chest 1990;98:672), and perhaps T-wave inversion corresponding to severe toxicity (Chest 1989;96:429).

Emergency Management:
- Activated charcoal 1 gm/kg po (Crit Care Med 1984;12:113), with sorbitol.
- Airway control if seizing, for status epilepticus refer to p284, may need to move quickly to pentobarbital.
- Arrhythmias should follow standard protocols for atrial and ventricular arrhythmias; adenosine may precipitate bronchospasm; consider labetalol or esmolol (Ann EM 1990; 19:671) if β-blockade considered—caution in those with bronchospastic disease.
- Hemoperfusion/hemodialysis/plasmapheresis (Crit Care Med 1991;19:288) for acute toxicity and level > 100 μg/ml, or chronic toxicity and level > 60 μg/ml (Am J Med 1990; 88:567).

Chapter 26

Trauma

26.1 Burns

Cause: Thermal (majority of burn unit admissions), chemical (3-16% of burn unit admissions) or electrical (3-4% of burn unit admissions) (Clin Plast Surg 2000;27:133) injury with subsequent tissue damage.

Epidem: Annually, a minority of pts with massive ($> 75\%$ of total body surface area) burns, approximately 3% in children (Jama 2000;283:69). Major burns with worse outcomes in infants and the elderly (Burns 2000;26:49). Scald burns of the perineum and lower extremities are common and preventable injuries in infants and the elderly (Burns 2000;26:251).

Pathophys: Tissue (skin) damage from the three above mentioned causes is inherent in their physical properties—that of heat, acidic or alkaline extremes, or electrical destruction. Thermal burns can cause acute or subacute ocular and airway damage that is linked to the initial insult or steam generation with consequent inhalation. Steam injury to the lungs can be quickly overwhelming (Burns 1996;22:313). Chemical burns have a predisposition for ocular and oropharyngeal damage. Chemical burns to the lungs can occur from hydrocarbon source as seen in huffing, if linked with smoking (Burns 1996;22:566). For associated electrical injury problems, see p85.

Major burns are those involving $> 20\%$ total body surface area (TBSA) or any fourth degree burns; or those with associated airway, fracture, or other secondary injury problems. Burns in infants or the elderly are at higher risk for secondary complications; as well as burns that involve the hands, feet, perineum, cross major joints, or are circumferential.

Moderate burns are those involving 10-20% TBSA, with none of the aforementioned concerns of hands, feet, perineum, crossing a major joint, or circumferential locations. Moderate burns may be more concerning in infants, the elderly, or those with secondary medical concerns.

Minor burns are those with TBSA involvement of < 10% of second degree, < 2% of third degree, no fourth degree, and none of the concerns mentioned above.

Sx: Pain, hoarseness, dyspnea, visual problems.

Si: Tissue damage. Do a full evaluation, with particular attention to the head and neck looking for singed hair (including nasal), pharyngeal edema, soot deposits in oropharynx, and circumferential neck burns; look for circumferential burns on any extremities or for places where burns cross joints; inspect perineum, as this is very thin skin; look for burn patterns, and photograph, if any concern for abuse; look for secondary injuries, such as fractures. TBSA should be calculated with a burn chart [most accurate (Burns 2000;26:156), such as the Lund and Browder], rules of nines in adults, and modified for children. For adults, 9% (one portion or multiples) of body surface for each of the following areas:

1) Head and neck is 1 portion (9%)
2) Anterior torso is 2 portions (18%)
3) Posterior torso is 2 portions (18%)
4) Each upper extremity is one portion
5) Each lower extremity is 2 portions (18% each)
6) 1% for perineum

In children, may approximate burn size with dorsum of pt's hand, including digits, as approximately 1% or by referring to burn chart. An infant's head and neck is approximately 2½ portions (22%), and each lower extremity is one portion (9%).

1st Degree: Erythematous skin, no blisters, not part of the TBSA calculation.

2nd Degree: Blister formation, tender; superficial second is erythematous and blistered; deep second is with charring but not quite full thickness—may be leathery texture to the skin.

3rd Degree: Full thickness with anesthesia, venous thrombosis and extends down to the sc fat layer.

4th Degree: With involvement of sc fat, muscle or bone.

Crs: Burns with > 20% TBSA cause systemic inflammatory response.

Cmplc: Airway compromise, hypovolemia, systemic inflammatory response, later secondary infection, including tetanus, or aeromonas if immersion injury post burn (Burns 2000;26:478); ischemic bowel disease (Arch Surg 1997;132:440); aggressive fluid resuscitation with consequent pulmonary edema (Ann Surg 1977;185:100); electrolyte imbalance.

Diff Dx: Blistering skin diseases such as Toxic epidermolysis necrosis, Stevens-Johnson Syndrome, Staphylococcal scalded skin syndrome, and others that are all rare (Burns 2000;26:82) and should be differentiated by hx.

Lab: Those with minor and moderate burns usually do not require any laboratory evaluation, whereas those with major burns should receive the following: CBC with diff; metabolic profile; CO level; ABG, if airway involvement; PT/PTT; total CPK; UA; urine for myoglobin. Elevated serum calcitonin correlates with mortality and pulmonary injury, whereas elevated TNF-α and TNF receptor I and II levels also correlate with mortality; threshold values unknown (J Burn Care Rehabil 1992;13:605; Burns 2000;26:239).

- *X-ray:* CXR if airway involvement, although findings may be delayed (Brit J Radiol 1994;67:751); assessment for secondary fractures.

Emergency Management:

Major Burns:
- Secure airway if obvious or impending obstruction—ET intubation. Inhalation injuries need not have extensive obvious tissue involvement to be severe (J Emerg Med 1988;6:471), but look for evidence of insult, such as oral or nasal signs or carbanaceous sputum. Consider early intubation before edema makes this difficult.
- Wet chemical burns should be irrigated with water usually (J Burn Care Rehabil 2000;21:40) and use a mild liquid detergent if water solubility in question. Sodium metals, other metals, and phenol will do better with mineral oil. Dry chemicals should be brushed or lifted for removal. Cover burns with dry gauze or opt for synthetic semipermeable membrane, such as Biobrane (Plast Reconstr Surg 2000;105:62), Opsite, Tagaderm or Duoderm as barrier—avoid hypothermia by not wetting the dressings.
- Iv access and bladder catheter, Parkland formula: 4 cc of LR/kg/% TBSA, with half in the first 8 hr and half in the following 16 hr (Ann N Y Acad Sci 1968;150:874; Heart Lung 1973;2:707) for fluid resuscitation with urine output goal of 0.3-0.5 cc/kg/hr. Avoid excessive resuscitation if pulmonary involvement (J Trauma 1982;22:869). Sodium bicarbonate drip if rhabdomyolysis (see Compartment Syndrome p484).
- Iv narcotics/benzodiazepines for pain control and anxiolysis; splint fractures.
- Update tetanus and antibiotic eye ointment if ocular involvement.
- Do not debride intact blisters (Acad Emerg Med 2000;7:114).

- < 18 yr of age with burn > 40% of TBSA benefit from β-blocker treatment—this attenuates hypermetabolism (Nejm 2001;345:1223).
- Chest plate escharotomy, if trained to do so and cannot ventilate pt.

Moderate or minor burns:
- Moderate burns are major if occurring in infants, the elderly, or those with significant secondary medical problems.
- If isolated burn that crosses a joint in an otherwise healthy pt, may splint the joint in anticipation of next day follow-up (Burns 1998;24:493).
- Update Tetanus, if needed.
- Do not debride intact blisters (Acad Emerg Med 2000;7:114).
- Remove foreign body, cover wounds with ointment of choice—do not put silver sulfadiazine on the face because it will stain, and all ointments have equal efficacy. Topical neomycin may cause a contact dermatitis. May opt for synthetic semipermeable membrane, such as Biobrane (Plast Reconstr Surg 2000;105:62), Opsite, Tagaderm, or Duoderm. Perhaps topical octylcyanoacrylate as cover (Acad Emerg Med 2000;7:222; Burns 2000;26:388).
- Honey (Burns 1996;22:491; Infection 1992;20:227) and papaya fruit are appropriate wound salves (Burns 2003;29:15); honey better than Opsite (Brit J Plast Surg 1993;46:322).
- Ibuprofen [which increases tissue perfusion and limits burn extension (Burns 2000;26:341)] and oral narcotics for pain control, if needed.
- Follow-up in 24 hr for burn recheck, consider debridement if broken blisters at this time, and then in 5-7 d if no complications. Daily dressing changes at home if able, otherwise through health care provider.
- Topical heparin may have a future role (Burns 2001;27:349).

TRAUMA

26.2 C-spine

J Accid Emerg Med 1999;16:208; Orthop Clin N Am 1999;30:457

Cause: Trauma from any cause may cause fracture, subluxation, soft-tissue hyperextension injury, spinal cord trauma, or radiculopathy; increased risk in those with Down syndrome (Clin Neuropathol 1999;18:250) or other disease states that affect the integrity of the neck.

Epidem: Age-related injuries, with children having spinal cord injury without radiographic abnormalities—this only relates to plain radiographs, will be apparent on MRI (J Trauma 1989;29:654; Am J Emerg Med 1999;17:230), and the elderly having a lower incidence of C-spine fractures, but a higher group percentage of C1-C2 fractures (Spinal Cord 1999;37:560) and perhaps more difficult plain films to interpret secondary to arthritis. Blunt trauma fracture incidence is approximately 1-3%, with primarily males in their third or fourth decade of life. Pure subluxation is rare (J Trauma 2000;48:724). Those with blunt cervical trauma unlikely to have intra-abdominal pathology if not consistent with mechanism and if patient hemodynamically stable ($< 1\%$) (J Spinal Disord 1992;5:476).

Pathophys: The mechanism of injury can give information as to what type of injury to predict, with axial loading, such as seen in diving or football (spearing) (J Am Acad Orthop Surg 1999; 7:338) injuries at high risk for fractures.

Sx: Pain, paresthesias, paralysis, incontinence of bladder or bowel.

Si: Hypotension with spinal shock, midline neck pain, abnormal neurologic exam including loss of sphincter control.

Crs: Cannot predict in ER which neurologic deficits are reversible; upper rib fractures associated with C-spine fractures, especially first rib and C7 (Can Assoc Radiol J 1999;50:41).

Cmplc: Altered mental status, intoxication or distracting injuries (eg, head injury, hip fracture) precludes from clearing C-spine clinically, and conversely, have a high index suspicion for intracranial injury with C-spine trauma (Paraplegia 1986;24:97), especially if C1 or C2 injured (J Trauma 1999;46:450); in major trauma, any spinal fracture should prompt imaging of entire spine to look for other fractures; vertebral artery injury incidence unknown, and symptomatic injury appears to be low (J Trauma 1999;46:660).

Diff Dx: Erb's Palsy or other brachial plexopathy; atraumatic atlanto-axial subluxation secondary to severe arthritis (J Rheumatol 1999;26:687); metastatic disease to the C-spine (Clin Orthop 1999:89); physiologic C2-C3 pseudosubluxation in peds.

Lab: *X-ray:* NEXUS Criteria—radiographs perhaps not necessary in blunt trauma, if no midline tenderness, no focal neurologic deficit, normal mental status without intoxication, and no distracting injury—this will miss an injury in approximately 1 in 4000, and significant injury even more uncommon (Nejm 2000;343:94); high-energy cause may be other risk for fracture/spinal cord injury (Radiology 1999;211:759). NEXUS numbers low with respect to children < 8 yr of age, so use with caution (Peds 2001;108:E20). Canadian C-spine rules follow a different algorithm with mentation considerations similar to NEXUS, but mechanism of injury as key component with high risk energy transfer delineated from non-high risk energy transfer—algorithm more complicated without any compelling evidence of better x-ray screening criteria or better utilization of resources (Nejm 2003;349:2510).

Protective head gear and shoulder pads prevent adequate radiographs (Ann EM 2001;38:26) and ER/prehospital staff should have training to remove these—bending at the waist in the supine and conscious pt to 30°-40° of elevation while the head is stabilized is effective, and is a protocol put forth by the Nationals Athletic Trainers' Association (Spine 2002;27:995).

Begin with traditional 3-view (AP, lateral, odontoid) with collar on if x-rays needed and low to moderate risk of fracture; with CT or MRI (Radiology 1999;213:203) or tomography (Radiology 1999;211:882) if unable to interpret; or CT or MRI, if specific abnormality noted on neurologic exam or plain films. Specific classifications are referrable to excellent work by Harris et al (Orthop Clin N Am 1986;17:15).

May advocate that in those with high to moderate risk for C-spine fracture a lateral plain film with helical CT, helical CT with sagittal reconstruction (J Trauma 1999;47:896, 902; Radiology 1999;212:117) or MRI (J Neurosurg 1999;91:54) as the initial test. One set of high-energy risk factors includes the following (for those > 16 yr of age):

1) High speed MVA > 35 mph (56 km/h);
2) Crash with death at scene;
3) Fall from height > 10 ft (3 m);
4) Significant closed head injury or ICH on CT;
5) C-spine symptoms or abnormal neurologic exam; or
6) Pelvic or multiple extremity fractures (Am J Roentgenol 2000;174:713).

Also, if scanning other areas of the body, adding cervical spine CT as the screening test of choice is also more effective than trying to obtain plain films (J Trauma 2004;56:1022).

Advocate for MRI, if suspect ligamentous instability—this is rare (Am Surg 2000;66:326). Flexion/extension plain films (Am J Emerg Med 1999;17:504) considered to have a niche, but not advocated here.

Emergency Management:

- Prehospital care should begin with long board, collar, and head immobilization. Infants require an item 3-4 cm in thickness posterior to the scapula when supine to maintain neutral head position (about the thickness of an adult hand).

- Maintain airway, with intubation facilitated by gum elastic bougie or fiberoptic instrumentation (J Neurosurg Anesthesiol 1999;11:11). Cricothyrotomy, if airway needed and cannot intubate; remember in-line stabilization, not traction.
- In moving pt from the board, control spinal alignment, and move pt as a unit.
- High dose methylprednisolone at 30 mg/kg iv is controversial, but is used for spinal cord injury, see Spinal Cord Injury p288. Use of high dose steroids in these pts is to be determined by the trauma surgeon/neurosurgeon caring for the pt.
- Neurosurgery consult for abnormal neurologic exam or radiographic abnormalities.

26.3 Compartment Syndrome

Hand Clin 1998;14:335

Cause: Increased pressure in a tissue (muscle) compartment that is contained by fascial and bony planes, such that intercompartment muscle, nerve, and blood vessel viability is threatened or impaired. Various etiologies include fractures, blunt trauma, penetrating trauma, revascularization of ischemic extremity, venous occlusion, circumferential burns, chronic and repetitive exertion (Med Sci Sports Exerc 2000;32:S4), external compression by medical antishock trousers (pneumatic trousers) (J Trauma 1989;29:549), and prolonged limb compression from drug overdose (Clin Orthop 1975;81:81).

Epidem: Uncommon.

Pathophys: A function of the non-elastic properties of bone and fascia, with the critical mass found in medium sized compartments in the forearm and leg being most vulnerable, but possible at any site; thigh has been reported and is uncommon (Orthop Rev 1990;19:421; J Trauma 1998;45:395). Hypotension is a risk factor, since the diastolic pressure has to exceed the pressure in the compartment for flow to occur through that compartment.

Sx: Pain, swelling.

Si: Tense edema, pallor, distal hypesthesia or anesthesia, lack of distal pulses, distal paralysis, pain with distal passive range of motion testing.

Crs: Dependent on whether isolated injury or part of multisystem trauma; fasciotomy wounds associated with high infection rate.

Cmplc: Ischemic (Volkmann) contracture; renal failure, rhabdomyolysis, metabolic acidosis, hyperkalemia, multi-organ failure.

For Rhabdomyolysis: Consider this diagnosis in those with elevated total CPK and myoglobinuria. Rx consists of placing a urinary catheter and intravenous infusion of 2-3 amps of $NaHCO_3$ (88-132 mEq) in 1 L of D_5W to keep urine pH > 6.5 (J Biol Chem 1998:31731); mannitol of no proven value (Ren Fail 1997;273:283). Diff Dx of rhabdomyolysis includes trauma (any type—crush injury, penetrating, heat related, etc); prolonged immobility; drugs, such as statins (Jama 2004;292:2585), ethanol, opiates, cocaine or heroin; hypokalemia (acute tubular necrosis, diuretic use, Bartter's syndrome); acute intermittent porphyria (Ann Clin Biochem 2004;41:341); and licorice ingestion (Nejm 1966;247:602).

Diff Dx: Muscle contusion; DVT; rarely de novo compartment syndrome secondary to neoplasm (J Surg Oncol 1994;55:198) or ruptured aneurysm (J Vasc Surg 1993;18:295).

Lab: CBC with diff; metabolic profile; total CK; UA and urine for myoglobin.
- *X-ray:* To look for associated fracture.
- *Compartment pressure:* > 30 mm Hg at a minimum for fasciotomy (ortho consult for procedure)—exact threshold

number is controversial and depends on clinical exam (Clin Orthop 1975:43).

- *EMG:* May be useful if diagnosis uncertain (Acta Belg Med Phys 1990;13:195).

Emergency Management:
- Iv access with fluid resuscitation if hypotensive; iv narcotics.
- General or orthopedic surgery consult.

26.4 Multi-Trauma

Neck, chest, abdomen, pelvis, penetrating trauma of extremities and amputations considered here (not covered elsewhere in this handbook).

Cause: Blunt or penetrating trauma to either isolated body area or multisystem trauma—virtually possible in any activity.

Epidemiology: Common, composite number unknown.

Pathophys: Besides the obvious functional impediments, always remember the caveat that trauma may be a result of a medical problem—hypoglycemia, seizure, MI, CVA, syncope, or other etiology.

Sx: Loss of consciousness, pain, dyspnea, paralysis.

Si: Tachycardia; hypotension; GCS 14 or less; tenderness; deformity; loss of pulse(s); loss of motor/sensory function; seat belt sign conveys 3% risk for vascular injury in blunt trauma—usually either thoracic (majority) or carotid (J Trauma 2002;52:618). Blood at the urethra or pelvic injury necessitates a urethrogram and a digital rectal exam (DRE) in males to be sure that the prostate is "not floating"—DRE of questionable efficacy but some suggestion that abnormal neurologic exam, blood at urethral meatus, and > 65 yr of age as indicators of those who need DRE (Acad Emerg Med 2004;11:635).

Penetrating Trauma of Extremities (Am Surg 2002;68:269):
Consider arterial injury with injury to extremity that is either close to an artery or not (sometimes the course is not obvious).

Hard signs:
- Obvious arterial bleed
- Expanding hematoma
- Loss of pulse
- Bruit
- Thrill
- ABI < 1

Soft signs:
- Neurologic deficit

Crs/Complc: Besides the functional impairment for selected injuries, ischemia can cause end-organ dysfunction including ARDS, MI, CVA, ATN, hepatic necrosis, ischemic bowel, rhabdomyolysis, and consequent sepsis. Avoid T < 95°F to decrease chance of cold-induced coagulopathy. Complete physical exam empirically needed because pt's acute trauma may mask other injuries [such as testicular dislocation in those with blunt abdominal trauma (Ann EM 2004;43:371)].

Lab:
- *Neck:* C-spine evaluation with plain film lateral C-spine with CT of C-spine, if high-likelihood of fracture—may do CT sagittal reconstruction to obviate the need for single view lateral C-spine (see C-Spine p480); penetrating trauma may need great vessel evaluation which may be done with duplex ultrasound, helical CT angiography (Radiology 2000;216:356), MRA or angiography.
- *Chest:* CXR is not adequate screening for major blunt chest trauma—50% of injuries will be missed and a subset of these will of course be lifethreatening—CT is better (J Trauma 2001;51:1173). Those with blunt trauma, hemodynamic sta-

bility, and a normal physical examination do not require routine imaging (J Trauma 2002;53:1135)—contrary to this, those with penetrating trauma may develop hemopneumothoraces without obvious clinical findings.

- *Abdomen:* Abdominal evaluation with either bedside US or CT with iv contrast only. Bedside US effective for diagnosing hemoperitoneum and intra-abdominal injuries in those with hypotension (79% sensitive and 95% specificity), but a negative US does not preclude further evaluation or observation (Radiology 2004;230:661)—those with hypotension may need to have abdominal CT, diagnostic peritoneal lavage (DPL) or other evaluation for hypotension (Ann EM 2004;43:354). It is appropriate to CT scan abdomen without pelvis with upper quadrant injury only and no hematuria (essentially looking for liver or spleen laceration as leading diagnosis). Those with macroscopic hematuria or microscopic hematuria associated with shock or other major injuries need CT checking for renal or bladder fracture after clearance of urethra, if needed (EMJ 2002;19:322). May consider cystogram for ruptured bladder if you have the combination of gross hematuria with pelvic fracture (World J Surg 2001;25:1588).
- *Pelvis:* Pelvis x-ray will help explain obvious fractures here (see Fractures p 330). X-rays not necessary in neurologically and hemodynamically intact adults with blunt trauma, neg physical exam and no anemia (J Trauma 1995;39:722); pts with GCS > 13 and with or without intoxication need no x-ray if clinically no suspicion for pelvic fracture (sensitivity 93%) and missed fractures with this approach did not require surgical intervention (J Am Coll Surg 2002;194:121).
- Urethrogram, if blood at urethral opening.
- *Cardiac:* EKG. Cardiac Markers if contusion suspected (may not be pos for 9-12 hr). No real correlation between sternal fracture and cardiac contusion.

- *Blood or urine studies:* Blood glucose; H/H; type and cross as clinically indicated; ABG (J Trauma 2002;52:601); UA.
- Angiography for any "hard sign" for vascular injury (Am Surg 2002;68:269).

Diff Dx: Consider compartment syndrome for trauma to extremities.

Emergency Management:

Hinkle-Broselow tape/kit helpful in peds:

- O_2; airway; surgical cricothyrotomy, if massive facial trauma and intubate burn pts early if stridor, singed facial hair, or soot in nares or mouth.
- Chest tube(s), if penetrating chest trauma with hypoxia, shock or flail chest or evidence of pneumo/hemothorax.
- 2 ivs, NS preferred, LR OK.
- C-collar and board for transport, difficult to clinically clear (even with radiographs) C-spine unless pt is neurologically intact.
- Consult general surgery, trauma surgery, or other specialists.
- Keep warm, avoid significant hypothermia.
- Blood replacement, if > 20 cc/kg of crystalloid needed to treat hypotension.
- Splint all fractures; reduce fractures or dislocations if distal vascular or neurologic compromise; for open fractures update Td, if needed and iv antibiotics.
- Traction splint for femur fracture (Hare or Sager, eg).

Specific Considerations:

Neck:

- Penetrating trauma deep to the platysma necessitates surgical consult.

Chest:

- For penetrating injury, place chest tube and get CXR. Clamp chest tube if > 500 cc of blood drained in ER—get emergent surgical consult. If tension physiology (pneumothorax with shock), consider needle decompression first—place needle over second rib in midclavicular line on affected side, and then a chest tube. 24 hr of first generation antibiotic prophylaxis iv (eg, cefazolin 1-2 gm iv q 8 hr) reduces the risk of infection (EMJ 2002;19:553).

Abdomen:
- Major abdominal trauma necessitates an immediate surgical consult if pt is hypotensive (the resuscitation should take place in the operating theater) or if penetrating trauma.

Pelvis:
- Be prepared to resuscitate those with clinical or radiographic evidence of pelvic fractures, especially if they are "Open Book." Penetrating lesions to the buttocks should be evaluated by a surgeon. Pelvic stabilizing devices do help for unstable pelvic fractures, consider using the pelvic portion of MAST pants, if available.

Amputations:
- Completed amputation: An amputation that has been completed needs bleeding control and should be treated as an open fracture. Whether re-implantation of the distal part can be accomplished is determined by availability/condition of amputated part, regional availability for those surgical services, and medical condition of the pt.
- Field amputation: An amputation that is needed in the field can be accomplished with use of a Giggly saw for those who are trained in this. A possible scenario may be someone with entrapment—whether relieved of the entrapment (such as freeing someone from a mudslide or other compressive injury) or if field amputation, 2 L of LR or NS IV prior to procedure decreases mortality.

26.5 Pressure Injection Injuries

Am Surg 1989;55:714

Cause: Usually from industrial sources, high velocity liquids such as grease, paint, or other material is injected into the body from accident with "gun."

Epidem: Most commonly involves hand.

Pathophys: Mechanical obstruction of distal nerves, arteries, and veins is possible from pressure effects. Liquefaction necrosis, if grease gun injury.

Sx: Pain, swelling.

Si: Erythema, tenderness, range of motion deficits, abnormal distal neurovascular exam.

Crs: Ischemia, relieved with surgical debridement.

Cmplc: Ischemia leading to necrosis if not recognized.

Lab: None.

Emergency Management:

- Iv access, parenteral pain control. **N.B. Do not do a digital or local block.**
- Tetanus update, if needed.
- Surgical consult for debridement and open wound treatment (J Hand Surg [Am] 1993;18:125); early amputation may be unavoidable (J Hand Surg [Br] 1998;23:479); early treatment desirable before complications develop.

Chapter 27

Urology

27.1 Epididymitis

Sex Transm Dis 1984;11:173

Cause: Not always infectious, but infectious agents correlate with age of pt

Less than 40 yr of age: Chlamydia, occasionally gonorrhea or ureaplasma.

Greater than 40 yr of age: Gram-negative bacteria.

- Rarely from intravesical BCG instillation (Aust N Z J Surg 1993;63:70) or amiodarone (Can J Cardiol 1993;9:833).

Epidem: Rare < 18 yr of age; peak incidence at 32 yr of age. Perhaps increased risk with intact foreskin (J Urol 1998;160:1842).

Pathophys: Considered an STD in those young, reflux of infected urine if Gram-negative bacteria implicated; testes is spared. Considered a malfunction of the genitourinary tract in those ≤ 18 yr of age.

Sx: Gradual pain onset, with the possibility of first symptom coincident with minor trauma; nausea; dysfunctional voiding characteristics.

Si: Swollen and tender epididymis with normal testicle; Prehn's sign is neg (relief with elevation of testicle).

Crs: May last 7-10 d with rx.

Cmplc: Chronic epididymitis—consider non-infectious etiology (chemical inflammation from urine reflux); consider prostatitis or urethral obstruction of some degree in those > 40 yr of age; orchitis; abscess; rarely infarction (Acad Emerg Med 1998;5:1128).

Diff Dx: Testicular torsion; appendix testes torsion; symptomatic varicocele (Prehn's sign is positive—elevate the testicle and symptomatic relief); neoplasm.

Lab: UA; urine culture and sensitivity; do penile swab first for gc and chlamydia, if STD suspected.

Emergency Management:

Drugs 1999;57:743

- Scrotal support
- NSAID—ibuprofen 600 mg every 6 hr for 4-5 d; oral narcotics if needed; antiemetics, if needed.

Less than 19 yr of age (J Urol 1995;154:762):

- TMP/SMX DS 1 bid if pyuria, or consider for prophylaxis.
- Refer to urology outpatient for imaging and urodynamic studies.

20-40 yr of age:

- Ceftriaxone 250 mg im one dose; or ciprofloxacin 500 mg po one dose; or ofloxacin 400 mg po one dose—along with doxycycline 100 mg po for 10 d or azithromycin 1 gm po one dose.
- Condom use reviewed, and suggest partner testing.
- Counseling/testing for syphilis and HIV.
- 2-wk follow-up with primary physician.

More than 40 yr of age:

- TMP/SMX DS 1 tab po bid for 2 wks, increase to 4 wks if prostatitis present; may use ciprofloxacin 250-500 mg po bid instead for same length of time.
- 2- to 4-wk follow-up with primary physician.

27.2 Priapism

J Urol 1969;101:576; Acad Emerg Med 1996;3:810

Cause: Medications [eg, iatrogenic injection for impotence or abuse of cocaine (J Urol 1999;161:1817) or use of phenothiazines/trazodone], sickle cell disease, high spinal cord lesion, idiopathic, and leukemic infiltration.

Epidem: Uncommon from all causes.

Pathophys: Both corpora cavernosa engorged with blood.

Sx: Pain if not due to a neurologic lesion.

Si: Tense corpora cavernosa, the glans and corpus spongiosum may not be tense.

Crs: Some are irreversible, such as some medications, spinal cord lesions or if truly idiopathic.

Cmplc: Infection, impotence.

Lab: Dependent on cause—CBC with diff and O_2 sat in those with SCD or leukemia; CNS or vertebral body imaging if trauma, syrinx, or other CNS insult considered; urine toxicologic screen, if considering cocaine use.

Emergency Management:

All causes:
- Terbutaline 0.25-0.5 mg im (deltoid).
- Urology consult; oncology consult if leukemic infiltration.

SCD:
- Transfuse RBCs.
- Dilute epinephrine 1:1,000,000 (1 cc of 1:1000 concentration epinephrine in 1 L of NS) irrigation of corpora cavernosa with 10 cc of solution (Blood 2000;95:78).
- Hyperbaric O_2.

UROLOGY

Other causes except SCD and leukemic infiltration:
- Aspiration of engorged corpora cavernosa.
- Instillation of 10 mg neosynephrine.
- Unfractionated heparin instillation—poor data.

27.3 Testicular Torsion

Peds 1998;102:73

Cause: May be seen in trauma or spontaneously.

Epidem: Those < 18 yr of age appear to present later to ER and thus are at higher risk for orchiectomy (J Urol 1989;142:746).

Pathophys: Testicle is usually anchored inferiorly by the gubernaculum (Greek for helmsman). Rotation causing torsion is usually an inward (medial) rotation in reference to the anterior part of the testes, and the rotation may be $\frac{1}{2}$ a rotation or multiple rotations.

Sx: Acute pain onset, either abdominal or scrotal; nausea.

Si: Prehn's sign usually neg (pain relief with elevation of testes); high riding testicle; loss of affected side cremasteric reflex (Peds 1998;102:73).

Crs: Operate within 4-5 hr to save 70%; 15% saved if operative intervention within 10 hr.

Cmplc: Infarcted testicle; sterility.

Diff Dx: Torsion of appendiceal testes—a vestigial remnant on the superior/anterior aspect of the testis (look here for a blue dot = infarction); it is pedunculated and may infarct, conservative (pain meds, ice, support) and surgical treatment both appropriate; appendicitis; epididymitis.

Lab: UA; CBC with diff.
- X-ray (Clin Radiol 1999;54:343): Duplex US (Urology 1984; 24: 41) vs testicular (radionucleotide) scan (Brit J Urol;1995;

76:628) may be helpful if symptoms > 24 hr, but do not do this in pts with acute presentations and high likelihood in lieu of surgical consult (J Urol 1995;154:1508).

Emergency Management:

- Iv access, narcotic analgesia, and urologic/surgical consult (J Urol 1997;158:1196).
- May attempt manual detorsion using procedural sedation protocols (benzodiazepine and narcotic) with gentle lateral/outward rotation; stop/reverse course, if seems to worsen; endpoint is pain relief and does not obviate the need for surgical exploration.

Index

C

Trimethaphan in aortic dissection, 55
Tympanic membrane perforation, 343

U

Universal precautions, 112
Unstable angina, 22
Upper extremity DVT, 181
Upper gi hemorrhage, 127
Uremic pericarditis, 47
Urinary retention, 241
Urinary tract infection, 243
    and indwelling catheter, 244
Urticaria, 4
Uterine Rupture, 291

V

Vaginitis, 159
Vasopressin
    in Shock, 51
    in Vfib, 61, 63

Venous thrombosis, 179
Ventricular Fibrillation, 55
Ventricular shunt management, 408
Ventricular Tachycardia, 55
Vertigo, 365
Vitamin A in Encephalitis, 268

W

Wandering atrial pacemaker, 23
Water deficit calculation, 74
Wolff-Parkinson-White syndrome, 23
Word catheter, 146
Wound management, 392
Wound repair, 393

Y

Yaws, 216